Methods in Neurosciences

Volume 15

Photoreceptor Cells

Methods in Neurosciences

Editor-in-Chief

P. Michael Conn

Methods in Neurosciences

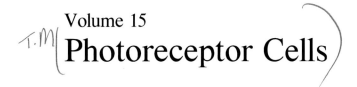

Volume 15
Photoreceptor Cells

Edited by
Paul A. Hargrave
Department of Ophthalmology
University of Florida
Gainesville, Florida

ACADEMIC PRESS, INC.
A Division of Harcourt Brace & Company
San Diego   New York   Boston   London   Sydney   Tokyo   Toronto

Front cover illustration: The rod cell phototransduction scheme as redrawn by Perry Dockins of Academic Press from the original drawn by Elizbieta Wozniewska-Krüger for Hermann Kühn to illustrate his article in *Aus Forschung und Medizin* **2,** 70 (1988). It shows rhodopsin (R) being activated by light (to R*), which in turn activates transducin (Tα•Tβγ), which activates phosphodiesterase (PDE). Hermann Kühn made significant contributions to our understanding of phototransduction. Thus it is fitting that this beautiful color drawing, which graced the poster for the 1990 International Symposium "Signal Transduction in Photoreceptor Cells" held in his honor, should again remind us of the color, beauty, and order of the visual system. Illustration courtesy of Dr. Wagenknecht and Dr. Friebel, Shering AG, Germany.

This book is printed on acid-free paper. ∞

Academic Press, Inc.
1250 Sixth Avenue, San Diego, California 92101-4311

United Kingdom Edition published by
Academic Press Limited
24–28 Oval Road, London NW1 7DX

International Standard Serial Number: 1043-9471

International Standard Book Number: 0-12-185279-2 (Hardcover) (alk. paper)

PRINTED IN THE UNITED STATES OF AMERICA
93 94 95 96 97 98   EB   9 8 7 6 5 4 3 2 1

Table of Contents

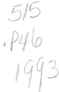

QH
515
.P46
1993

Section IV Molecular Biology of Photoreceptor Cells

Contributors to Volume 15

Article numbers are in parentheses following the names of contributors. Affiliations listed are current.

GRAZYNA ADAMUS (9), Robert S. Dow Neurological Sciences Institute, Portland, Oregon 97209

DON H. ANDERSON (1), Neuroscience Research Institute, University of California, Santa Barbara, Santa Barbara, California 93106

DEAN BOK (25), Department of Anatomy, Jules Stein Eye Institute, University of California Los Angeles School of Medicine, Los Angeles, California 90024

JANINA BUCZYŁKO (15), Department of Ophthalmology, University of Washington School of Medicine, Seattle, Washington 98195

NEIL J. COOK (19), Molekulare Membranbiologie, Max-Planck-Institut für Biophysik, D-6000 Frankfurt am Main 71, Germany

JOHN CRABB (17), W. Alton Jones Cell Sciences Center, Lake Placid, New York 12946

LIEVEKE L. J. DECALUWÉ (22), Department of Biochemistry, University of Nijmegen, 6500 HB Nijmegen, The Netherlands

WILLEM J. DEGRIP (22), Department of Biochemistry, University of Nijmegen, 6500 HB Nijmegen, The Netherlands

DUSANKA DERETIC (6), Department of Pathology, The University of Texas Health Science Center at San Antonio, San Antonio, Texas 78284

WILLIAM J. DINEHART (26), Departments of Immunology and Medical Microbiology, University of Florida School of Medicine, Gainesville, Florida 32610

LARRY A. DONOSO (23), Retina Service, Wills Eye Hospital, Philadelphia, Pennsylvania 19107

PAGE A. ERICKSON (1), Neuroscience Research Institute and Department of Biological Sciences, University of California, Santa Barbara, Santa Barbara, California 93106

STEVEN K. FISHER (1), Neuroscience Research Institute and Department of Biological Sciences, University of California, Santa Barbara, Santa Barbara, California 93106

JOHN G. FLANNERY (26), Departments of Ophthalmology and Neuroscience, University of Florida School of Medicine, Gainesville, Florida 32610

STEVEN J. FLIESLER (5), The Eye Institute, St. Louis University School of Medicine, St. Louis, Missouri 63104

SHAO-LING FONG (23), Department of Ophthalmology, Indiana University, Indianapolis, Indiana 46202

WEI-BAO FONG (23), Department of Ophthalmology, Indiana University, Indianapolis, Indiana 46202

YOSHITAKA FUKADA (10), Department of Pure and Applied Sciences, College of Arts and Sciences, The University of Tokyo, Tokyo 153, Japan

STEVEN B. GOLDIN (11), Department of Biochemistry, University of Illinois at Chicago, Health Sciences Center, Chicago, Illinois 60612

CHRISTOPHER J. GUÉRIN (1), Neuroscience Research Institute, University of California, Santa Barbara, Santa Barbara, California 93106

IRENE L. HALE (3), Department of Biological Sciences, University of California, Santa Barbara, Santa Barbara, California 93106

WILLIAM W. HAUSWIRTH (26), Departments of Ophthalmology and Immunology and Medical Microbiology, University of Florida School of Medicine, Gainesville, Florida 32610

FUMIO HAYASHI (16), Department of Biology, Faculty of Science, Kobe University, Nada, Kobe 657, Japan

YEE-KIN HO (11), Departments of Biochemistry and Ophthalmology, University of Illinois at Chicago, Health Sciences Center, Chicago, Illinois 60612

LARA D. HUTSON (16), Program in Neurobiology, University of Washington, Seattle, Washington 98195

JACQUES J. M. JANSSEN (22), Department of Biochemistry, University of Nijmegen, 6500 HB Nijmegen, The Netherlands

MICHAEL W. KAPLAN (13), Robert S. Dow Neurological Sciences Institute and Devers Eye Institute, Good Samaritan Hospital and Medical Center, Portland, Oregon 97209

AKIO KISHIGAMI (16), Kresge Eye Institute, Department of Ophthalmology, Wayne State University School of Medicine, Detroit, Michigan 48201

CHAO-HUNG LEE (23), Department of Pathology, Indiana University, Indianapolis, Indiana 46202

REHWA H. LEE (12), Department of Anatomy and Cell Biology, University of California Los Angeles School of Medicine, Los Angeles, California 90024, and Molecular Neurology Laboratory, Veterans Administration Medical Center, Sepulveda, California 91343

GEOFFREY P. LEWIS (1), Neuroscience Research Institute, University of California, Santa Barbara, Santa Barbara, California 93106

KENNETH A. LINBERG (1), Neuroscience Research Institute, University of California, Santa Barbara, Santa Barbara, California 93106

RICHARD N. LOLLEY (12), Department of Anatomy and Cell Biology, University of California Los Angeles School of Medicine, Los Angeles, California 90024, and Developmental Neurology Laboratory, Veterans Administration Medical Center, Sepulveda, California 91343

BRIAN MATSUMOTO (3), Neuroscience Research Institute, University of California, Santa Barbara, Santa Barbara, California 93106

J. HUGH MCDOWELL (7), Department of Ophthalmology, University of Florida College of Medicine, Gainesville, Florida 32610

LAURIE L. MOLDAY (8), Department of Biochemistry and Molecular Biology, The University of British Columbia, Vancouver, British Columbia, Canada V6T 1Z3

ROBERT S. MOLDAY (8), Department of Biochemistry and Molecular Biology, The University of British Columbia, Vancouver, British Columbia, Canada V6T 1Z3

T. ALLEN MORRIS (23), Department of Biological Sciences, Purdue University, West Lafayette, Indiana 47907

SEIJI NAGAO (16), Department of Clinical Oncology, Nagoya Memorial Hospital, Nagoya 486, Japan

ALEXANDRA C. NEWTON (18), Department of Chemistry, Indiana University, Bloomington, Indiana 47405

BRIAN E. NICHOLS (27), Department of Ophthalmology, The University of Iowa, College of Medicine, Iowa City, Iowa 52242

PAUL J. O'BRIEN (4), Health Research Associates, Rockville, Maryland 20850

DANIEL D. OPRIAN (21), Graduate Department of Biochemistry, Brandeis University, Waltham, Massachusetts 02254

KRZYSZTOF PALCZEWSKI (13, 14, 15, 17), Departments of Ophthalmology and Pharmacology, University of Washington School of Medicine, Seattle, Washington 98195

DAVID S. PAPERMASTER (6), Department of Pathology, The University of Texas Health Science Center at San Antonio, San Antonio, Texas 78284

ARTHUR S. POLANS (17), Robert S. Dow Neurological Sciences Institute and Department of Ophthalmology, Good Samaritan Hospital and Medical Center, Portland, Oregon 97209

VAL C. SHEFFIELD (27), Department of Pediatrics, The University of Iowa, College of Medicine, Iowa City, Iowa 52242

EDWIN M. STONE (27), Department of Ophthalmology, The University of Iowa, College of Medicine, Iowa City, Iowa 52242

CHRISSIE STREET (26), Department of Immunology and Medical Microbiology, University of Florida School of Medicine, Gainesville, Florida 32610

ANAND SWAROOP (20), Departments of Ophthalmology and Human Genetics, W. K. Kellogg Eye Center, University of Michigan, Ann Arbor, Michigan 48105

TUOW D. TING (11), Department of Biochemistry, University of Illinois at Chicago, Health Sciences Center, Chicago, Illinois 60612

GABRIEL H. TRAVIS (25), Department of Psychiatry, University of Texas, Southwestern Medical Center, Dallas, Texas 75235

JIRO USUKURA (2), Department of Anatomy, Nagoya University School of Medicine, Nagoya 466, Japan

JENNY VANOOSTRUM (22), Department of Biochemistry, University of Nijmegen, 6500 HB Nijmegen, The Netherlands

KIMBERLIE VANDENBURGH (27), Department of Ophthalmology, The University of Iowa, College of Medicine, Iowa City, Iowa 52242

AKIO YAMAZAKI (16), Kresge Eye Institute, Departments of Ophthalmology and Pharmacology, Wayne State University School of Medicine, Detroit, Michigan 48201

Tôru Yoshizawa (10), Department of Information Systems Engineering, Osaka Sangyo University, Osaka 574, Japan

Donald J. Zack (24), Wilmer Eye Institute, Departments of Ophthalmology, Molecular Biology and Genetics, and Neuroscience, The Johns Hopkins University School of Medicine, Baltimore, Maryland 21209

Preface

Advances in the study of photoreceptor cells have proceeded at a rapid pace during the past decade. Our increased understanding of cell functions has benefited from and been driven by new methods of analysis, which have rapidly rendered previous approaches obsolete and required investigators to adopt new techniques in order to remain at the "cutting edge" of their field.

This volume will aid researchers in their quest for appropriate methods to solve their problems. It includes up-to-date biochemical, cell and structural biological, and molecular biological techniques needed for the study of photoreceptor cells. The book begins with methods for observing the structure of photoreceptor cells and for studying their metabolism. Procedures for photoreceptor cell isolation are also included. It continues with chapters describing the preparation of proteins involved in rod cell metabolism, with particular emphasis on proteins of the visual transduction cascade. Finally, chapters are included that describe the application of molecular biological techniques for the examination of molecular components of the visual system and their structure, distribution, and function. Methods that have appeared previously in other publications have been updated and described in greater detail in this volume. Others are completely new and are presented for the first time.

I would like to thank the many investigators who gave advice concerning subjects to include. Particular thanks are due to the authors who conscientiously met tight deadlines so that this volume could reach the reader in a timely fashion.

PAUL A. HARGRAVE

Methods in Neurosciences

Section I

Structure of Photoreceptor Cells

[1] Light and Electron Microscopy of Vertebrate Photoreceptors
Including a Technique for Electron Microscopic Autoradiography

Steven K. Fisher, Don H. Anderson, Page A. Erickson, Christopher J. Guérin, Geoffrey P. Lewis, and Kenneth A. Linberg

Introduction

Light and electron microscopy continue to play fundamental roles in the development of our understanding of photoreceptor cell function. The purpose of this chapter is to acquaint the reader with the tools necessary to produce high-quality tissue preservation and tissue contrast so that photoreceptors may be studied by these techniques. The chapter provides an introduction to photoreceptor cell structure and step-by-step procedures for the preservation of retinal tissue by the standard technique of primary fixation in aldehydes, secondary fixation in osmium tetroxide, and embedment in resin along with the subsequent staining of tissue sections for transmitted light and electron microscopy. A method is also provided for producing autoradiograms that can be observed by electron microscopy, thus providing a high-resolution technique for the subcellular localization of radiolabeled molecules. Illustrations, derived from mammalian retinas prepared by the procedures described here, serve to familiarize readers with the appearance of each anatomical compartment of the photoreceptor cells in tissue generally considered to be "well preserved" for ultrastructural study.

Overview of Photoreceptor Cell Structure

Fundamental anatomical differences between rod and cone photoreceptors as observed by light microscopy are demonstrated in Fig. 1, which shows an example from the parafoveal region of a rhesus monkey retina. Cone outer segments, although somewhat tapered, are not really conical in mammalian retinas; rather, it is the large size of the cone inner segment relative to the outer segment that gives the cones an apparent conical shape. Figure 2

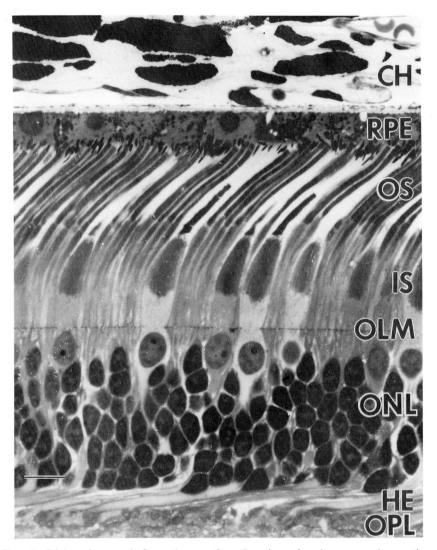

FIG. 1 Light micrograph from the parafoveal region of a rhesus monkey retina. The uppermost cellular layer is the choroid or choriocapillaris (CH). Nutrients and metabolic products must be exchanged between the choroidal capillaries and the layers of photoreceptor cells (OS through OPL) by way of the second cellular layer, the retinal pigment epithelium (RPE). The long, thin rod outer segments (OS) interdigitate directly with the apical border of the RPE, whereas the much shorter cone outer segments are, in primates, contacted by thin villuslike processes from the RPE [F. S. Sjöstrand, *Rev. Mod. Phys.* **31,** 301 (1959)]. The layer of inner segments (IS) can be divided into the densely stained ellipsoid and lightly stained myoid regions.

presents, in diagrammatic form, the basic structural features of vertebrate photoreceptors, and Figs. 3 and 4 are electron micrographs showing these general features.

In most species, rod outer segments are longer than cone outer segments, although this difference can be minimal, for example, in various species of diurnal squirrels or in the fovea (1–3). The highly ordered structure of the outer segment was clearly defined by early electron microscopic observations of rod outer segments (4–6), which demonstrated that they are composed of a stack of bimembranous disks separate from a surrounding plasma membrane. Although structural connections between the disks and the plasma membrane were shown later (7), the fundamental observation in rods remains that the molecular events in visual transduction associated with the disk membranes are physically isolated from the ion channels located on the plasma membrane.

In cone outer segments, however, the disks (although more properly referred to as "lamellae," disks is used here for convenience) are in continuity with the plasma membrane (5, 8–10). In nonmammalian species this fact is easily demonstrated by electron microscopy of thin sections, where patency of the disks occurs along the length of the cone outer segment in any given section. In mammalian cones, outer segment disks often appear patent only at the basal one-third of the outer segment; above this region the outer segment appears rodlike, with disks separate from the plasma membrane (10, 11; Fig. 5). This ultrastructural appearance probably results from the fact that as cone outer segments develop the "disks" become only partially enveloped by a rim separate from the plasma membrane, resulting in a narrow region of disk–plasma membrane continuity that may not be apparent in a single 90-nm-thick section (10). In fact, the issue of how many, if any, cone disks occur isolated from the plasma membrane remains unresolved. In rod outer segments, only the basalmost, newly forming disks are open to the extracellular space, and this compartment may be infiltrated with extracellular tracer molecules (8). Indeed, this phenomenon has been used, as an alternative, higher resolution, less time-consuming method to autoradiography for studying outer segment membrane renewal (12).

Outer segment disks in both rods and cones develop from evaginations of the membrane of the cilium that connects the inner and outer segments (13, 14). These evaginations can be seen as outgrowths of the connecting cilium

---

The outer limiting membrane (OLM) divides the layer of inner segments from the layer of photoreceptor cell bodies (ONL, outer nuclear layer). In the micrograph, the cell bodies connect to the layer of synaptic terminals that form the outer border of the outer plexiform layer (OPL) by way of relatively long "axons" called fibers of Henle (HE). Bar, 10 μm.

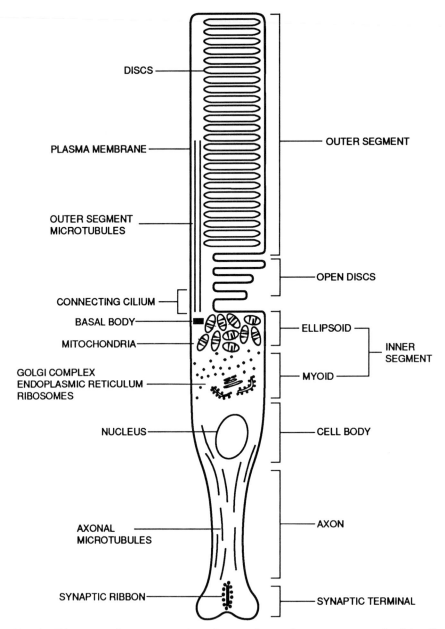

DISCS

PLASMA MEMBRANE

OUTER SEGMENT
MICROTUBULES

OUTER SEGMENT

OPEN DISCS

CONNECTING CILIUM

BASAL BODY

MITOCHONDRIA

ELLIPSOID

INNER
SEGMENT

GOLGI COMPLEX
ENDOPLASMIC RETICULUM
RIBOSOMES

MYOID

NUCLEUS

CELL BODY

AXONAL
MICROTUBULES

AXON

SYNAPTIC RIBBON

SYNAPTIC TERMINAL

FIG. 2   Diagrammatic representation of a vertebrate photoreceptor emphasizing the
high degree of polarity and compartmentalization in these cells. A rod photoreceptor
is represented; in cones, many (perhaps all, see text) of the outer segment disks

that grow toward the margin of the outer segment (Fig. 5). Each surface of an evagination will form the uppermost and lowermost surfaces of two adjacent disks. As the disks mature, a secondary event occurs: the rim of the disk and new outer segment plasma membrane form by growth of the ciliary membrane in a "zippering-like" process between adjacent disk-surface evaginations (14, 15). When this process is completed in rods, the disk becomes isolated from the plasma membrane; in cones, it is incomplete, such that the disks remain patent to varying degrees depending on species.

The process of outer segment disk formation occurs throughout the life of an organism, providing a mechanism for continual renewal of outer segment components. This process was first described in an elegant series of studies using light and electron microscopic autoradiography after labeling of the organism with tritiated amino acids (16; see Ref. 17 for a review). The autoradiographic studies also demonstrated a fundamental difference in the labeling pattern of rods and cones (16, 17). Rod outer segments always show the formation of an isolated "band" of radioactive protein at their base. This band of newly formed membrane then migrates toward the outer segment apex, where it is shed and phagocytosed by the adjacent retinal pigment epithelium (18). Cones, on the other hand, show a diffuse pattern of labeling in which silver grains are scattered over the length of the outer segment. The labeling pattern in rods can be explained as the literal "entrapment" of new molecular components in the disk membranes as the disks mature and become isolated from the plasma membrane. The diffuse labeling pattern in cones is generally interpreted as reflecting the fact that the "disks" of cone outer segments are in continuity with the plasma membrane, allowing the free diffusion of newly inserted protein molecules throughout the outer segment length (18, 19). Consistent with this hypothesis is the demonstration that with short labeling times a gradient of label does occur from the base to the tip of cone outer segments (20).

The connecting cilium emerges from the inner segment early in photoreceptor development and provides the only intracellular pathway for the movement of molecular components between the inner and outer segments. There have been rare observations of "cytoplasmic bridges" between the inner and outer segment (21), and Besharse and Horst (22) have presented a model in which vesicles budding from the apex of the inner segment may deliver molecular components to the outer segment. Examples of these nonmotile

---

would be in continuity with the plasma membrane. The region of open disks represents the new disk surface evaginations as they grow to their full width. In rods, these will become isolated disks by the growth of the disk rim and plasma membrane.

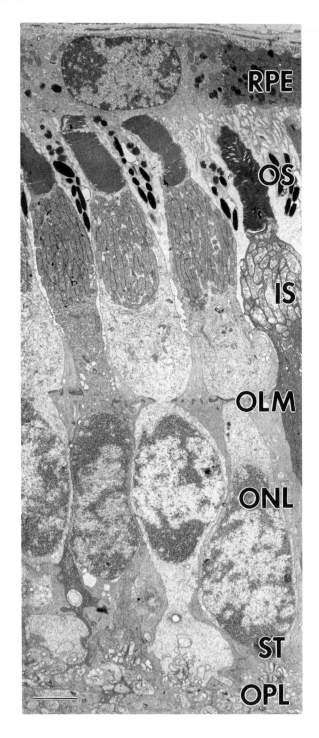

cilia are shown in Figs. 5 and 6. For a discussion of their specialized properties, readers are referred to Besharse and Horst (22).

The compartment of the photoreceptor inner segment from which the cilium arises is known as the ellipsoid and contains structures associated with the cilium (basal body, striated rootlet), vesicles of various sizes, cytoskeletal elements such as microtubules and actin filaments (22–24), and a large, densely packed population of mitochondria. Intermediate (10 nm) filaments and "wavy" filaments occur in this region of photoreceptors in at least some species, although the composition of the filaments has not yet been determined (Figs. 5 and 6).

Vesicles are often seen congregated around the basal body of the connecting cilium (13, 22) in a region known as the periciliary ridge complex (25). At least some of these vescicles, as well as those found elsewhere in the inner segment, are presumed to be transport vesicles for delivery of molecular components (e.g., opsin) destined for the outer segment (26). Others, however, are known to be endocytic vesicles (27).

Just proximal to the ellipsoid is the myoid region of the inner segment (Fig. 7). This compartment contains most of the subcellular machinery for protein synthesis, posttranslational modification of proteins, and their packaging and transport (ribosomes, rough endoplasmic reticulum, Golgi apparatus, etc.). It is also rich in cytoskeletal elements, especially microtubules. It is from this region that newly synthesized proteins must be transported to other locations in the cell (17).

The myoid region connects to the cell body of the photoreceptor cell. At the transition between the two compartments, photoreceptors are joined to each other and to the apical processes of Müller cells by adhering junctions that form a line along the outer border of the layer of photoreceptor nuclei (Figs. 1, 3, and 4; see Ref. 28 for immunocytochemical studies of these junctions). This is a landmark easily recognizable by light microscopy and is termed the outer limiting membrane, a misnomer left over from early light microscopic studies. This array of junctions may function as more than simply points of cell–cell adhesion. It may act as a molecular sieve because molecules with a Stokes radius of greater than 36 Å (about 44,000 molecular

FIG. 3   Low-power electron micrograph showing the cone photoreceptors of a California ground squirrel fixed by perfusion of mixed aldehydes. The very dark-staining photoreceptor on the right is found in regular arrays in the retina of several species and may represent a subclass of cones that are sensitive to short-wavelength light [i.e., blue-sensitive cones; P. K. Anhelt, H. Kolb, and R. Pflug, *J. Comp. Neurol.* **255**, 18 (1987)]. ST, Synaptic terminal. Bar, 2 μm.

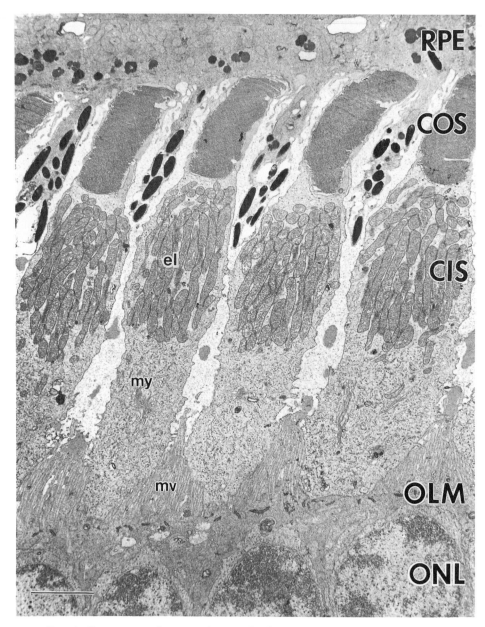

FIG. 4 Low-power electron micrograph of an array of cone photoreceptors (COS, cone outer segments; CIS, cone inner segments) in the retina of a ground squirrel fixed by mixed-aldehyde perfusion. el, Ellipsoid region of inner segment; my, myoid region of inner segment; mv, Müller cell microvilli. Bar, 2 μm.

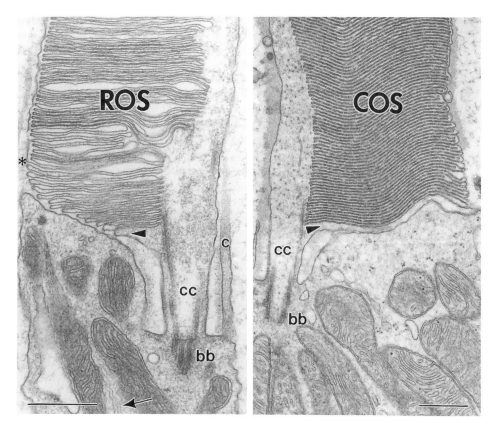

FIG. 5   Basal regions of rod (ROS) and cone outer segments (COS) from rhesus monkey and ground squirrel retina, respectively. Arrowheads indicate the cytoplasm of the evaginations that give rise to new disk surfaces. The asterisk indicates the beginning of the plasma membrane that encloses the rod disks; below that point the disks are open. Calycal processes (c) are slender, cytoplasmic, actin-filled processes that arise from the inner segment and extend along the outer segment. They occur in different numbers and lengths in different species. Note the accumulation of mitochondria in the apical inner segment, the membraneous vesicles near the basal body (bb), and the small cluster of 10-nm-diameter wavy filaments (arrow). cc, Connecting cilium. Bar, 0.5 μm.

weight) cannot diffuse through the junctions when applied to the photorecep-tor side of an isolated retina (29).

   The photoreceptor nucleus resides in the cell body, and a so-called axon arises from the distal end of the cell body (Fig. 8). The axon can be essentially absent, with the synaptic terminal being directly adjacent to the cell body

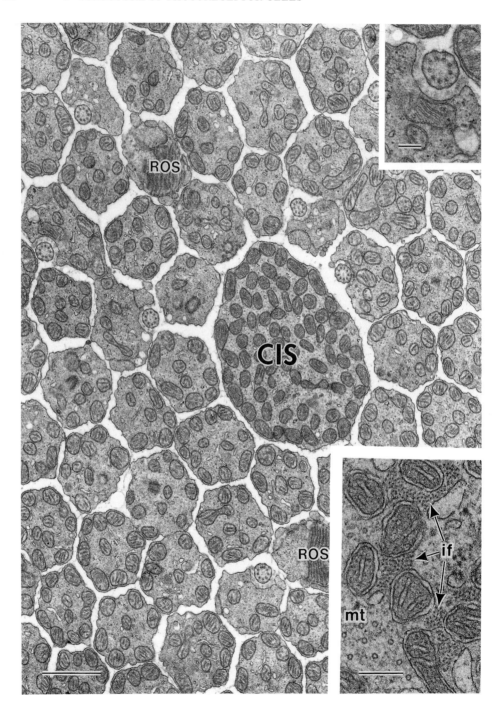

(2), or it can be quite long, as in the fibers of Henle that occur in the macula (see Fig. 1, for example). When present, these fibers have the ultrastructural appearance of axons elsewhere in the nervous system, that is, they contain few organelles other than microtubules and membranous vesicles presumably associated with the transport of proteins to and from the synaptic terminal (Fig. 8) (17, 30). Photoreceptors are often interconnected by gap junctions; in some species these occur between cytoplasmic "fins" that radiate from the inner segment of the cell (31), and in other species they occur between processes that extend from the synaptic terminals (Fig. 9; 32, 33).

The complex nature of information processing that must occur at the first-order synapse in the visual system was revealed by the pioneering ultrastructural studies of Sjöstrand and Missotten (34, 35) in which it was demonstrated that photoreceptors make numerous and complex contacts with their postsynaptic cells, the bipolars and horizontal cells (Fig. 10). In general, cones terminate as large pedicle-shaped endings with multiple synaptic invaginations and basal contacts, whereas rods terminate in spherule-shaped endings with a single synaptic invagination (35). These distinctions, however, are less clear in some species like the diurnal squirrels (2).

These synapses have received considerable attention in ultrastructural studies, especially those designed to disentangle their elaborate connectivity with secondary neurons (33, 36–38). It should be noted that the morphology of these synapses may also change depending on the adaptive state of the eye or time of day (39, 40). The reader is also referred to Chapter 9 of *Histology of the Human Eye* by Hogan *et al.* (41) for exquisite micrographs of photoreceptors from the human eye, and to books by Rodieck (42) and Dowling (43) for invaluable introductions to photoreceptor physiology, structure, and synaptic architecture.

FIG. 6   Electron micrograph of a section cut transversely across the ellipsoid region of a cat retina fixed by immersion in mixed aldehydes. A large cone inner segment (CIS) is surrounded by smaller rod inner segments. The plane of section is at a level that cuts through the base of two rod outer segments (ROS). Many connecting cilia occur in the field. The upper right inset demonstrates that the pattern of microtubules in the cilia is mirrored in the extracellular matrix trapped between the ciliary stalk and the inner segment. The lower right inset shows three clusters of intermediate (10 nm diameter) filaments (if) in a rod inner segment from a rhesus monkey retina. Also note the numerous microtubules (mt) that occur in the cytoplasm. Bar, 1 μm; inset bars, 0.2 μm.

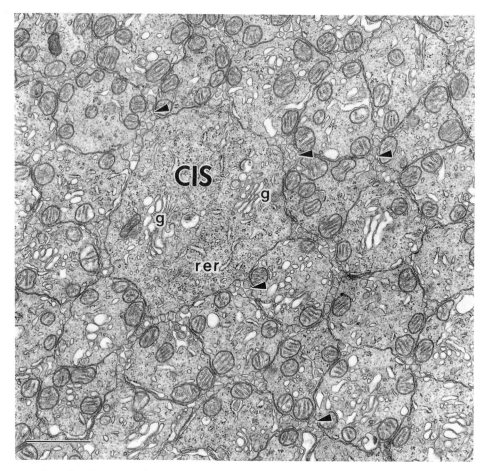

FIG. 7   Electron micrograph of a section cut transversely across the myoid region of a cat retina. A large cone myoid (CIS) is surrounded by smaller rod inner segments. Compare the tight packing that occurs in this region to that in the ellipsoid region (Fig. 6). The myoid area contains the majority of the metabolic machinery of the cell. Note the numerous cisternae that lie adjacent to the plasmalemma of the inner segments. Müller cell microvilli interdigitating between the inner segments are indicated with arrowheads. g, Golgi apparatus; rer, rough endoplasmic reticulum. Bar, 1 μm.

Methods

Fixation of retinal tissue can be accomplished either by immersion of an eye whose anterior and posterior segments have been separated or by intracardiac

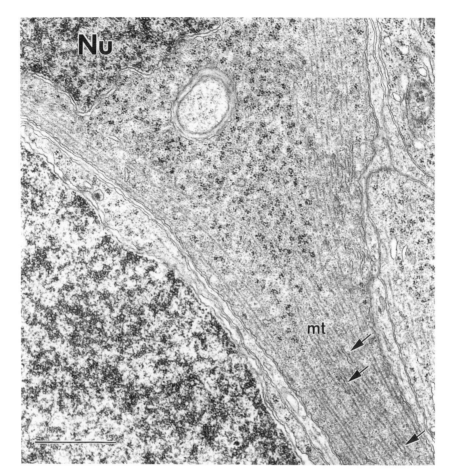

Fig. 8   Electron micrograph showing the emergence of an axon from a cone cell body in a rhesus monkey retina. Note the funneling of microtubules (mt) into the axon and the paucity of other organelles in that region. The small vesicles indicated by arrows may be associated with the transport of material through the axon. Nu, Nucleus. Bar, 1 μm.

perfusion of fixative. The choice of method will depend somewhat on the species (e.g., squirrels must be fixed by perfusion to obtain acceptable ultra-structure) and on the needs of the particular experiment. In our experience the best ultrastructure is obtained by fixation in mixed aldehydes and postfix-ation in osmium tetroxide. However, glutaraldehyde is often used alone, and osmium tetroxide can be used itself as a fixative. Again the choice of (plastic)

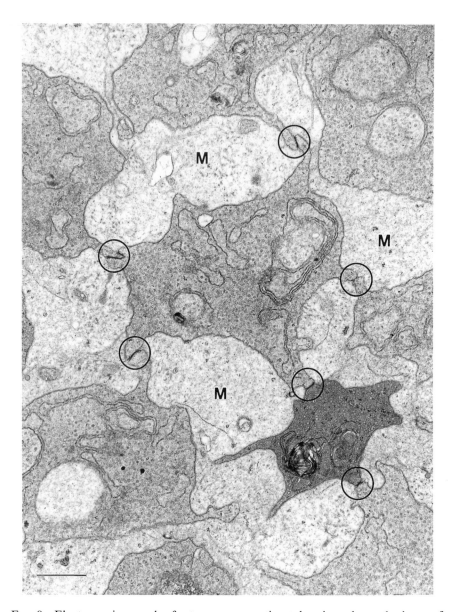

FIG. 9   Electron micrograph of a transverse section taken just above the layer of photoreceptor terminals in a ground squirrel retina. The photoreceptors are electrically linked at this point by gap junctions that occur between projections of the terminals (circles). The terminals are surrounded by Müller cell cytoplasm (M). Bar, 1 μm.

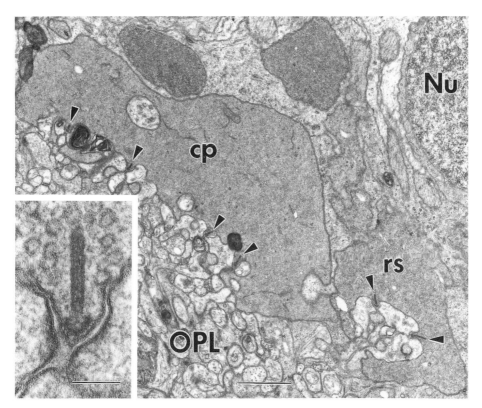

Fig. 10   Electron micrograph through the synaptic terminal layer of a human retina fixed by immersion in glutaraldehyde and postfixed in osmium tetroxide. Note the difference in shape between the rod spherule (rs) and cone pedicle (cp). Arrowheads indicate synaptic ribbons that demark the synaptic complexes of these terminals. Not apparent at this magnification are the basal junctions that occur between "flat" bipolar dendrites and the cone terminals. The inset shows a synaptic ribbon in a human rod spherule. The ribbon is surrounded by synaptic vesicles, and an electron-dense structure, known as the "arciform density," occurs between the ribbon and the photoreceptor membrane. Bar, 1 μm; inset bar, 0.1 μm.

resin for tissue embedment will be dictated by the specifics of the experiment as well as the preference of the individual. Hydrophobic epoxy resins such as Spurr's (Polysciences, Washington, PA) and Araldite (Polysciences) have superior sectioning qualities and increased stability in the electron beam compared to hydrophilic methacrylate plastics like London Resin White (LR White; Ted Pella, Redding, CA).

Preparation of Stock Solutions

Sodium Phosphate Stock Buffer

The basic buffer solution is 0.172 M sodium phosphate adjusted to a pH of 7.2. For each 100 ml of buffer stock, use 0.68 g of monobasic sodium phosphate ($NaH_2PO_4 \cdot H_2O$) and 1.73 g of dibasic sodium phosphate (Na_2HPO_4). Add sequentially to double-distilled water while stirring vigorously. Begin with less than the target volume. After dissolving the phosphate salts, dilute to the final volume and then adjust the pH with 1 N HCl or 1 N NaOH. Isotonicity approximately equal to that of mammalian blood will be achieved later by dilution with double-distilled water or, in the case of the fixative, with 2% paraformaldehyde dissolved in double-distilled water.

2% Paraformaldehyde

Into a volume of double-distilled water that is one-half of the volume of fixative needed, add fresh paraformaldehyde crystals to create a 2% (w/v) solution (i.e., 2 g per 100 ml). The water needs to be heated to approximately 80°C to help dissolve the paraformaldehyde. Do not allow the temperature to rise much beyond 80°C or potential degradation of the formaldehyde may occur. The best way to accomplish this without overheating, which causes turbidity, is to immerse the paraformaldehyde solution in a boiling water bath and heat it, with frequent swirling, until it dissolves (about 20–30 min). Remember to keep the flask loosely covered (a 2-inch square of aluminum foil is good), so that loss by evaporation is minimized. Beware of vapors since they are highly toxic. An alternative method is to heat the water to 80°C with a Bunsen burner, transfer to a hot plate with a magnetic stirrer, and stir while dissolving the paraformaldehyde. A few drops of 1 N NaOH will assist in dissolving the paraformaldehyde (which is clear when dissolved). It is important to make the solution well in advance so it can cool to room temperature before use. The 2% paraformaldehyde solution can be stored at 4°C but should be brought to room temperature before use.

2% Glutaraldehyde in Stock Buffer

Into a volume of stock 0.172 M phosphate buffer that is one-half that of the final volume of fixative desired, dilute enough 70% (v/v) electron microscopy (EM) grade glutaraldehyde to yield a concentration of 2% (v/v) (use 2.9 ml of 70% glutaraldehyde for each 100 ml buffer). The solution is very toxic so gloves and a fume hood are recommended.

1:1 Aldehyde Fixative

To prepare the final fixative, mix equal volumes of the cooled 2% paraformaldehyde and 2% glutaraldehyde solutions to yield a mixture containing 1% paraformaldehyde and 1% glutaraldehyde in 0.086 M buffer.

2% Osmium Tetroxide

Osmium tetroxide (OsO_4) is very toxic so always handle it under a fume hood. *Always wear latex gloves* since OsO_4 can penetrate vinyl gloves.

   1. Dissolve 2.0 g of OsO_4 crystals in 50 ml double-distilled water (in a hood with a magnetic stirrer or sonicator).
   2. To 50 ml of 0.172 M sodium phosphate buffer add the 50 ml of 4% OsO_4. This yields 2% (w/v) OsO_4 in 0.086 M sodium phosphate, pH 7.2.

   Alternately, prepared OsO_4 solutions that are ready to use may be purchased; they are, however, more expensive. The 2% OsO_4 fixative can be stored for several months at 4°C if the storage bottle is free of contaminants and well sealed (double seal over the cap with Parafilm). Osmium tetroxide vapors are difficult to contain, so it is recommended that the fixative solution not be kept in the same refrigerator with sensitive materials (antibodies, cells, etc.).

Wash Buffer (0.137 M)

Isotonic wash buffer (~315 mOsmol) used in the tissue processing steps is prepared by diluting 4 parts of 0.172 M sodium phosphate stock buffer with 1 part of double-distilled water.

Immersion Tissue Fixation

   1. Following enucleation, wash the globe in 0.137 M wash buffer, then make a small slit just behind the iris to allow fixative access to the inside.
   2. Immerse the globe in fixative at room temperature for 5 to 10 min.
   3. Remove the globe from the fixative and carefully cut around the perimeter of the globe by enlarging the original slit, until the anterior segment structures are removed. Although not as critical in smaller eyes, we routinely remove the vitreous body from larger eyes, such as those of the cat, to allow faster penetration of the fixative.
   4. Reimmerse the eye cup in the fixative for 12 to 24 hr at 4°C.

An alternative method is to leave the globe in the fixative while enlarging the original slit and removing the anterior segment structures and vitreous body. This technique is very gentle on the globe, but it requires some practice to cut the globe while it is immersed in fixative. An additional benefit to this procedure is that the globe can be bisected right away after immersion in fixative, thus allowing more rapid penetration of the fixative to the retina.

Fixation by Cardiac Perfusion

Figure 11 illustrates a simple apparatus that can be used for perfusion fixation.

1. The animal is euthanized by an overdose of appropriate anesthetic and then placed on its back in a sink or other receptacle which can serve to catch the blood and excess fixative. After opening the chest cavity, the descending aorta is clamped with a hemostat.

2. Air is infused into a flask above the level of primary fixative. The flask also has a second line extending to the bottom of the flask and leading to an 18-gauge blunted/beveled needle. The needle is placed in the left ventricle of the heart and secured with a small hemostat if necessary. A manometer is connected to the air line before it enters the flask in order to monitor the air pressure. Perfusion pressure should never exceed normal blood pressure

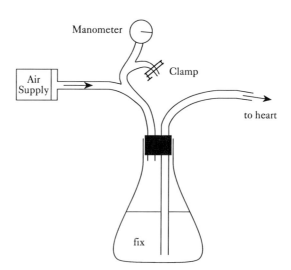

FIG. 11   Diagram of apparatus for use in perfusion fixation.

for the species being perfused or artifactual vacuolization can occur, particularly in the basal half of the retinal pigment epithelium.

3. Air pressure is adjusted by means of a clamp installed in a small side line between the air source and the fixative flask. Opening or closing the clamp will regulate the pressure until it reaches the desired level. A small slit is made in the right atrium to allow for drainage. Continue perfusing until there is only a small amount of blood in the fixative draining from the heart, then turn off the air and enucleate the eye. Remove the anterior structures as for immersion tissue fixation (see above) and immerse in the same fixative at 4°C for 12 to 24 hr.

Dissection of Retinal Tissue after Fixation

For optimal dehydration and embedment, eyes larger than 1.5 cm in diameter should be dissected into at least four pieces. We regularly cut the posterior pole into superior and inferior hemispheres, then into temporal and nasal quadrants. Tissue pieces of that size or smaller will dehydrate and embed properly.

It is a good idea to keep track of retinal quadrants and their orientation. Most tissues become completely black after OsO_4 fixation, and tissue landmarks may be difficult to find. A notch may be cut in the periphery of each quadrant or in the eyecup at an identifying location to allow orientation after OsO_4 fixation. After disection, transfer the tissue to small vials; glass scintillation vials work well.

Postfixation in 2% Osmium Tetroxide

Postfixation in 2% buffered OsO_4 is virtually required for routine study of tissue by electron microscopy to optimize membrane stability as well as to increase membrane density in the electron beam. (*Note:* There are procedures, such as postembedding immunocytochemistry, in which this step must be omitted; see Refs. 45 and 46.)

1. After overnight fixation, rinse the tissue using three changes of 0.137 M sodium phosphate buffer for 15 min each rinse.
2. Immerse the tissue pieces for 1 to 2 hr in a volume of 2% OsO_4 solution sufficient to cover. The tissue will usually darken or turn black. Fixation with OsO_4 hardens the tissue, preventing osmotic damage during subsequent exposure to solutions that are far from isotonic.

Dehydration

1. Make the following percentage ethanol solutions using 100% ethanol and double-distilled water as the diluent: 30, 50, 70, 85, and 95% (v/v).

2. Wash the osmicated tissue in double-distilled water three times for 15 min each. To be safe, treat the wastewater as a dilute OsO_4 solution and exercise appropriate precautions and disposal procedures.

3. Dehydrate the tissue sequentially through the 30, 50, 70, 85, and 95% ethanol solutions, each time leaving the tissue for 10 min in a volume of ethanol sufficient to cover the tissue twice over. (*Note*: During dehydration there is the option of staining the tissue *en bloc* with 2% uranyl acetate dissolved in 70% ethanol to increase tissue contrast. This is particularly valuable when embedding in Spurr's resin or LR White since they impart low contrast in the electron beam. Simply add one change in the uranyl acetate solution for 1 hr after the 50% ethanol solution and then continue the series with the 70% ethanol step. See Ref. 45 for details.)

4. Complete the dehydration process with three changes of 100% ethanol, for 20 min each. For the final two changes, the vials should be capped so that the alcohol will not absorb water from the air.

5. Process the tissue through two 10-min changes of propylene oxide, a transitional solvent between alcohol and resin.

Embedment

Embedding resins are usually bought as kits containing the different components. The following are slight modifications of the standard instructions.

Embedment in Araldite Resin

Araldite 6005 is usually the most brittle of the epoxy resins; however, for thin sectioning many find its stability and hydrophobicity an advantage. One batch of resin (made according to the following recipes) is sufficient to infiltrate or to embed tissue from one cat eye. Resins are toxic and potential carcinogens, so use gloves and a fume hood.

1. Into a 100-ml disposable beaker weigh out 25 g of Araldite 6005 resin.

2. Add 22.25 g of DDSA (dodecyl succinic anhydride). A convenient way to make this mixture is to weigh out the Araldite and then slowly add the DDSA from a large syringe (12–20 ml) to a total weight of 47.25 g. Use a disposable pipette to add 1.09 ml of BDMA (benzyldiethylamine).

3. Mix the components thoroughly using a glass rod. The resulting mixture will be very viscous.

4. Add an equal volume of propylene oxide to the resin mixture and stir until well incorporated.

5. Cover the tissue with enough of the 1:1 (v/v) propylene oxide–resin mixture to cover the tissue twice over. For good infiltration place the vials, uncapped, overnight on a rotating platform at about a 40° angle.

6. For embedment make up another batch of resin mixture and stir until well mixed. Try not to incorporate too much air as it can prevent proper infiltration. Air bubbles can be reduced by placing the mixture in a 45°C oven for 15 min. Remove the tissue from the resin–propylene oxide mixture (by now much of the solvent should have evaporated). Place the tissue pieces on Whatman (Clifton, NJ) No. 4 filter paper and place into a 45°C oven for 10–15 min to remove residual solvent–resin mixture. Place the tissue pieces in small aluminum weighing pans and cover with fresh resin. Place the pans in a 45°C oven for 12 to 24 hr and then transfer to a 60°C oven for an additional 12 hr.

Embedment in Spurr's Resin

Spurr's resin is a low-viscosity resin, suitable for embedding large specimens (47). However, this plastic has a number of idiosyncrasies which can make it difficult to work with. First, it is toxic and may be a potent carcinogen. Consequently, all work should be done with gloves, under a fume hood. Second, the plastic tends to be harder than either Araldite or Epon, and it is usually best to work with either the "soft" or even the "softer" version of the plastic formulation (Table I). Third, thin sections of this plastic are difficult to stain, and it is recommended that the specimens be stained *en bloc* with uranyl acetate. Finally, when mixing the components, add the

TABLE I Formulas for Spurr's Resin

Component[a]	Amount (g)			
	Hard	Firm	Soft	Softer
ERL 4206	10.0	10.0	10.0	10.0
DER 736	4.0	6.0	8.0	9.0
NSA	26.0	26.0	26.0	26.0
DMAE	0.4	0.4	0.4	0.4

[a] ERL, vinylcyclohexane dioxide; DER, diglycidyl ether of polypropylene glycol; NSA, nonenyl succinic anhydride; DMAE, dimethylaminoethanol.

accelerator DMAE (dimethylaminoethanol) last and only after the previous components have been thoroughly mixed.

1. Infiltrate the tissue in 2 parts propylene oxide and 1 part Spurr's resin for 30 min with rotation at room temperature. Special platforms for rotating samples during infiltration can be purchased from most EM supply companies (e.g., Ted Pella). See Table I for formulas for various Spurr's mixtures. Note that the hard, firm, and soft formulations are from the manufacturer's recommendations, while the softer formulation was provided by Dr. Brian Matsumoto (personal communication, 1991).

2. Infiltrate in 1 part propylene oxide and 2 parts Spurr's resin for 30 min with rotation at room temperature.

3. Remove the infiltration mixture and replace with fresh Spurr's resin. Rotate for 2.5–24 hr.

4. Transfer specimens to fresh vials or pans containing the resin. Polymerize between 60 and 80°C at least overnight.

Embedment in London Resin White

LR White can be used for conventional light and electron microscopy. In addition, with some tissue processing modifications LR White is suitable for postembedding immunocytochemistry owing to its slightly hydrophilic nature. This is a single component resin that does not require propylene oxide as a transitional solvent. For complete details on tissue processing and embedment, see Erickson *et al.* (46).

Microtomy

All of the resins may be cut either as 0.5- to 1-μm-thick sections for light microscopy or 60- to 90-nm-thick sections for transmission electron microscopy (for complete details, see Ref. 48).

Staining Sections

Staining for Light Microscopy

The following stains are suitable for resin-embedded sections. The stains may be used either alone or in combination. The staining effect can be tailored to the particular needs of an experimenter. Basic fuchsin, which primarily stains extracellular matrix, connective tissues, and nuclei, is useful when visualizing silver grains in autoradiograms. The blue stains allow for easier visualization of nuclei, although they may obscure labeling on autora-diograms or sections used for immunocytochemistry. Lipophilic stains such as *para*-phenylenediamine (PPDA) stain photoreceptor outer segments nicely and can be used along with either of the above stains.

Azure II–Methylene Blue–Toluidine Blue

1. To make 400 ml of stain, start with 350 ml of double-distilled water in a 16-ounce (~480 ml), screw-capped bottle.
2. While stirring add 1.0 g sodium borate (0.25%) and stir until dissolved.
3. Add 1.0 g azure II (0.25%), 1.0 g methylene blue (0.25%), and 1.0 g toluidine blue (0.25%).
4. Add 50 ml double-distilled water, cap the bottle tightly, and shake. Remove the cap and stir until dissolved.

Basic Fuchsin

1. To make 400 ml of stain, start with 380 ml of double-distilled water in a 16-ounce (~480 ml), screw-capped bottle. Add 20 ml of 50% ethanol and stir.
2. Add 2.0 g basic fuchsin (0.5%), cap the bottle tightly, shake, remove the cap, and stir until dissolved.

para-Phenylenediamine

para-Phenylenediamine is used as a saturated solution; we usually make 200 ml at a time. Crystalline PPDA should be added to double-distilled water until it no longer goes into solution. Care should be used when handling PPDA since it is carcinogenic.

Staining Procedure

The following procedure is applicable for staining using any of the reagents mentioned above.

1. Pipette a small drop of stain onto the sections (we usually stain on a hot plate at 100–125°C to speed up the process). Staining times will vary with temperature, thickness, tissue type, and resin. Do not let the stain dry, or precipitates will form.
2. Wash the sections thoroughly in double-distilled water and let dry.
3. Coverslip with a mounting medium (e.g., Permount from Fisher Scientific, Pittsburgh, PA).

Note: Various combinations of stains can be used in sequence to achieve different effects. In addition, if precipitates form, filter the stains through filter paper.

Staining for Transmission Electron Microscopy

The most common problems encountered in the staining of thin sections are dirt and salt precipitates. To avoid the former, always store grids covered in a petri dish or grid box. To avoid the latter, which is caused primarily by exposure to CO_2, we highly recommend Grid Sticks (Ted Pella). In this system, grids are attached to a grid holder and inserted into a glass pipette. Stains are then drawn into the pipette, minimizing exposure to air. Alternatively, the grids can be floated on drops of stain placed on a wax substrate or immersed in small pools of stain in depression slides.

The most common stains used for transmission electron microscopy (TEM) are Reynolds lead citrate (49) and uranyl acetate (50). Caution is advised in handling either of these heavy metal salts as both are dangerous if inhaled.

Lead Citrate

1. To make 100 ml of lead citrate, start with 60 ml of double-distilled water and, with stirring, add 2.66 g of lead nitrate, $Pb(NO_3)_2$, and stir until completely dissolved.

2. Add 3.52 g of trisodium citrate, $Na_3(C_6H_5O_7) \cdot 2H_2O$, and shake for 1 min.

3. Let stand for 30 min with intermittent shaking. The solution is milky white during this stage.

4. Add 16 ml of 1 N NaOH to clear the solution.

5. Bring the final volume to 100 ml with double-distilled water. Store tightly capped at 4°C.

1% Uranyl Acetate

1. To make 100 ml of uranyl acetate, add 1 g of uranyl acetate, $UO_2(C_2H_3O_2)_2 \cdot H_2O$, to 85 ml of double-distilled water and stir for about 5 min.

2. Bring the final volume to 100 ml with double-distilled water, store tightly capped in a brown or foil-wrapped bottle at room temperature.

Use of Grid Sticks

1. Attach grids to the holder and insert into a glass pipette.

2. Slowly draw uranyl acetate into the pipette; leave for the recommended time (see Table II).

TABLE II   Staining Times for Various Embedding Media

Stain	Staining time (min)		
	Araldite	Spurr's	LR White
Uranyl acetate	10	15	5
Lead citrate	15	20	7

3. Rinse several times with double-distilled water and then repeat the process using lead citrate.

Note: Staining times will vary depending on the type of resin and tissue. We have found that the times listed in Table II work well for mammalian photoreceptors. Carbon coating of the grids in a vacuum evaporator may be necessary to stabilize and electrically ground the sections for viewing (for full details, see Ref. 48).

Electron Microscopic Autoradiography

Autoradiography, the process of detecting radioactive isotopes in a section of tissue by the use of an overlying photographic-type emulsion, is a powerful technique that can be used at either the light or electron microscopic level. Although time consuming, this procedure can provide high-resolution localization of labeled molecules and results that can be quantified. It has proved useful in a variety of studies of photoreceptor metabolism (see Refs. 17 and 20). Bok (51) provides a complete technique for light microscopic autoradiography especially tailored to studies on photoreceptors. The method presented below is a modification of that described by Young and Droz (52). This modified technique should result in the recovery of over 90% of the sections as usable autoradiograms. Typical results that can be expected from this technique are illustrated in Fig. 12.

Slide Preparation

1. Prepare a 2% (w/v) solution of Parlodion (purified pyroxylin, Ted Pella) in isoamyl acetate. Stirring overnight often is required for the resin to dissolve completely.
2. Mark frosted glass slides with a diamond scribe as shown in Fig. 13. Scribe two + marks in the location indicated on the back, that is, the nonfrosted side of the slide. These will be used as guides in the placement of

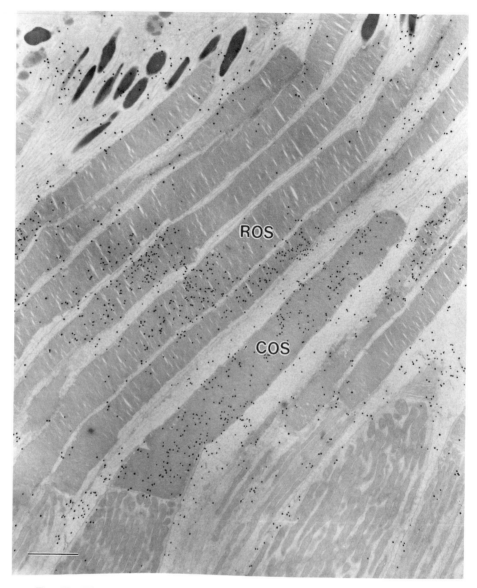

FIG. 12   Electron microscopic autoradiograph of photoreceptors from a rhesus monkey retina. The animal was labeled with [³H]fucose 96 hr before perfusion fixation by the method described in the text. The label is accumulated in restricted "bands" in the rod outer segments (ROS) but occurs diffusely scattered over the cone outer segment (COS). Bar, 2 μm.

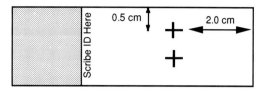

F<small>IG.</small> 13   Appropriate marking of glass microscope slides for the location of the sections to be used in EM autoradiography.

the sections later on. Also scribe an identification of some sort on the front of the slide just below the frosted part. You can also write on the frosted glass to further identify the specimen.

   3. Clean the slides as follows:

      a. Wash each slide in Liquinox or 7X detergent (Ladd Research Industries, Burlington VT) for a few minutes by rubbing the slides between your fingers (its a good idea to wear rubber gloves during this procedure). Overcleaning can result in films that stick so well they will never float off. It is strongly suggested that you go all the way through Step 5 and then try to get some films off. If you have trouble, try again.

      b. Rinse each slide several times in double-distilled water.

      c. Dip each slide in 95% ethanol and wipe dry with a lint-free cloth or Kimwipe.

      d. Store in a dust-free environment until use.

   4. Conduct the first Parlodion dip as follows:

      a. Dilute the 2% parlodion 1:1 with isoamyl acetate to produce a 1% (v/v) solution.

      b. Dip the nonfrosted end of the slide into the Parlodion to a point just below the identification marking.

      c. Dry the slides in a clean place at about a 30° angle. This layer of Parlodion will provide a substrate on which to place the thin sections.

   5. Conduct the second Parlodion dip as follows: Using the 2% Parlodion, redip only the bottom 1 cm of each slide and dry as before. This provides an "anchor" that will assist in getting the Parlodion to come off the slide at the end of the procedure.

Transferring Sections to Slides

   1. Make a plastic or wire loop that is the same size as the diameter of an EM grid (e.g., about 3 mm inside diameter). It will also be best if the loop is quite thin. (*Note*: Several EM supply houses, such as Ted Pella, sell section transfer loops. They work well but have inside diameters of 2 mm

or less, thus restricting the size of the sections that can be used. For this reason we make our own out of very thin but flexible plastic. Plastic rulers are good for this if they are not more than 0.5 mm thick. If you have made a loop it will be necessary to attach it to a handle, such as a pair of forceps, using some method; premade loops will come with a handle.)

2. Take very thin sections of the tissue (silver to pale gold at the thickest), then group a bunch of sections, enough to fill the loop, away from the other sections in the knife boat.

3. Gently lower the loop over the sections until you touch the surface of the water surrounding the sections.

4. *Very* gently withdraw the loop, carrying the sections in the film of water remaining in the center of the loop.

5. Place the loop over one of the scribed + marks (Parlodion-coated side up and scribed + on the underside) and slowly lower the loop until the water touches the Parlodion-coated glass surface. Be careful here that you do not touch the loop to the Parlodion coating as this may rupture it, causing the film to lift off during later stages in the procedure.

6. While holding the loop steady, wick away the water from beneath its edge using a wedge of filter paper. Be careful not to touch the sections or draw the water away too quickly, or the sections may end up on the filter paper.

7. Repeat the process so that there is one group of sections over each scribed + mark on the slide. (*Note*: Once the sections have dried onto the coated slide they will be nearly invisible!)

8. Store in a clean dust-free place.

Staining with Heavy Metals

1. Prepare a 5% aqueous solution of uranyl acetate.

2. Filter the solution and dilute with an equal volume of absolute ethanol.

3. Using a Pasteur pipette, place drops of this solution, about twice the diameter of the loop (e.g., 6 mm) over each + mark on the slides. Let sit for about 20 min. As with any heavy metal staining do not breathe onto the drops if possible as this may cause precipitates (more important with the lead citrate).

4. Wash the slides (gently), under running deionized water for 10 or 15 sec each.

5. Dry slides thoroughly and protect from dust and other contaminants.

6. Prepare a standard solution of Reynolds lead citrate as described above.

7. Place a drop of lead citrate, the same size as before, over each group of sections. Stain for 5–7 min.

8. Wash and dry as before.

Carbon Coating

Coat slides with a thin layer of carbon using a vacuum evaporator. Exact procedures are described by Hyatt (48). Too thick a layer will make the film brittle and difficult to remove. Carbon is necessary to provide subsequent stability in the electron beam and to prevent an undesirable interaction between any OsO_4 in the tissue and the nuclear track emulsion applied later.

Coating with Emulsion

The following is done in a darkroom under dim red (No. 4) or sodium vapor (recommended) illumination. These instructions are for ^3H- and ^{14}C-labeled specimens specifically; check the suitability of the emulsion before using these methods for other isotopes.

1. Coat about 50 clean slides with a single layer of 1% Parlodion. These will be used for removing bubbles from the emulsion and checking for proper thickness of the emulsion layer.

2. Stabilize a water bath at 40°C.

3. In a container (a 100-ml Tri-Pour beaker is good for this) that will remain stable in the water bath (e.g., not float around), mark lines with a permanent marker at 60 and 75 ml. This will be used to obtain a 1 : 4 dilution of emulsion in water.

4. Fill the container up to the lower (60 ml) line with deionized water, cover with Parafilm, and place in the water bath to stabilize at 40°C. This will take about 30 min.

5. Assemble the following materials: aluminum foil, black electrician's tape, porcelain spoon, slide boxes lined with filter paper, and small packages (about 4 cm × 2 cm × 2 cm) of desiccant wrapped in a couple layers of cheesecloth.

6. Under safe illumination, open a bottle of Ilford L4 nuclear track emulsion (Polysciences) and spoon chunks of it into the beaker of warmed deionized water until the level reaches the 75 ml mark. Return the beaker to water bath to melt the emulsion. Use fresh emulsion only, or high background can result.

7. After 15 min, stir the emulsion gently with the porcelain spoon. Repeat after another 15 min, and if there are still lumps repeat once more.

8. After the final stir, dip some of the blank, Parlodion-coated slides into the emulsion until no bubbles can be seen on the surface of the slide after dipping. Then dip several more slides to just below the scribed identification area and let dry at a fixed angle (about 30°).

9. Wait until the test slides dry (about 10 min in normal humidity) and then take a couple of slides out into the light to examine. You should have

an even surface, free of bubbles, and the coating over the area where the + marks are located should have a purple-green interference color when held at about a 45° angle to a light source. This will assure a proper thickness for producing a monolayer of silver grains. If the color is too dark (e.g., blue) then the emulsion needs to be diluted. If the color is too light (e.g., greenish-gold), then the emulsion is too thin and more should be added. When the thickness is correct go to Step 10.

10. Dip each slide containing the tissue into the emulsion to just below the scribed area, then blot the end onto filter paper to remove excess emulsion from the slide. Allow to dry for 1 or 2 hr at the same angle as the test slides.

11. When dry, place the slides into slide boxes, making sure you have several small groups of slides to use as test boxes for determining the proper exposure. Each test box should contain at least one slide from each experiment. There should be enough test boxes so that the proper exposure time can be safely determined. For example, if the estimated exposure time is 10 weeks, then there should be enough test slides to develop one at 8 weeks, one at 9 weeks, etc. Into each slide box place a couple packages of desiccant, using a blank slide to separate them from the dipped slides. Close the slide boxes and tape shut with black electrical tape, then place them into light-tight plastic bags (e.g., the kind Ilford photographic paper comes in) and wrap them with aluminum foil. Store at 4°C.

Note: A good rule of thumb is that the electron microscopic autoradiographic exposure time will be approximately equal to 10 times the exposure time for light microscopic autoradiograms cut from the same tissue sample (e.g., light microscopy, 7 days; electron microscopy, 10 weeks).

Development

The following development procedure uses phenidone (Lauder Chemicals, San Mateo, CA), which produces small round grains. If it is desired to visualize the entire track (worms), then elon development is suggested (53).

1. Prepare an ice bath that is large enough to hold the containers of fixer and developer.

2. Prepare fresh fixer (recipe makes 600 ml). Dissolve 180 g of crystalline sodium thiosulfate in 500 ml of double-distilled water and bring up to 600 ml. This fixer does not harden the gelatin or remove the stain.

3. Prepare phenidone developer as follows:
   a. In 300 ml deionized water dissolve in sequence 6.0 g ascorbic acid and 1.0 g 1-phenyl-3-pyrazolidone (phenidone).
   b. Vacuum filter (will take time), then add 2.4 g potassium bromide,

5.2 g sodium carbonate, and 80 g sodium sulfite (will saturate the solution and make it cloudy).

   c. Vacuum filter the solution (will take time), then add 24 g potassium thiocyanate (Mallinckrodt, St. Louis, MO, recommended).

   d. Bring the volume to 400 ml with double-distilled water, stir, vacuum filter, and use at once.

4. Bring a beaker of developer and two beakers of fix to 15°C. (*Note*: The temperature is critical to control of grain size; warmer developer means larger grains.)

5. Remove a slide or slides from the box and immerse into the developer to a level above the sections but below the edge of the Parlodion coating. This is to give the film an anchor so that it will not float off of the slide during processing. Plastic holders (Peel-A-Way, Polysciences, Warrington, PA) that can accommodate five slides are convenient for this and are available from most EM supply companies.

6. Develop for 1 min.

7. Rinse in the first beaker of fixer for 5 sec and then transfer into another beaker of fix for 5 min.

8. Wash in three sequential double-distilled water baths (at room temperature), for 1 min each.

9. Let the slides sit in double-distilled water for 5 to 10 min. Watch for signs of the film coming loose at the top of the slides, and if this occurs take them out at once.

Removing Films

1. Let slides dry for 1 to 2 min, then remove the bottom 3–4 mm of coating from the slide with a fresh razor blade, using a fresh blade for each slide. Score around the sides and top of the film with a razor blade.

2. Holding the frosted end of the slide, slowly immerse it into a large dish of deionized water at about a 45° angle. In the best of all possible situations the film should be loosened and float onto the surface of the water. They may need some encouragement: use a paper clip bent into an L shape to support the loose end of the film and gently pull the slide down and back while holding the film steady. (This is one of these steps you have to practice. It is not easy.)

3. Carefully place an EM grid over the sections on the floating Parlodion film. You should be able to see them if the film is dry and the light is just right.

4. Gently lay a strip of Parafilm onto the surface of the film, then slowly lift it up steadily from one end while rolling it over (thus inverting the film)

at the same time. With luck, the film and grids will come with the Parafilm. Place it, inverted (wet side of the Parlodion film up), onto a flat surface to dry thoroughly.

5. Using a pair of fine forceps punch all around the edges of the grid and then carefully lift the grid away from the surrounding Parlodion film and off of the supporting Parafilm.

6. View in the electron microscope.

Miscellaneous Notes

Electron microscopic autoradiography is not a trivial procedure. If you attempt it you can expect a trying time, but with some luck and caution you should be able to get through it the first time. Many of the steps require much time. For example, plan on 1–2 hr just to make the developer. The isoamyl acetate used for the Parlodion should be used in a fume hood. Peeling the films is an acquired skill. The first time you try, expect to lose up to 85% of the sections. As you become proficient you can expect up to 95% recovery. The thickness of the sandwich (e.g., Parlodion–section–emulsion) is very important, but some allowances can be made for the capacity of the microscope to deal with thicker (e.g., >90 nm) sections. In general, do not use sections thicker than necessary, in order to maximize resolution (i.e., start with silver sections).

A good reference for the theory and techniques of autoradiography is *Techniques of Autoradiography* (53).

Acknowledgments

The authors thank Dr. Dean Bok for time and patience in teaching the EM autoradiography technique described here in modified form, and Dr. Brian Matsumoto for many helpful hints and discussions. Dr. Richard Young provided the original design for the perfusion apparatus. The original data presented here were obtained as part of studies supported by research grants from the National Eye Institute (EY00888 and EY02082).

References

1. D. H. Anderson and S. K. Fisher, *J. Ultrastruct. Res.* **55**, 119 (1976).
2. S. K. Fisher, G. H. Jacobs, D. H. Anderson, and M. S. Silverman, *Vision Res.* **16,** 875 (1976).
3. D. H. Anderson and S. K. Fisher, *J. Ultrastruct. Res.* **67**, 23 (1979).
4. F. S. Sjöstrand, *J. Cell Comp. Physiol.* **33**, 383 (1949).
5. F. S. Sjöstrand, *Rev. Mod. Phys.* **31**, 301 (1959).

6. A. I. Cohen, *Exp. Eye Res.* **1**, 128 (1961).
7. D. I. Roof and J. E. Heuser, *J. Cell Biol.* **95**, 487 (1982).
8. A. M. Laties, D. Bok, and P. Liebman, *Exp. Eye Res.* **23**, 139 (1976).
9. A. I. Cohen, *J. Cell Biol.* **37**, 424 (1968).
10. D. H. Anderson, S. K. Fisher, and R. H. Steinberg, *Invest. Ophthalmol. Visual Sci.* **17**, 117 (1978).
11. A. I. Cohen, *in* "Handbook of Sensory Physiology" (M. G. F. Fuortes, ed.), Vol. VII/2, p. 63. Springer-Verlag, New York, 1972.
12. I. L. Hale, S. K. Fisher, and B. Matsumoto, *Invest. Ophthalmol. Visual Sci.* **32**, 2873 (1991).
13. M. S. Kinney and S. K. Fisher, *Proc. R. Soc. London B* **201**, 149 (1978).
14. R. H. Steinberg, S. K. Fisher, and D. H. Anderson, *J. Comp. Neurol.* **190**, 501 (1980).
15. K. Arikawa, L. L. Molday, R. S. Molday, and D. S. Williams, *J. Cell Biol.* **116**, 659 (1991).
16. R. W. Young, *J. Cell Biol.* **33**, 61 (1967).
17. D. Bok, *Invest. Ophthalmol. Visual Sci* **26**, 1659 (1985).
18. R. W. Young, *J. Cell Biol.* **49**, 303 (1971).
19. P. A. Liebman and G. Entine, *Science* **185**, 457 (1974).
20. D. H. Anderson, S. K. Fisher, and D. J. Breding, *Exp. Eye Res.* **42**, 267 (1986).
21. T. M. Richardson, *Vision Res.* **9**, 727 (1969).
22. J. C. Besharse and C. J. Horst, *in* "Ciliary and Flagellar Membranes" (R. A. Bloodgood, ed.), p. 389. Plenum, New York, 1990.
23. W. S. Sale, J. C. Besharse, and G. Piperno, *Cell Motil. Cytoskeleton* **9**, 243 (1988).
24. D. K. Vaughan, S. K. Fisher, S. A. Bernstein, I. L. Hale, K. A. Linberg, and B. Matsumoto, *J. Cell Biol.* **109**, 3053 (1989).
25. K. R. Peters, G. E. Palade, B. S. Schneider, and D. S. Papermaster, *J. Cell Biol.* **96**, 265 (1983).
26. D. S. Papermaster, B. S. Schneider, and J. C. Besharse, *Invest. Ophthalmol. Visual Sci.* **26**, 1386 (1985).
27. J. G. Hollyfield and M. E. Rayborn, *Exp. Eye Res.* **45**, 703 (1987).
28. D. S. Williams, K. Arikawa, and T. Paallysaho, *J. Comp. Neurol.* **295**, 155 (1990).
29. A. H. Bunt-Milam, J. C. Saari, I. B. Klock, and G. G. Garwin, *Invest. Ophthalmol. Visual Sci.* **26**, 1377 (1985).
30. R. Vallee and G. Bloom, *Annu. Rev. Neurosci.* **14**, 59 (1991).
31. G. L. Fain, G. H. Gold, and J. E. Dowling, *Cold Spring Harbor Symp. Quant. Biol.* **40**, 547 (1976).
32. E. Raviola and N. B. Gilula, *Proc. Natl. Acad. Sci. U.S.A.* **70**, 1677 (1973).
33. K. A. Linberg and S. K. Fisher, *J. Comp. Neurol.* **268**, 281 (1988).
34. F. S. Sjöstrand, *Ergeb. Biol.* **21**, 128 (1958).
35. L. Missotten, "The Ultrastructure of the Human Retina." Arscia Uitgaven, Brussels, 1965.
36. H. Kolb and R. Nelson, *Prog. Retinal Res.* **3**, 21 (1984).
37. A. P. Mariani, *Int. Rev. Cytol.* **86**, 285 (1984).
38. B. B. Boycott and J. M. Hopkins, *Visual Neurosci.* **7**, 49 (1991).

39. M. D. McCartney and D. H. Dickson, *Exp. Eye Res.* **41,** 313 (1985).
40. M. Kirsch, M. B. A. Djamgoz, and H.-J. Wagner, *Cell Tissue Res.* **260,** 123 (1990).
41. M. J. Hogan, J. A. Alvarado, and J. E. Weddell, "Histology of the Human Eye." Saunders, Philadelphia, Pennsylvania, 1971.
42. R. W. Rodieck, "The Vertebrate Retina." Freeman, San Francisco, 1973.
43. J. E. Dowling, "The Retina: An Approachable Part of the Brain." Harvard Univ. Press, Cambridge, Massachusetts, 1987.
44. P. K. Anhelt, H. Kolb, and R. Pflug, *J. Comp. Neurol.* **255,** 18 (1987).
45. P. A. Erickson, D. H. Anderson, and S. K. Fisher, *J. Electron Microsc. Tech.* **5,** 303 (1987).
46. P. A. Erickson, G. P. Lewis, and S. K. Fisher, *in* "Methods in Cell Biology" (D. Asai, ed.), in press. Academic Press, New York, 1992.
47. A. R. Spurr, *J. Ultrastruct. Res.* **26,** 31 (1969).
48. M. A. Hyatt, "Principles and Techniques of Electron Microscopy," 2nd Ed. Univ. Park Press, Baltimore, Maryland, 1981.
49. E. S. Reynolds, *J. Cell Biol.* **17,** 208 (1963).
50. M. L. Watson, *J. Biophys. Biochem. Cytol.* **4,** 475 (1958).
51. D. Bok, *in* "Methods in Enzymology" (L. Packer, ed.), Vol. 88, p. 763. Academic Press, New York, 1982.
52. R. W. Young and B. Droz, *J. Cell Biol.* **39,** 169 (1968).
53. A. W. Rogers, "Techniques of Autoradiography," 3rd Ed. Elsevier/North-Holland, Amsterdam, 1979.

[2] Rapid Freezing and Subsequent Preparation Methods in Retinal Cell Biology

Jiro Usukura

Introduction

Recent progress in molecular biology has greatly advanced vision research, permitting explanation of the mechanism of phototransduction and several retinal diseases at the molecular level (1–3). In particular, progress in gene manipulation has made it possible to create transgenic animals for determination of the total function of certain genes and the proteins they encode. Current biological analysis also requires an exact morphological counterpart that is close to the living state while maintaining high resolution. In recent years, rapid freezing followed by freeze-substitution and production of freeze-etching replicas has emerged as the method of choice for sample preparation for electron microscopy, because it is able to preserve delicate structures that are difficult to fix by conventional chemical techniques. Although the results largely depend on the quality of rapid freezing, at optimum, rapid freezing is able to arrest cellular metabolism instantaneously without chemical alteration or redistribution of proteins while preserving the structure in the living state. In other words, this approach has the potential to avoid possible morphological artifacts induced by chemical fixation.

In this chapter, we describe our method of rapid freezing for tissue fixation followed by freeze-substitution, freeze-etching, freeze-drying, and related methods. We illustrate these techniques with applications to the retina.

Rapid Freezing

Cryofixation techniques, including primitive rapid freezing, are methods in which cooling is done quickly so that water molecule migration in the biological sample is arrested prior to appreciable ice crystal formation. Cryofixation has been in use for several decades (4–6). The needs for improved resolution have increased along with the development of freeze-etching methods and progress in neurobiology. Several rapid freezing methods such as rapid quench-freezing (7–9), propane jet freezing (10–12), metal contact freezing using liquid nitrogen (13, 14) or liquid helium (15, 16), and high-pressure freezing (17) have been utilized so far. Each method has its specific advantages and disadvantages depending on the nature of the sample. In general, simple metal contact freezing, in which the sample is applied to a polished surface of copper block cooled by liquid cryogen, has been the most popular method to date and has given reliable results. In this chapter we present a practical protocol for metal contact freezing using a recently developed apparatus.

Practical Method

An eyeball enucleated from a double-pithed bullfrog (*Rana catesbeiana*) is opened along the ora serrate and dissected into small pieces about 3 mm square. For observation of photoreceptor cells, neural retinas are carefully detached from the pigment epithelium and then mounted on a circular filter paper (about 4 mm in diameter) wetted with Dulbecco's phosphate-buffered saline (PBS: 10 mM phosphate buffer containing 0.9% NaCl adjusted to pH 7.4) with the ganglion cell layer against the paper surface. The specimen on the filter paper is placed in the shallow hole of the specimen holder and inserted in the tip of the plunger as illustrated in Fig. 1. Immediately, the specimen is smashed against the polished surface of a copper block cooled with liquid helium which is contained within our recently developed rapid freezing apparatus (16) (now commercially available as RF 20 from EIKO Engineering, Mito, Japan).

The rapid freezing device is schematically illustrated in Fig. 2. It consists of two concentric Dewar vessels. The inner Dewar vessel contains the main freezing chamber, which is suspended from the shroud on three stainless steel poles and filled with liquid helium. The outer Dewar vessel is filled with liquid nitrogen and surrounds the inner vessel for cooling. A copper block with a mirror-polished surface is located in the center receptacle in the main (inner) chamber. It can be replaced for each freezing experiment, assuring a clean, frost-free contact surface. The specimen is protected from damage due to prefreezing in the stream of cold helium gas generated in the guide tube by an electrical heater and automatic shutter located at the end of the guide tube.

After freezing, specimens can be stored temporarily in a separate liquid nitrogen container prior to further processing.

Freeze-substitution

Specimens are dehydrated and fixed simultaneously in the frozen state by the freeze-substitution method. In this way, elution and rearrangement of soluble and structural proteins are extremely limited as compared with con-

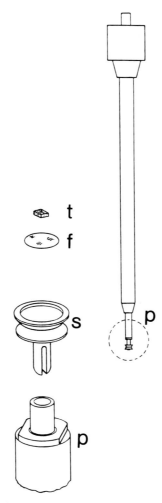

FIG. 1 Schematic illustration showing attachment of the specimen onto the tip of the plunger. t, Tissue specimen; f, filter paper; s, specimen holder; p, plunger.

ventional chemical fixation. Specimens prepared by this method are suitable for immunocytochemistry, hybridization histochemistry, and other investigations.

Practical Method

After freezing, specimens are quickly transferred with prechilled forceps into 10 ml of acetone with or without fixative, precooled to just above the

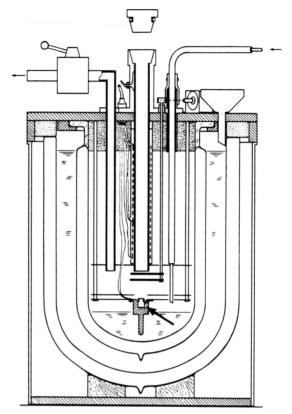

FIG. 2   Schematic diagram of an improved rapid freezing device. The copper block (arrow) can be exchanged by using a special pickup tool.

melting point. Samples are then kept for 2 days in a freezer at $-80°C$ or in a bath containing a slush of equal parts of solid dry ice and acetone (about $-80°C$).

Several classic fixative reagents can be used for freeze-substitution by dissolving them in acetone. Our experiment employed four fixatives: pure acetone, 2% OsO_4 in acetone, 2% tannic acid in acetone, and 2% glutaraldehyde in acetone as substitution media. Substitution media containing OsO_4 or tannic acid are easily made by dissolving the crystals in absolute acetone. In the case of substitution media containing glutaraldehyde, 400 μl of 50% glutaraldehyde is dissolved in 10 ml pure acetone and then dehydrated with a molecular sieve (No. 9882, 3 Å, 1/16", Sigma, MO).

After incubation for 2 days at $-80°C$, the specimens are warmed gradually to room temperature by placing them in a freezer at $-20°C$ for 2 hr and then in a refrigerator at 4°C for 1 hr. Subsequently, the specimens are washed 3 times with fresh pure acetone. For morphological study, the specimens (substituted chiefly with the OsO_4–acetone medium) are routinely embedded in Polybed 812 epoxy resin. For immunocytochemistry, the specimens (substituted with pure acetone or acetone containing glutaraldehyde or tannic acid) are embedded in Lowicryl K4M resin or London Resin White (LR White) after being washed once with pure resin. Finally, they are cured in the fresh resin under UV light (Lowicryl K4M) or thermally (LR White). For added contrast, some specimens are substituted with the medium containing tannic acid and further soaked in 1% OsO_4 in acetone for 5–20 min at room temperature, then washed well with pure acetone and conventionally embedded in Polybed 812. The specimens osmicated in this way showed excellent image contrast while maintaining antigenicity as described below.

Immunocytochemistry of Freeze-Substituted Retina

To examine the antigenicity of the specimens freeze-substituted with various substitution media, thin sections mounted on Formvar-coated grids are subjected to electron microscopic (EM) immunocytochemical labeling with anti-opsin antibody using the two-stage labeling method described in previous papers (18, 19). In all cases, the grids are floated with sections down on droplets containing appropriate solutions in PBS. The section surface is first blocked with 40 μl of 4% BSA (bovine serum albumin) in PBS (pH 7.4) for 5 min. Then the sections are incubated with 40 μl of a 1:200 dilution of the antiopsin antibody (antiserum) for 1 hr and washed 6 times with 500 μl PBS (1 min each) at room temperature. Subsequently, the grids are incubated for 1 hr with 40 μl of gold-conjugated anti-rabbit immunoglobulin G (IgG) (Auroprobe GARG 10 or G15, Amersham, Arlington Heights, IL), diluted 1:30 with 1% BSA in PBS. After being washed 7 times with 500 μl of PBS (1 min each), the sections are fixed with 100 μl of 2% glutaraldehyde in PBS for 15 min and then washed 8 times with 500 μl of Milli-Q (Millipore, Bedford, MA) water for 1 min each. The sections are stained with an aqueous solution of 5% uranyl acetate for 10 min prior to observation in the electron microscope.

Observation and Discussion

Morphological Aspect

Freeze-substituted photoreceptor cells show excellent preservation of membrane and cytoplasmic fine structure, including several filaments. In particular, rod and cone outer segments substituted with tannic acid followed by poststaining with OsO_4 reveal extremely regular stacking of disks with high contrast and definition. The disk-to-disk spacing in cones (35.8 ± 0.6 nm) is

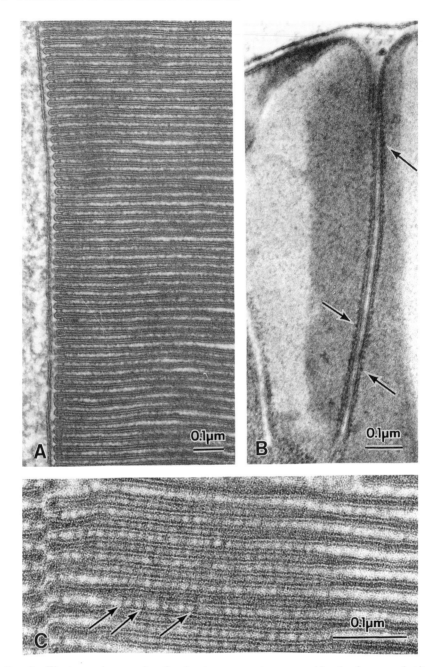

FIG. 3   Electron micrographs of rod outer segments prepared by the freeze-substitution method using tannic acid and OsO_4. (a) Longitudinal section showing regularly

obviously wider than that in rods (30.1 $\pm$ 0.3 nm) (compare Figs. 3 and 4). The disks appear to be flat and collapsed except at the marginal rim region. In rod outer segments, the filamentous substances connecting between disks at the neck of the hairpin loops (20, 21) are also observed much more clearly with this improved freeze-substitution technique using tannic acid than with conventional fixation (Fig. 3a). A grazing section through the disk margin reveals the filaments to be regularly spaced at intervals of about 15 nm (Fig. 3c). When sections are successively obtained in exact cross section, many electron-dense blobs are found along both the rim and the disk incisure, which may represent special large membrane proteins (Fig. 3b).

In contrast to the rod, the luminal space of a substituted cone disk is slightly variable in detail in spite of being almost collapsed. The lumen is more compressed near the open terminal opposite the ciliary side: the upper and lower disk membranes appear to be in direct contact, closing the lumen completely just before opening (Fig. 4). After opening, each disk membrane turns sharply and continues to the adjacent disk membrane as shown in Fig. 4a,c. Characteristic glycocalyal processes extend into the extracellular space from such membrane folds, with some reaching the surface of calycal processes coming from the inner segment (Fig. 4a).

Immunocytochemical Aspect

Freeze-substitution is able to preserve the antigenicity of proteins as well as the structure. Outer segments freeze-substituted with acetone alone retain high antigenicity. Although membrane images are negative, probably because of lipid extraction during acetone treatment, general morphology is good. To compare the immunocytochemical antigenicity of freeze-substituted tissue with that of conventionally fixed ones, tissues prepared by each method are labeled simultaneously with antiopsin antibodies. As shown in Fig. 5, the freeze-substitution method seems to be superior to conventional fixation using immunogold labeling.

In the future, freeze-substitution may become most useful in immunocytochemical investigation of delicate and/or unstable structures. However, the low image contrast of specimens substituted with acetone alone remains a problem in spite of the good preservation of antigenicity. Improvements in the substitution media, the staining method, and embedding resins will be required to overcome this problem. Indeed, tannic acid and glutaraldehyde

---

stacked disk membrane. (b) Cross section of disk membranes showing electron-dense blobs aligned along the rim (arrows). (c) Grazing section through the hairpin loops of the disk rims. Arrows indicate filamentous structures connecting disks to each other, which are arranged at regular intervals.

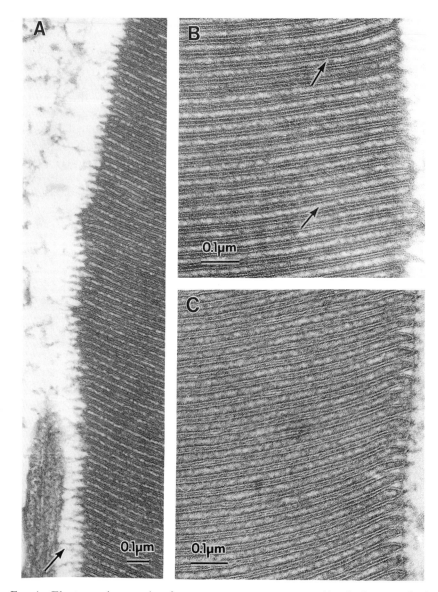

FIG. 4 Electron micrographs of cone outer segments prepared by the freeze-substitution method using tannic acid and OsO$_4$. (a) Low-power view of a longitudinal section. The arrow indicates the glycocalyx linking the calycal process and the open end of the disks. (b) Longitudinal section slightly oblique to the marginal region opposite the ciliary side. Arrows indicate that the luminal space of the disk becomes progres-

dissolved in acetone are useful as substitution media. The general morphology and immunocytochemical labeling appearance in samples substituted with these media resemble those substituted with acetone alone, except for a slightly improved image contrast.

On the other hand, poststaining with 1% OsO_4 in acetone after freeze-substitution with 2% tannic acid in acetone raises contrast while retaining the specific immune response to antiopsin (Fig. 6a,b), but the labeling intensity is significantly reduced in comparison to tissues incubated without osmium. However, morphological contrast and accuracy are excellent; actin filaments in calycal processes and the trilamellar structure of the membrane are observed more clearly. Antigenicity may be kept high by reducing the incubation time with osmium or by performing the incubation with osmium at low temperature. Brief incubation with osmium is found to increase the binding density of antiopsin antibodies with a minimum loss of morphological contrast (Fig. 6c).

Biochemical Aspect

Retinal homogenates freeze-substituted with several substitution media may be analyzed by sodium dodecyl sulfate–polyacrylamide gel electrophoresis (SDS-PAGE) and immunoblotting. The SDS-PAGE patterns of the samples substituted with acetone alone or tannic acid in acetone are almost identical to the pattern shown in unfixed material (J. Usukura, unpublished, 1986). This result suggests that no aggregation of proteins by strong chemical cross-linking occurs in the substitution process using acetone and tannic acid. In addition, immunoblotting of the samples shows good preservation of opsin antigenicity. Materials substituted or conventionally fixed with glutaraldehyde or OsO_4 cannot be analyzed by SDS-PAGE because they do not dissolve in the SDS sample buffer.

Freeze Replicas

To date, creation of freeze replicas combined with rapid freezing has been the only way to observe fine structure in three dimensions or the internal

---

sively more compressed from the closed to the open end. (c) Longitudinal section of the open end of the cone disks. The disk membrane is continuous with the adjacent disks and shows the characteristic sharp turn from which glycocalycal processes extend into the extracellular space.

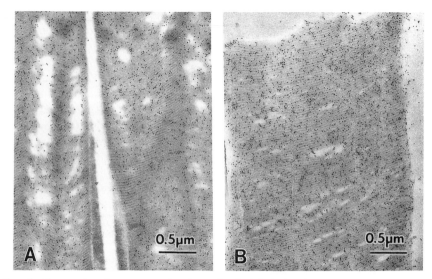

FIG. 5   Comparison between antiopsin antibody-labeled rod outer segments prepared by conventional chemical fixation (a) and by freeze-substitution with acetone alone (b). The specimens were labeled in the same procedure using the same antibody.

structure of the membrane at high resolution without chemical fixation. In a strict sense, freeze replica techniques are divided into two similar methods, freeze-fracture and freeze-etching replicas. Freeze-fracture reveals exclusively fractured membrane faces (P and E faces). In contrast, freeze-etching is able to reveal the cytoplasmic matrix and true surfaces of the membrane, which can be exposed only by sublimation (etching) of the ice filling the spaces between structures. This is a key method for a morphological investigation of the cytoskeleton and the extracellular matrix.

Practical Method

Fresh tissues are placed on the specimen holder and quickly frozen as described above. In our freezing device, the specimen holder is identical to that used in the freeze-fracture apparatus. In general, the same specimen holder should be used in the freezing device and the freeze-fracture apparatus, because it is difficult to transfer frozen specimens between holders. Frozen specimens are transferred to the freeze-fracture apparatus and fractured with a razor blade (a cutting knife is part of the apparatus) cooled at $-130°C$ or below under a reduced pressure of $3–5 \times 10^{-7}$ mmHg and at a specimen temperature of $-110°C$. After freeze-fracturing, the fracture planes

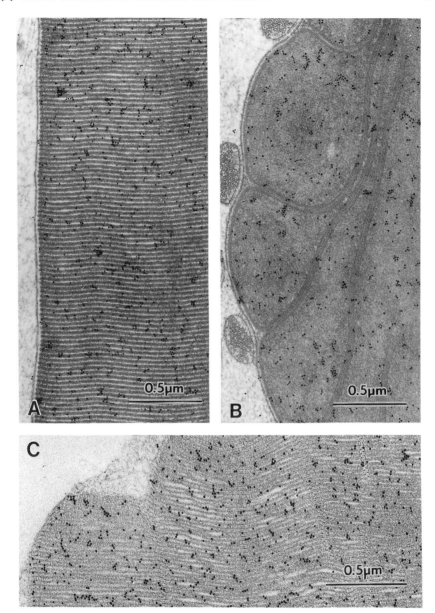

Fig. 6   Antiopsin labeling of rod outer segment prepared by the freeze-substitution method using tannic acid and OsO_4. (a, b) Immunogold-labeled longitudinal and cross section of the rod outer segment osmicated for 20 min at room temperature after freeze-substitution with 2% tannic acid in acetone. (c) Immunogold-labeled longitudinal section osmicated for 5 min at room temperature after freeze-substitution with 2% tannic acid in acetone. The labeling density obviously increased with the shorter OsO_4 treatment time without much loss of contrast.

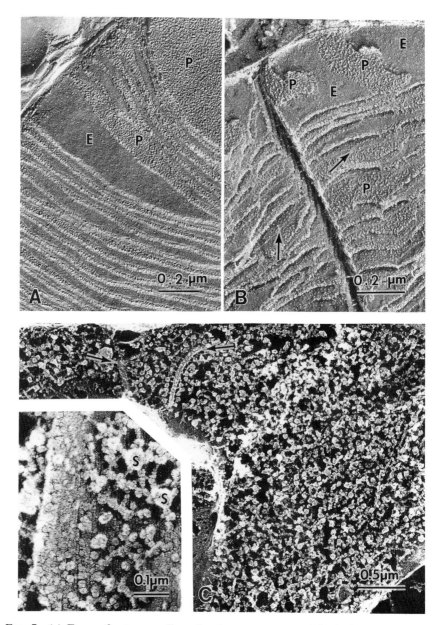

Fig. 7   (a) Freeze-fracture replica of rod outer segment. The P face (P) contains many more membrane particles than the E face (E). (b) Freeze-etched replica of rod outer segment. The cytoplasmic true surfaces (the ES face; arrows) are observed in addition to the P and E faces, which contain several particles presumed to be peripheral membrane proteins. (c) Deeply freeze-etched replica of the synaptic region of are immediately shadowed with platinum using an electron gun positioned at a 30° angle to the tissue surface, then coated with a film of carbon produced by electrical heating of carbon rods positioned at a 90° angle to the tissue surface. For freeze-etching, the temperature of the specimen must be raised to −90°C to enhance the sublimation of ice between the structures after fracturing the specimen, and the specimen must remain for several minutes at high vacuum to generate enough etching. Subsequently, the etched (slightly dried) surface is coated with platinum and carbon as mentioned above while being rotated. The thickness of platinum and carbon films deposited is 3 and 10 nm, respectively. Film thickness is determined with a quartz monitor.

Because the ice crystals on the fractured surface are evaporated completely in deeply freeze-etched replicas, an alternative fracturing method for frozen tissues has been developed by Ishikawa *et al.* (22). Slices several microns in thickness are removed from the initial frozen surface with a prechilled glass knife in a cryomicrotome at −130°C. The specimen is then transferred to the freeze-fracture apparatus. The etching time is slightly longer (10–20 min at −90°C) than in fracturing under vacuum. In our experience, this method is convenient for preparing deeply freeze-etched replicas of the retina, because a well-preserved region can be precisely chosen with the accuracy of a microtome.

All platinum-coated samples are removed from the vacuum and then carefully floated for 1 hr on detergent including sodium hypochlorite (kitchen bleach) to digest the tissue. Resulting replicas are subsequently transferred to two changes of distilled water for further cleaning, with meticulous care, using a platinum wire loop or molybdic mesh. Finally, the replicas are mounted on copper grids (No. 100) coated with Formvar.

Observation and Discussion

Morphological Aspect

Freeze-fracture replicas of rod outer segments reveal the asymmetric structure of the disk membranes; a large number of membrane particles presumed to be intrinsic membrane protein (mostly opsin) are found on the P fracture face but not on the E fracture face (Fig. 7a). In general, however, many more membrane particles are found on the P face than on the E face in

---

the photoreceptor cell. Numerous synaptic vesicles connecting one another with fine filaments are arrested in three dimensions. Arrows indicate synaptic ribbons. The inset shows the cytoplasmic surface of the synaptic ribbon on which synaptic vesicles (S) are attached with a few thin filaments.

various membranes. In freeze-etching replicas, the cytoplasmic surface (PS face) and the external surface (ES face) of the membrane become observable in addition to the P and E faces. The PS face of disk membranes contains several large particles estimated to be peripheral membrane proteins such as G proteins and phosphodiesterase (PDE) (Fig. 7b) (21). In particular, the use of freeze-etching replicas permits the observation of cytoskeletal architecture. Figure 7c shows freeze-etching images of the photoreceptor synaptic terminal in which synaptic vesicles are connected to one another with short filaments presumed to be synapsin I. Some synaptic vesicles are clearly attached to the surface of the synaptic ribbon with three to four thin filaments. Etching replicas also reveal substructures of the synaptic ribbon surfaces formed by a regular arrangement of elementary particles 4–6 nm in diameter (see inset of Fig. 7c).

Freeze-Drying

Freeze-drying is another innovative preparation method that provides tissue samples for morphological analysis of soluble proteins and ions. Freeze-dried tissues are amenable to current probing techniques such as immunocytochemistry, *in situ* hybridization, autoradiography of soluble proteins, and energy dispersive analysis of elements. In general, however, it is believed to be difficult to dry whole tissues without damaging the fine structure, because cellular water is able to form crystalline ice during the drying process as readily as during the freezing process. Therefore, a well-programmed drying sequence is needed to prevent devitrification of ice in frozen tissues during drying. More recently, a freeze-drying apparatus called a molecular distillation device, which removes water molecules from frozen specimens over a programmed drying cycle that minimizes ice crystal formation, is available commercially (RMC, Tucson, AZ) (23). Here, we describe a simple freeze-drying method that may not be molecular distillation in a strict sense. However, in application to EM autoradiography using [³H]ouabain, localization of the sodium pump was detected precisely with excellent morphological background.

Practical Method

Radioactive Labeling with [³H]Ouabain
The labeling is carried out mostly as described previously (24). Frog retinas excised into small pieces together with sclera are preincubated for 15 min in modified Ringer's solution (MRS) consisting of 82.5 mM NaCl, 27.5 mM

NaHCO$_3$, 2 mM KCl, 1 mM MgCl$_2$, 1.8 mM CaCl$_2$, and 10 mM glucose adjusted to pH 7.4 by equilibration with 95% O$_2$/5% CO$_2$ at 20°C. The tissues are then incubated for 90 min in MRS containing 1.7 μM [^{3}H]ouabain (35 μCi/ml) (NEN Research Products, Boston, MA). For control preparations, samples are preincubated for 15 min in MRS containing 10^{-4} M nonradioactive ouabain (Sigma Chemical Co., St. Louis, MO). They are then transferred to medium containing 10^{-4} M nonradioactive ouabain together with 1.7 μM [^{3}H]ouabain and incubated for 90 min. All solutions are kept at room temperature and are gassed with 95% O$_2$/5% CO$_2$ to pH 7.4 during incubation. After the incubation, the samples are washed twice with fresh MRS for 5 min each time, then rapidly frozen as described above.

Freeze-Drying Method

A bronze block in the shape of a cube (7.5 × 7.5 × 7.5 cm) with a deep cavity machined into the center (5 cm deep × 4 cm long × 1.2 cm wide) is used for freeze-drying of samples. Frozen samples are transferred to the cavity of the block in liquid nitrogen, then covered with a bronze plate (7.5 cm long × 7.5 cm wide × 2 mm thick). The cold block containing the samples is immediately brought into a vacuum evaporator in which the block is thermally insulated from the metal plate at the bottom of the evaporator with three folded Kimwipes. The block and specimens are gradually warmed to room temperature (about 48 hr) under high vacuum (10^{-7} to 10^{-6} mmHg), owing to the great heat capacity of the massive bronze block. Dried specimens are carefully removed to a glass vial that is saturated with OsO$_4$ vapor and are then fixed for 30 min in it. Dried and fixed samples are infiltrated and embedded with Spurr's epoxy resin according to the manufacturer's protocol (Polysciences, Warrington, PA). Subsequent autoradiography is carried out conventionally as described previously (25).

Observation and Discussion

Freeze-dried tissues embedded in the epoxy resin produce an extremely high contrast image in the electron microscope with adequate resolution. These properties are also retained in hydrophilic resins such as Lowicryl K4M (not discussed here). Because freeze-dried tissues preserve antigenicity well, this method will be suitable for immunocytochemistry of soluble substances.

Ouabain binds to the active sodium pump (Na$^+$,K$^+$-ATPase) too weakly to be retained through the chemical fixation procedure or freeze-substitution. As shown in Fig. 8, however, [^{3}H]ouabain binding sites are retained during freeze-drying and can be observed as silver grains. Most of the silver grains are localized in the inner segment plasma membrane of the photoreceptor cells. The density of silver grains is highest in the ellipsoid region. It is

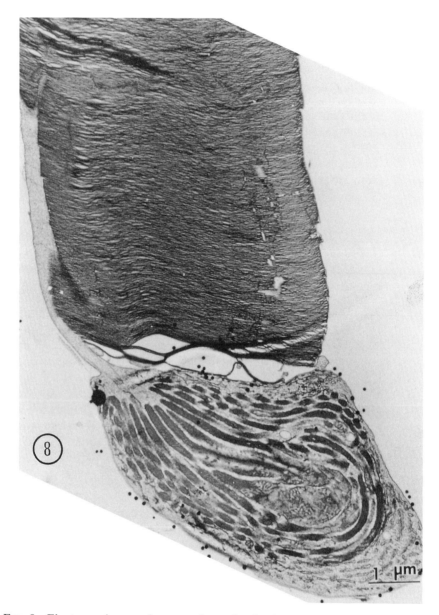

FIG. 8   Electron microscopic autoradiograph of a freeze-dried rod photoreceptor cell incubated in Ringer's solution containing [³H]ouabain. Grains are found exclusively over the plasma membrane of the ellipsoid region in the inner segment.

possible that the Na^+,K^+-ATPase is present in the plasma membrane or in some other location in the photoreceptor cell. However, from this experiment and other published data, it seems reasonable to conclude that most of the active Na^+ transport in the photoreceptor cell occurs across the plasma membrane of the ellipsoid region into the subretinal space.

References

1. T. Shinohara, L. Donoso, M. Tsuda, K. Yamaki, and V. K. Singh, *Prog. Retinal Res.* **8,** 51 (1988).
2. C. Bowes, T. Li, M. Dancinger, L. C. Baxter, M. L. Applebury, and D. B. Farber, *Nature (London)* **347,** 677 (1990).
3. G. H. Travis, J. G. Sutcliffe, and D. Bok, *Neuron* **6,** 61 (1991).
4. O. Eranko, *Acta Anat.* **22,** 331 (1954).
5. H. Fernandes-Moran, *Ann. N.Y. Acad. Sci.* **85,** 689 (1960).
6. K. M. Kretzschmar and D. R. Wilkie, *J. Physiol. (London)* **202,** 66 (1969).
7. M. J. Costello and J. M. Corless, *J. Microsc.* **112,** 17 (1978).
8. D. A. Handley, J. T. Alexander, and S. Chien, *J. Microsc.* **121,** 273 (1981).
9. H. Y. Elder, C. C. Gray, A. G. Jardine, J. N. Chapman, and W. H. Biddlecombe, *J. Microsc.* **126,** 45 (1982).
10. L. Bachmann and W. W. Schmitt, *Proc. Natl. Acad. Sci. U.S.A.* **68,** 2149 (1971).
11. H. Plattner, W. M. Fischer, and L. Bachmann, *J. Cell Biol.* **53,** 116 (1972).
12. R. Van Venetie, W. J. Hage, J. G. Bluemink, and A. J.Verkleij, *J. Microsc.* **123,** 287 (1981).
13. A. Van Harreveld and J. Crowell, *Anat. Rec.* **149,** 377 (1964).
14. H. D. Coulter and L. Terracio, *Anat. Rec.* **187,** 477 (1977).
15. J. E. Heuser, T. S. Reese, and D. M. D. Landis, *Cold Spring Harbor Symp. Quant. Biol.* **40,** 17 (1976).
16. J. Usukura, H. Akahori, H. Takahashi, and E. Yamada, *J. Electron Microsc.* **22,** 180 (1983).
17. H. Moor, *in* "Cryotechniques in Biological Electron Microscopy" (R. A. Steinbrecht and K. Zierold, eds.), p. 175. Springer-Verlag, Berlin, Heidelberg, New York, London, Paris, and Tokyo, 1987.
18. D. S. Papermaster, P. M. Reilly, and B. Schneider, *Vision Res.* **22,** 1417 (1982).
19. J. Usukura and D. Bok, *Exp. Eye Res.* **45,** 501 (1987).
20. J. Usukura and E. Yamada, *Biomed. Res.* **2,** 77 (1981).
21. D. J. Roof and J. E. Heuser, *J. Cell Biol.* **95,** 487 (1982).
22. H. Ishikawa, J. Usukura, and E. Yamada, *J. Electron Microsc.* **31,** 198 (1983).
23. J. G. Linner, S. A. Livesey, D. S. Harrison, and A. L. Steiner, *J. Histochem. Cytochem.* **34,** 1123 (1986).
24. J. Usukura, G. L. Fain, and D. Bok, *Invest. Ophthalmol. Visual Sci.* **29,** 606 (1988).
25. R. W. Young and D. Bok, *J. Cell Biol.* **42,** 392 (1962).

[3]   Preparation of Retinas for Studying
       Photoreceptors with Confocal Microscopy

Brian Matsumoto and Irene L. Hale

Introduction

Fluorescent antibody staining is a standard method for localizing specific proteins within photoreceptors. For high-resolution studies, the major limitation is its inability to detect small structures and intricate detail within thick specimens. Under such conditions, fluorescence arising outside the plane of focus reduces image contrast by creating a background haze. Thus, it is necessary to reduce light emanating from outside the plane of focus in order to obtain maximum contrast and resolution for epifluorescence microscopy.

The most direct means of increasing image contrast is to use thin preparations. For example, isolated cell preparations reduce background haze by limiting specimen thickness to the diameter of the cell. Vaughan and Fisher (1) used enzymatic digestion to separate individual photoreceptors, whereas Sale and co-workers (2) mechanically separated the cells. The technique is analogous to staining a monolayer of cells grown in culture in that it enables the microscopist to detect submicroscopic objects (smaller than 200 nm). Weber and co-workers (3) showed that single microtubules, only 25 nm in diameter, can be studied in cultured cells by immunofluorescence microscopy. Normally, a microscopist would use electron microscopy (EM) to visualize such small structures; however, fluorescence microscopy is a useful alternative since it enables the cell biologist to detect, for example, single microtubules while examining their relationship to other cellular organelles. By using epifluorescence microscopy, Vaughan and Fisher showed the presence of F-actin in the connecting cilium of photoreceptors, and Sale and co-workers showed that microtubules within the cilium and elliposid of the photoreceptor are acetylated (1, 2).

Although cell isolation is an obvious approach for obtaining photoreceptors for fluorescent antibody staining, few laboratories use this technique routinely. There are three factors that limit its general application. First, the isolation and staining of individual cells is time consuming and technically difficult. Photoreceptors must be separated from the retina, harvested, and then stained. Second, the structural relationship between photoreceptors and other retinal cells is disrupted. Obviously, it is impossible to study the interdigitation between the outer segment of rods and the apical villous

Methods in Neurosciences, Volume 15

processes of the retinal pigmented epithelium if the two are separated. Third, the isolation of cells can induce structural changes within the photoreceptor. For example, mechanical trituration of photoreceptors can result in the isolation of incomplete cells that have broken just distal to the nucleus (4).

To avoid these problems, it is necessary to prepare thin samples for observation by sectioning the intact retina. These preparation techniques include, but are not limited to, embedding tissues in paraffin and cutting the wax-infiltrated tissue (5), embedding in epoxy resins and cutting the plastic-infiltrated tissue (6–8), or freezing and then cutting the frozen tissue (9–12). In these procedures, it is often necessary to remove the support matrix so that antibodies have access to tissue epitopes. In the case of paraffin embedding, tissue sections are treated with xylene (5). Retinas embedded in epoxy plastics are treated with sodium methoxide (6–8). Finally, frozen sections are often treated with cold acetone. This organic solvent exposes cellular epitopes to antibodies by extracting lipid from the cell plasma membrane (9–12).

An alternate method is now available for obtaining the optical equivalent of thin fluorescent sections, namely, laser scanning confocal microscopy (LSCM). The optical principle of confocal microscopy is simple, but a large investment in hardware and software is required. By positioning an aperture within the optical path of an epifluorescence microscope, the contribution of light emitted from structures outside the plane of focus is reduced (13). It is impossible to remove 100% of the fluorescence from out-of-focus structures; nevertheless, a dramatic improvement in image contrast can be obtained. LSCM optically isolates fluorescence emission to the image plane, providing a means of obtaining high-resolution images of photoreceptor cells in thick sections.

This chapter describes the procedures and techniques that our laboratory uses for preparing retinas for confocal microscopy. We first provide a general description of the protocol, followed by a detailed paradigm for each procedure. Our laboratory has successfully stained a variety of proteins with these techniques, including cytoskeletal proteins (actin, tubulin, vimentin, and glial fibrillary acidic protein), integral membrane proteins (opsin, high molecular weight rim protein, and peripherin/rds), and soluble cytoplasmic proteins [glutamine synthetase, cellular retinaldehyde-binding protein (CRALBP), and transducin]. In addition, the basic procedure has been applied with lectins (Concanavalin A, wheat germ agglutinin, and peanut agglutinin) as well as fluorescent phalloidins and phallotoxins. The ability to stain a diverse population of retinal proteins with a variety of fluorescent probes shows the general applicability of this technique for localizing any protein within the retina (Fig. 1).

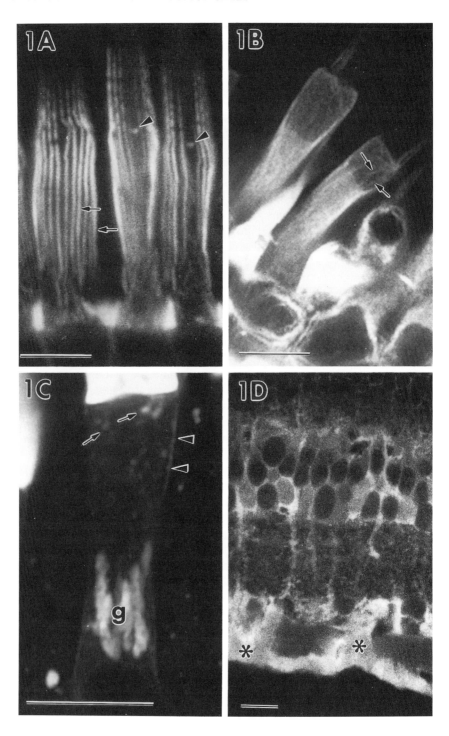

Overview of Methodology

The techniques for preparing tissues for laser scanning confocal microscopy are similar to those developed for the histological preparation of tissues for either light or electron microscopy. An investigator first preserves tissue structure with chemical fixation. Tissues are then supported by embedding in a support matrix, cut into sections, and finally stained with fluorescent probes.

Fixation

For optimum imaging, it is important to employ the most effective techniques for the preservation of photoreceptor structure. Because the investigator has the potential to reveal structures that normally require examination with an electron microscope, it is not surprising that the procedures and reagents developed for ultrastructural studies can be used effectively by the confocal microscopist.

Photoreceptors are preserved by placing the retina into a solution containing an aldehyde (fixative) that kills the photoreceptor cell and maintains its structure. As in histological procedures for electron microscopy, the goal is to reduce the ultrastructural damage that results from cellular death. Thus, it always is desirable to minimize the time between death of the organism

---

FIG. 1   Illustration of the variety of cellular proteins that can be visualized with fluorescent antibody staining and laser scanning confocal microscopy. (A, B, C) Micrographs showing the subcellular structure of the rod photoreceptor of *Xenopus laevis*. (A) Photoreceptor stained with rhodamine phalloidin. Arrows point to the parallel cables of F-actin in the inner segment of the cell. Arrowheads point to the concentration of F-actin found in the connecting cilium of the rod. (B) Sensitivity of the confocal microscope in detecting cytoskeletal filaments. A rod photoreceptor stained with an antibody specific for β-tubulin shows single microtubules (arrows); although these structures are only 25 nm in diameter, the optical characteristics of the light microscope make them appear 0.2 μm wide. (C) Photoreceptor stained with an antibody specific to opsin. Opsin is present in the Golgi apparatus (g) of the rod. In addition, opsin can be localized to the inner segment plasma membrane (arrowheads) and to vesicles within the ellipsoid (arrows). (D) Cat retina stained with an antibody specific to CRALBP. Müller cell end feet are intensely fluorescent (asterisks). CRALBP is a soluble cytoplasmic protein, and positive staining of the cells shows that such proteins are not extracted by the preembedding staining techniques described in this chapter. The staining of cytoskeletal proteins (A, B), of integral membrane proteins (C), and finally of soluble proteins (D) shows that preembed staining protocols can be applied to a variety of proteins within the retina. Bars, 10 μm.

and retinal fixation. Fortunately, the investigator has easy access to the retina and can quickly expose its cells to the aldehyde solution. Fixation is accomplished by taking an eye and flooding the vitreal cavity with a solution containing formaldehyde. In our work with cultured frog eyes, we routinely remove the anterior segment before placing the eye in culture medium and immediately after incubation place the eye into fixative. Anuran eyes are unusually convenient for specimen fixation since their rigid, cartilaginous sclera maintains the curvature of the retina, eliminating the torsional forces that can separate the retina from the retinal pigmented epithelium (RPE).

In contrast, it is more difficult to maintain the photoreceptor–RPE interface in the mammalian eye. We have found that the removal of the anterior segment before fixation causes artifactual retinal detachment and retinal wrinkles. Presumably, this is caused by the distortion of the spherical shape of the eye when it loses intraocular pressure. Normal apposition between the photoreceptor and RPE can be maintained by removing the eye from the animal and making a small incision in the limbus with a No. 11 scalpel blade (Bard-Parker, Franklin Lakes, NJ). The eye is then immersed in fixative, and the 5- to 10-mm slit allows the diffusion of this solution into the posterior segment. After 10 to 20 min of fixation at 4°C, the anterior segment of the eye is removed to allow for the diffusion of additional fix into the posterior segment.

The most generally useful fixative for this purpose is formaldehyde. This aldehyde rapidly penetrates tissue and, if properly applied, can preserve ultrastructural detail for electron microscopy (14, 15). More importantly, formaldehyde is a mild fixative, and proteins from tissues preserved in this reagent may better retain their antigenicity.

Fixatives containing glutaraldehyde should be used with caution. It is well known that this dialdehyde is superior to formaldehyde in the preservation of subcellular structure; however, as pointed out by Sabatini et al. (16), there is an inverse relationship between the ability of the fixative to preserve fine structure and protein enzymatic activity. Thus, a change in the conformation of a protein and loss of its antigenicity may accompany the improved visualization of structural detail. Besides the potential reduction of antibody binding, glutaraldehyde can further reduce the ability of the microscopist to detect low levels of labeled antigens by causing nonspecific tissue fluorescence (17). Taken together, these factors contraindicate using glutaraldehyde as the sole fixative.

Occasionally, the disadvantages of glutaraldehyde fixation are outweighed by its superior capabilities for preserving structure. Microtubules fixed in formaldehyde can appear fragmented while similar preparations preserved in fixatives containing glutaraldehyde appear intact (18). It is noteworthy that most electron microscopists have standardized on a primary fixative that contains glutaraldehyde for routine ultrastructural studies. We have observed that the ability of the photoreceptor plasma membrane to exclude extracellular dye molecules, such as Lucifer yellow, is retained following glutaraldehyde fixation but is lost following paraformaldehyde fixation.

Scientists who perform preembedding immunocytochemistry have observed that the deleterious effects of glutaraldehyde are concentration dependent. Many investigators use this fixative effectively at low concentration and in combination with formaldehyde. For experiments that require plasma membrane integrity or intact microtubules, we use a glutaraldehyde–formaldehyde fixative (0.08 to 0.1% glutaraldehyde, 4% formaldehyde in 0.1 M sodium cacodylate buffer, pH 7.4). The low glutaraldehyde concentration minimizes the formation of nonspecific tissue fluorescence and the loss of protein antigenicity. We have observed, however, that glutaraldehyde fixation, even at low concentrations, reduces antibody binding. The investigator also should be aware that glutaraldehyde will form polymers and degradation products during prolonged storage (19). It has been our experience that impure glutaraldehyde can cause increased nonspecific tissue fluorescence and loss of protein antigenicity. In our laboratory, we have standardized on electron microscope grade, 8% glutaraldehyde from Polysciences (Warrington, PA). This reagent is sold in small nitrogen-filled ampules that can be opened just before an experiment. Freshly opened vials are used to make the combination fixative.

In summary, 4% formaldehyde fixation is generally applicable for LSCM studies. The combination of formaldehyde and glutaraldehyde may be necessary to maintain either plasma membrane integrity or delicate cytoskeletal structure. The latter should be used with caution, however, because it may either reduce antibody binding or induce tissue fluorescence.

Embedding and Sectioning

Because the confocal microscope is used to obtain the optical equivalent of thin sections, it is neither necessary nor desirable to section the retina into slices thinner than 50–100 μm. We have observed that thinner sections are easily damaged during tissue processing. Sections of 100 μm thickness are easily cut with a Vibratome (Technical Products International, Kansas City, MO). This instrument advances a single-edge razor blade with a rapid reciprocating motion into tissue blocks. The major limitation is its inability to cut dense tissue containing large amounts of collagen (i.e., sclera or the optic nerve). This handicap can be avoided by separating the neural retina with attached RPE from the sclera at the level of the choroidal–scleral junction. If the resultant tissue preparation is surrounded by an agarose matrix, it can

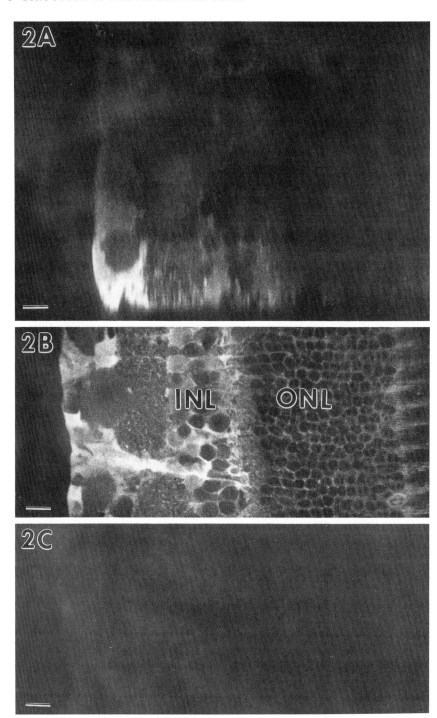

be cut easily with the Vibratome. Because agarose is made up as an aqueous solution in phosphate-buffered saline (PBS), tissue samples are not dehydrated but are immersed directly into melted agarose. The tissues blocks are then sectioned in PBS. Sections are usuable for antibody staining without further processing.

Staining

The purpose of cutting sections is to expose retinal cells to staining reagents. Antibodies do not rapidly diffuse through fixed tissues and, even in Vibratome sections, will be restricted to regions near the surface (Fig. 2). Vibratome sections are placed in a solution of PBS containing the primary antibody, 0.5% bovine serum albumin, and 0.1% Triton X-100. The detergent facilitates the diffusion of antibody into the sections. We have found that antibodies can penetrate about 10–25 μm with this detergent solution. Increased depth of antibody staining is advantageous, as it effectively provides a larger sample size. The microscopist can study more cells by simply focusing on different planes within the thick section. We have successfully used Triton X-100 at concentrations of 0.1 and 1.0% (Sigma, St. Louis, MO), lysophosphatidyl choline at a concentration of 0.1% (Sigma), and saponin at a concentration of 0.1% (Sigma). Antibody penetration into the tissue slice can be enhanced by increasing the amount of detergent in the staining solution; however, we

---

FIG. 2 Illustration of the limited diffusion of antibodies into a Vibratome section of the retina. To illustrate the general pattern of antibody penetration, sections from a cat retina were stained with anti-CRALBP. (A) Cross-sectional view of a Vibratome section lying flat on a glass slide. In this preparation, antibodies in buffered solutions containing 0.1% Triton X-100 penetrated only the first 20 μm of the section surface. Only one side of the section is stained, presumably the face opposite to the floor of the staining container. Under such conditions, it is important for high-resolution imaging that the stained half of the Vibratome section be placed next to the cover glass. Failure to do this will limit the achievable sensitivity, resolution, and contrast of the confocal microscope. (B) View of the same section, oriented 90° from the first image. The most intensely stained regions of the section reveal the Müller cell end feet, and faint staining occurs between the nuclei in the inner nuclear layer (INL) and the cell processes of the outer nuclear layer (ONL). Contrast this image with the equivalent image (C) obtained from the middle of the Vibratome section. In terms of electronic imaging, the gain and contrast settings of the confocal microscope are identical to those used to obtain the images in (B). This demonstrates the importance of collecting images near the surface of Vibratome sections. Bar, 10 μm.

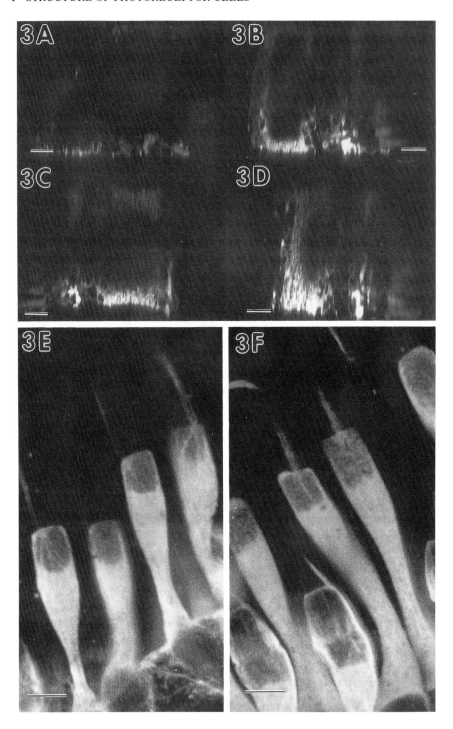

do not use more than 0.1% Triton X-100 (Fig. 3) because of the possibility that higher detergent concentrations will extract soluble proteins. We have successfully labeled CRALBP (Fig. 1D). It is significant that this soluble cytosolic protein can be effectively stained, since this is evidence that proteins of this type are not extracted during either fixation or staining.

Mounting Specimens

A variety of mounting media have been recommended for use with the confocal microscope. Media can range from aqueous solutions such as PBS for live cell work to methyl salicylate (20). We have abandoned the use of PBS because the fluorochromes fluorescein and rhodamine rapidly lose their fluorescence (bleach) in this medium when irradiated with light of the excitation wavelength. Although oil of wintergreen clears the tissue and permits deeper views within the retinal slice, we do not routinely use it as a mounting agent because it is water immiscible and the sample first must be dehydrated with ethanol. Dehydration is a potential problem, since it can cause tissue shrinkage. In addition, alcohol dehydration can extract certain fluorescent stains from the tissue. For example, fluorescent phalloidin will be extracted from cells exposed to either ethanol or methanol. Indeed, methanol treatment has been proposed as a method for quantitatively extracting fluorescent phalloidin from stained cells in order to assay the F-actin content with fluorometry (21).

We routinely mount tissues in 5% n-propyl gallate in 100% glycerol. n-Propyl gallate (Sigma) is an antioxidant that retards the bleaching of fluorescent dyes when they are irradiated with light of the excitation wavelength (22). Glycerol provides a nonaqueous environment that can enhance the

---

FIG. 3 Effects of detergents on the diffusion of tubulin antibodies into Vibratome sections. (A) Lateral view of a section in which antibodies were in a buffer solution without detergent. There is only a superficial band of staining at the surface of the Vibratome section. The addition of either 0.1% saponin (B) or 0.1% Triton X-100 (C) to the antibody solution increased the intensity and extent of fluorescent staining. The most intense staining occurred when 1% Triton X-100 was added to the staining solutions (D). (E) High-magnification image of photoreceptors stained with a β-tubulin antibody in 0.1% Triton X-100. (F) Photoreceptors stained with a β-tubulin antibody in 1.0% Triton X-100. The microtubule distribution for both photoreceptors appears normal when retinas are exposed, after fixation, to either 0.1% or 1.0% Triton X-100. Bar in (A–C), 20 μm; bar in (E, F), 10 μm.

fluorescent emission of fluorochromes, and this reagent does not extract phalloidin from F-actin.

Because the objective lens of the light microscope has a small working distance (130 μm for a 63× lens with a numerical aperture of 1.40), the investigator must ensure that the cover glass does not interfere with the downward focus of the microscope. Two precautions should be observed. A thin cover glass should be used, and the space between cover glass and specimen should be reduced to a minimum. It is possible to purchase cover glasses thinner than No. 1 thickness (0.13–0.19 mm range in thickness). For example, zero-thickness cover glasses (0.11–0.15 mm range in thickness) can be special ordered from many scientific supply houses. The space between specimen and cover glass can be minimized by mounting the sections on the cover glass and then inverting it onto a glass slide.

Confocal Microscopy

Obtaining images with LSCM can be an intimidating experience. An investigator must not only be a skilled light microscopist, but also a video microscopist who understands image processing paradigms. This chapter does not attempt to provide a general introduction to video imaging other than to caution the investigator to be aware that this technology can provide deceptive data. The reader is strongly urged to read Inoué's *Video Microscopy* (23) as it has an excellent description of image processing and the proper use of the light microscope. However, we discuss briefly two aspects of LSCM that should be considered for studying the photoreceptor.

Limits of Resolution

The interpretation of confocal microscope images can be difficult. It should be noted that a light microscope is more efficient at detecting the presence of small structures than it is in resolving those structures as separate entities. As mentioned earlier, epifluorescence microscopy can detect a single microtubule, 25 nm in diameter, but distinguishing individual microtubules as distinct entities requires that they be separated by almost 10 microtubule diameters. If two microtubules lie closer than 200 nm, they will appear as a single fluorescent strand.

A consequence of this optical limitation is that minute structures can be studied most effectively when they are present in low density. This is shown in Figs 1 and 3. A single microtubule that traverses the ellipsoid can be detected as an individual filament, but in the myoid, where microtubule density is much greater, the filamentous nature of the proteins is indiscernible. Under such conditions, a confocal microscope can only detect the presence of fluorescently stained tubulin.

From the description of this limitation, it is evident that there are advantages in studying the largest cells in the confocal microscope. In this regard, amphibian photoreceptors are valuable models for studying subcellular domains or cytoskeletal organization. A rod photoreceptor from *Xenopus laevis* has an outer segment that is 8 μm in diameter and 40 μm in length. In contrast, mammalian photoreceptors have outer segments that are only 1 μm in diameter and 15 μm in length. Photoreceptors from mammals, reptiles, fishes, and birds are so small that, following fluorescent antibody staining, the density of stained structures may make the entire inner or outer segment appear fluorescent. Under such conditions, LSCM can only provide evidence for the presence of a given protein within the photoreceptor.

Orientation of Planar Structures

The microscopist should be aware that a laser scanning confocal microscope image is not infinitely thin but has a significant depth of field. Although the LSCM allows optical sectioning of thick specimens, the depth of the image plane is of the order of 0.5 μm (63$\times$ oil-immersion lens with a numerical aperture of 1.40). As a result, the fluorescence intensity of a planar or linear structure varies with its orientation to the optical axis of the microscope.

Membranes whose surface is perpendicular to the optical axis of the microscope have a lower fluorescence intensity than membranes whose surface runs parallel to that axis. In the latter condition, the LSCM integrates the fluorescence of approximately 0.5 μm of stained membrane. Membranes that are oriented at right angles to the optical axis of the microscope appear fainter, because the LSCM can only collect light emitted from a single thickness of the plasma membrane ($\sim$0.1 μm). This is illustrated in Fig. 4. In Fig. 4A, a photoreceptor is stained for opsin and sectioned along its longitudinal axis. Opsin staining of the inner segment plasma membrane, endoplasmic reticulum, Golgi apparatus, and post-Golgi vesicles is present. Inner segment plasma membrane staining is very faint along the sides of the photoreceptor and is not evident in membranes whose plane is running perpendicular to the optical axis of the photoreceptor. In contrast, Fig. 4B shows a photoreceptor cross-sectioned optically at the plane of the connecting cilium, so that the bore of the connecting cilium and the ciliary plasma membrane run parallel to the optical axis of the microscope. Opsin staining is obvious in the plasma membrane of the connecting cilium. This variation in fluorescence intensity necessitates the examination of the photoreceptor from two orthogonal planes (i.e., in both longitudinal and cross sections).

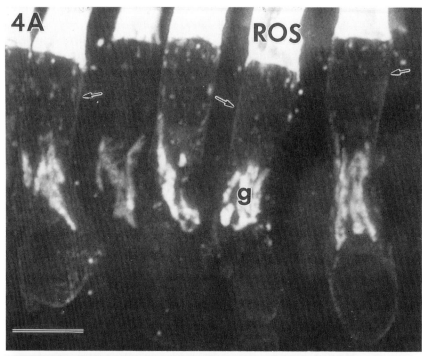

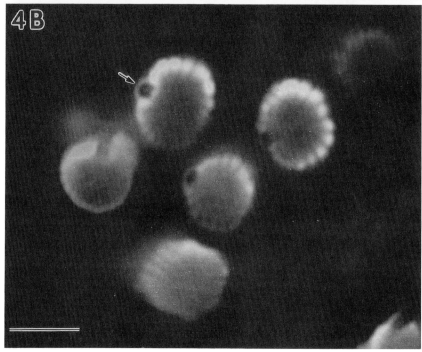

In conclusion, the investigator must evaluate whether the LSCM can provide useful information for the specific studies undertaken. In certain instances, the selection of the suitable animal model is predicated on the necessity of using a cell whose size is sufficiently large to provide useful information. Additionally, no matter what species of photoreceptor is selected, the investigator must analyze preparations from two orthogonal axes.

Reagents

Fixative

1. Prepare 100 ml of 0.2 M sodium cacodylate buffer solution (4.28 g/100 ml).
2. Add 8 g paraformaldehyde.
3. Heat the mixture on a hot plate in a fume hood. Stir continuously until paraformaldehyde powder goes into solution. Exercise extreme caution, as toxic formaldehyde vapors are generated by heating. As soon as the paraformaldehyde is dissolved, remove the solution from the hot plate.
4. Add distilled water to bring the volume to 180 ml. Allow the solution to cool to room temperture.
5. Adjust the pH by addition of 1 N HCl until the pH is between 7.2 and 7.4.
6. Bring the final volume to 200 ml. The solution is ready to be used as a fixative. The solution can be stored for long periods at 4°C. This composition

FIG. 4 Importance of orientation for visualizing membrane proteins in the confocal microscope. (A) Longitudinal view of rod photoreceptors stained for opsin. There is a low level of fluorescence (arrows) in the inner segment plasma membrane. The rod outer segment, post-Golgi vesicles, endoplasmic reticulum, and Golgi complex all show intense opsin fluorescence. ROS marks the rod outer segment of one photoreceptor, and g marks the region of the Golgi complex of that photoreceptor. (B) If photoreceptors are cut in cross section so that the plane of the ciliary plasma membrane runs parallel to the optical axis of the microscope, opsin staining is obvious in its plasma membrane (arrow). Because of the orientation, opsin staining appears more intense in the ciliary plasma membrane here than in the plasma membrane of the inner segment of the photoreceptor (A). In the cilium, a long section of the plasma membrane lies within the optical path of the microscope. Conversely, owing to the curvature of the photoreceptor inner segment, only a small portion of its plasma membrane in (A) is aligned along the optical axis of the microscope. Bars, 10 μm.

of the fixative is 4% paraformaldehyde in 0.1 M cacodylate buffer, pH 7.2–7.4.

Note: To supplement the fixative with glutaraldehyde, add 2 ml of 8% glutaraldehyde (EM grade, Polysciences) after Step 4. This will make a solution with final concentrations of 0.08% glutaraldehyde, and 4% formaldehyde in 0.1 M sodium cacodylate buffer. This solution should be used immediately.

Staining Buffer

1. Prepare 1 liter 10× phosphate-buffered saline (PBS stock). Dissolve the following salts in double-distilled water: A, 13.8 g $NaH_2PO_4 \cdot H_2O$ and 85.0 g NaCl in double-distilled water to 1 liter; B, 14.2 g Na_2HPO and 85.0 g NaCl in double-distilled water to 1 liter. Mix 280 ml of A with 720 ml of B.
2. To make 100 ml PBS with bovine serum albumin (BSA) and Triton X-100, take 10 ml 10× PBS stock and added 80 ml H_2O. Then add 0.5 g bovine serum albumin (Sigma) and 1 ml 10% Triton X-100 stock (Sigma). Stir gently to avoid frothing. Check the pH and adjust with 1 N HCl or 1N NaOH, and bring to a final volume of 100 ml.

Embedding Medium

Preparation of embedding medium requires 100 ml PBS and 5.0 g low gelling temperature agarose (Sigma, type VI). Place 5 g of agarose in 100 ml PBS and heat in an Erlenmeyer flask suspended in a water bath. As the water bath comes to a boil, the agarose goes into the solution. Aliquot the agarose solution to test tubes and then cap with Parafilm; store in a refrigerator. These test tubes can be heated in a water bath as needed to remelt the agarose for embedding.

Mounting Medium

Add 5g *n*-propyl gallate to 100 ml glycerol. The powder will not immediately dissolve in glycerol; however, overnight stirring at room temperature will result in a homogeneous medium. The solution is stable at room temperature and can be maintained for 2 or 3 months.

Procedures

Fixation

Eyes are first removed from an anesthetized animal. In the case of amphibian eyes, it is possible to remove the anterior segment by first inserting an 18-gauge hypodermic needle in the area of the limbus. A pair of iridectomy scissors is used to enlarge the incision until iris, cornea, and lens are detached from the sclera. The rigid cartilaginous sclera of the frog eye prevents the collapse of the posterior segment of the eye. The eyecups can simply be placed in fixative since the removal of the anterior segment allows paraformaldehyde to diffuse rapidly into the retina. One obtains a neural retina that is closely apposed to the RPE. For long-term storage, eyes can be maintained in 4% paraformaldehyde in 0.1 M cacodylate buffer at 4°C.

For mammalian eyes, a No. 11 scalpel blade is inserted at the region of the limbus. The blade is removed and the eye placed in chilled fixative (4°C). We have found that mechanical trauma of the photoreceptor–RPE interface can occur if an attempt is made to remove the anterior segment of an eye that has not yet been hardened by fixation. Under these conditions, the neural retina can be thrown into folds that separate the photoreceptor outer segments from the RPE. Eyes are fixed for at least 10 min to harden the tissue. Then the initial incision is enlarged until the anterior segment is removed. The eyecup is fixed overnight at 4°C and then rinsed the next day in chilled PBS, 3 times for 5 min each. All solutions are kept cooled by leaving on ice. If desired, it is possible to rinse overnight at 4°C with agitation.

Embedding and Sectioning

Because it is difficult to cut both the rigid sclera and the soft neural retina, we separate the retinas and attached RPE from the sclera at the plane of the choroidal–scleral interface. Large retinas are cut into 5 mm by 10 mm rectangles. Solid agarose is liquefied by heating in a boiling water bath. Once melted, the agarose is cooled to 40°C before pouring into disposable plastic weighing cups. Tissue is placed in the melted 5% agarose. The resultant agarose blocks are hardened by placing them in a refrigerator (4°C). If it is necessary to store tissues overnight in the agarose, the agarose must be placed in a humidified chamber. An absorbent paper, wet with water, should be placed at the bottom of a petri dish. Agarose blocks are then added and the petri dish covered. Failure to store the tissue in this manner will result in desiccation of the blocks, making them unusable for either sectioning or staining.

Agarose cubes containing the neural retina are made by slicing the hardened gel with a single-edged razor blade. The investigator should avoid cutting the tissue directly since this can rend the tissue from its support matrix. A small border of agarose should always surround the specimen. The cube is blotted dry with a Kimwipe, and a small drop of cyanoacrylate (Krazy Glue) is applied to an anodized aluminum block. The agarose cube is placed on the glue and will bind to the block in a few seconds. Blocks are then placed in a Vibratome for cutting 100-μm-thick sections. A camel's hair brush is used to remove sections from the boat of the Vibratome.

Staining

Vibratome sections are transferred to a solution of primary antibody diluted in staining buffer (PBS with 0.5% BSA and 0.1% Triton X-100). Sections are stained overnight at 4°C with gentle agitation. The antibody solution is then removed, and sections are rinsed 3 times in staining buffer. Secondary antibodies conjugated to either florescein or rhodamine can be used; however, it should be noted that tissue autofluorescence is a greater problem when shorter wavelengths of light are used to illuminate the specimen. Thus, structures stained with fluorescein are more susceptible to being masked by tissue autofluorescence than those stained with rhodamine.

Mounting

1. Transfer tissue sections to the surface of a No. 1 or 0 thickness cover glass.
2. Wick away excess PBS with a No. 1 filter paper until the section is closely apposed to the cover glass.
3. Invert the cover glass with specimen and gently lower onto a glass slide that has a small drop of glycerol containing n-propyl gallate. Seal the edges of the coverglass with nail polish. These slides are temporary mounts, and sections should not be stored for long periods of time before being used for confocal microscopy. Usually, we mount and view the specimen the same day. We discard slides after 1 week.

Acknowledgment

The authors thank Drs. Don H. Anderson, Geoffrey A. Lewis, and Steven K. Fisher for critically reading the manuscript and providing helpful suggestions. In addition, we are indebted to Robert Gill for expert technical assistance. Finally, the following investigators are gratefully acknowledged for providing high-quality antiserum for staining the cells of the retina: Dr. Robert Molday provided a monoclonal antibody to rhodopsin (rho 4D2), Dr. John Saari provided a polyclonal antibody to CRALBP, and Dr. Michael Klymkowsky provided a monoclonal antibody to β-tubulin. Research was supported by National Institute of Health Research Grant EY-07191.

References

1. D. K. Vaughan and S. K. Fisher, *Exp. Eye Res.* **44**, 393 (1987).
2. W. S. Sale, J. C. Besharse, and G. Piperno, *Cell Motil. Cytoskeleton* **9**, 243 (1988).
3. K. Weber, P. C. Rathke, and M. Osborne, *Proc. Natl. Acad. Sci. U.S.A.* **75**, 1820 (1978).
4. M. Spencer, P. B. Detwiler, and A. H. Bunt-Milam, *Invest. Ophthalmol. Visual Sci.* **29**, 1012 (1988).
5. G. P. Lewis, P. A. Erickson, D. H. Anderson, and S. K. Fisher, *Invest. Ophthalmol. Visual Sci.* **53**, 629 (1991).
6. J. G. Wood, J. C. Besharse, and L. Napier-Marshall, *J. Comp. Neurol.* **288**, 299 (1984).
7. J. G. Wood and L. Napier-Marshall, *Histochem. J.* **17**, 585 (1985).
8. P. Röhlich, G. Adamus, J. H. McDowell, and P. A. Hargrave, *Exp. Eye Res.* **49**, 999 (1989).
9. L. V. Johnson, G. S. Hageman, and J. C. Blanks, *Invest. Ophthalmol. Visual Sci.* **27**, 129 (1986).
10. M. M. Dewey, P. K. Davis, J. K. Blasie, and L. Barr, *J. Mol. Biol.* **39**, 395 (1966).
11. I. Vigh-Teichmann, P. Röhlich, P. Vigh, and B. Aros, *Z. Mikrosk. Anat. Forsch.* **95**, 624 (1980).
12. L. V. Johnson and J. C. Blanks, *Curr. Eye Res.* **3**, 969 (1984).
13. E. H. K. Stelzer and R. W. Wijnaendts-van-Resandt, *in* "Cell Structure and Function by Microspectrofluorometry" (E. Cohen, ed.), p. 131. Academic Press, San Diego, 1989.
14. D. C. Pease, *Anat. Record* **142**, 342 (1962).
15. D. C. Pease, "Histological Techniques for Electron Microscopy." Academic Press, New York, 1964
16. D. D. Sabatini, K. Bensch, and R. J. Barrnett, *J. Cell Biol.* **17**, 19 (1963).
17. M. Osborn and K. Weber, *Methods Cell Biol.* **24**, 97 (1982).
18. B. S. Eckert and J. A. Snyder, *Proc. Natl. Acad. Sci. U.S.A.* **75**, 334 (1978).
19. R. Gillett and K. Gull, *Histochemie* **30**, 162 (1972).
20. P. C. Cheng and R. G. Summers, *in* "Handbook of Biological Confocal Microscopy" (J. B. Pawley, ed.), p. 179. Plenum, New York, 1990.
21. T. H. Howard and C. O. Oresajo, *Cell Motil.* **5**, 545 (1985).
22. H. Giloh and W. Sedat, *Science* **217**, 1252 (1982).
23. R. J. Walter, Jr., and M. W. Berns, *in* "Video Microscopy" (S. Inoue, ed.), p. 327. Plenum, New York, 1986.

Section II

Metabolic Studies

[4]   *In Vivo* Labeling of Retinal Components by Intraocular Injection

Paul J. O'Brien

Introduction

Advantages of Intraocular Administration

Because of the critical dependence of photoreceptors on the pigment epithelium both for nutrition and for vital processes such as phagocytosis of shed outer segment tips and reisomerization of retinoids, it is advantageous to study the cell biology of photoreceptors with the retina attached to the pigment epithelium. This can be done conveniently in amphibians with *in vitro* eye cup preparations. Unfortunately, in mammalian eye cup preparations the retina readily detaches, frustrating further study.

An alternative for mammalian studies is *in vivo* metabolic labeling. This method, however, can consume inordinate quantities of radioactive substrates if the labeled materials are introduced systematically, particularly in larger species. In addition to the expense of the isotopes, this approach also creates the problem of disposal of the radioactive animals. A convenient and much less expensive alternative is intraocular injection of the isotopes. The quantity of isotope needed is reduced by a factor of about 1000; for example, a 125-g rat has a vitreous volume of about 100 μl, resulting in a 1250-fold smaller dilution volume, assuming uniform distribution of the isotope in the body of the animal. The savings can be highly significant when one is working with larger animals such as cats, dogs, or primates.

An additional advantage of intraocular injection is the ability to use each eye independently, since there is very little crossover of radiolabeled precursor from one eye to the other. An example of the lack of crossover is an experiment in which reserpine was injected into one eye of each of a group of rats to block rod outer segment shedding. The shedding peak was abolished in the reserpine-injected eyes, whereas normal shedding was observed in the noninjected as well as in sham-injected eyes (1). Injected isotopes not taken up by the retina are eventually released into the blood, but, because of the dilution factor and the competition for uptake by other tissues, little if any of the isotope ever reaches the contralateral eye. As a result two different labeling protocols can be carried out in the same animal, a distinct advantage when working with large animals or scarce genetic mutants.

Advantages of Pulse Labeling

In attempting to follow intracellular transport of macromolecules or metabolic processing of precursor molecules, it is important that the pool of molecules be labeled relatively quickly and that no further labeling take place, that is, the pool should be pulse labeled. This permits uncomplicated analysis of further migration or metabolism of the pool. Intraocular injection accomplishes pulse labeling of retinal components when viewed on the scale of a few hours. Experience with rat retina labeling has shown that the uptake of a variety of compounds such as sugars, amino acids, glycerol, fatty acids, retinol, or inorganic phosphate is complete in 2 hr. Thereafter, the metabolic fate of these molecules can be studied without concern that new labeled molecules are entering the pools. In larger animals such as dogs, the uptake is delayed slightly because of the somewhat greater distance that the precursor molecules must diffuse through the vitreous body.

Mode of Uptake of Isotopes

Intraocular injection would appear to introduce labeled precursors by an abnormal route, but this may not be the case. Photoreceptors receive nutrients from the choroidal circulation through the pigment epithelium. Nutrients are transported through the pigment epithelial cells and across the interphotoreceptor space. Three cell types line this space: (1) the pigment epithelium, (2) photoreceptor inner and outer segments, and (3) the microvillous processes of Müller cells. In view of the fact that cellular retinol-binding protein and cellular 11-cis-retinal-binding protein are both found in pigment epithelium as well as Müller cells, one must assume that Müller cells are directly involved in the transport of the retinoids to photoreceptors. Furthermore, the large stores of glycogen in Müller cells suggest a role in supplying glucose to adjacent photoreceptors and inner retinal cells. The large surface area of the Müller cell microvillous processes in the interphotoreceptor space ideally suits this cell for a major role in the absorption and transport of nutrients coming from the pigment epithelium and destined for the photoreceptors.

Thus, it may be that nutrients reach the photoreceptors primarily through the Müller cells. The importance of this route becomes significant when one considers the architecture of the vitreal surface of the retina, which is composed almost exclusively of Müller cell end feet. As a consequence, labeled precursor molecules injected into the vitreal cavity are in a position to be taken up primarily by Müller cells, which are in intimate contact with the inner segments of photoreceptors through junctional complexes. Thus, there may be a direct pipeline from the vitreous body to all retinal cells nourished by Müller cells, and labeled molecules introduced by intraocular injection could reach the photoreceptors by the same route that they would follow if introduced systemically, but with the advantages cited above. It is known, however, that smaller macromolecules can cross the external and internal limiting membranes and gain access to the intercellular space. Presumably, small molecules can do the same. Regardless of the route, experience has shown that many different radioactive precursors rapidly label photoreceptors.

Methods

Intraocular Injection in Small Eyes: Rats or Mice

Anesthesia

The most convenient technique for rapidly anesthetizing a series of rats or mice for sequential injections involves the use of an inhalation chamber. This can be a desiccator with a gauze or cotton pad below the false bottom or a similar commercially available chamber with a side funnel that permits easy introduction of the anesthetic. Ether is very rapid, but methoxyflurane can also be used. Once the animal is unconscious, it can be removed from the chamber and maintained at a suitable level of anesthesia with the use of a nose cone. This can be a test tube with a gauze or cotton wad soaked with the anesthetic. Procedures using volatile, explosive anesthetics such as ether should be carried out in an approved hood.

Equipment

The eyes of rats and mice must be supported during the injection because they have so much mobility that they retract into the orbit when pressure is applied with the needle. To accomplish this, a pair of gently curved smooth-tipped forceps is used, with each tip ensheathed in fine polyethylene tubing. When the eyelids are gently separated, the eye can be proptosed with the forceps without abrasion of the extraocular tissues. The tips of the forceps are then used to cradle the eye during the injection (Fig. 1).

For the injection of radiolabeled compounds a 10-μl Hamilton (Reno, NV) syringe is used. The needle is $\frac{3}{8}$ inch in length and is cemented in place by the manufacturer, thus virtually eliminating any dead volume. A 30- or 33-gauge needle with a No. 4 needle style is suitable for both rats and mice. The syringe can be decontaminated with detergent after use and both dried and sterilized with alcohol. Maintenance of the tip with a sharpening stone permits indefinite reuse of the syringe and needle.

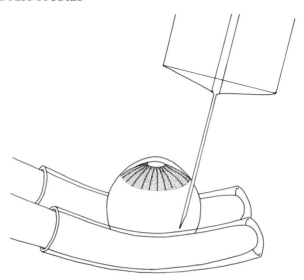

FIG. 1   Insertion of a needle into the eye of a rat. Note that the tip of the needle must be kept close to the sclera to avoid contact with the lens, which nearly fills the vitreous cavity. The tips of the forceps cradle the eye to prevent retraction of the globe into the orbit. (Original art work by Michael O'Brien.)

Procedures

For initial attempts at intraocular injection the use of a dissecting or operating microscope can be helpful. With experience the microscope is not necessary for injecting rat eyes, but it is essential for mice. With the eye held in place by the forceps, the needle is brought into contact with the sclera over the pars plana, being careful to avoid the vascular ring that is plainly visible, particularly in albino animals. The needle is inserted as nearly parallel to the sclera as possible to avoid contact with the lens (Fig. 1). In albino rats, the needle can be seen through the lens without dilation of the pupil after it has penetrated about one-third of its length. It is then positioned near the posterior pole, and a typical 2-μl injection can be made. Up to 5 μl can be injected into rat eyes, but only 1–2 μl into mouse eyes, without significant backflow. The quantity of isotope injected into each eye is usually 10–20 μCi but can be as high as 80 μCi, depending on the competing pathways.

Many labeled compounds are shipped at lower concentrations than needed for these injections. It is convenient to evaporate stock solutions to dryness in a beem capsule (used for tissue embedment). Beem capsules are used for all injections since an aliquot of isotope can be removed from the stock container and used in its entirety without risk of contamination of the stock. The capsule is conical at the bottom, permitting withdrawal of all but 2 or

3 μl, is wide enough to accommodate the barrel of the syringe, and can be capped to prevent evaporation. Large volumes of stock solutions can be evaporated with a stream of nitrogen while the capsule is held in a warm water bath. This procedure permits the mixing of two isotopes for double-labeling experiments. When one is a lipid, such as a fatty acid, and the other is water soluble, such as an amino acid, the lipid is redissolved in half the desired final volume of ethanol, and saline is then added to dissolve the amino acid and bring the solution up to the desired volume. The retina and vitreous body tolerate the 50% ethanol quite well.

Intraocular Injection in Large Eyes: Dogs or Cats

Anesthesia

Dogs are anesthetized with thiopental sodium for the injection. Inhalation anesthetics or long-acting barbiturates are not necessary as the preparation of the animal and the duration of the anesthesia are considerably longer than the injection procedure. Anesthesia with ketamine is contraindicated as it frequently results in increased intraocular pressure which produces backflow following the injection.

Equipment

Hamilton microsyringes with a volume of 0.5 ml and equipped with 26-gauge needles 1.25 cm long are used for the injection. A pair of toothed forceps is essential to grasp the conjunctiva and hold the eye steady during the injection. Because the globe retracts into the orbit with anesthesia and the sclera is difficult to penetrate with the needle, firm fixation is essential for atraumatic injection.

Determination of Dose and Vitreous Volume

To compensate for the variation in the size of large eyes, a determination of vitreous volume is made from the vertical corneal diameter according to the method developed by Aguirre (2). By adjusting the dose, comparable levels of labeling can be achieved in eyes of different sizes.

Procedures

The globes are massaged digitally for 45–60 sec through the closed eyelids to reduce intraocular pressure prior to the injection and to prevent backflow. The needle is inserted through sclera over the pars plana, taking care to avoid obvious blood vessels. The injection volume is 50–200 μl containing 50–200 μCi of isotope, depending on the size of the eye.

Selected Results

Labeling of Rat Rhodospin with Leucine and Palmitic Acid

Following the procedures described above, groups of four rats were injected with a mixture of 2 μCi [^{14}C]leucine and 20 μCi [^{3}H]palmitic acid per eye. The injection volume was 2 μl of 50% ethanol in physiological saline. At selected intervals rhodopsin was extracted from four pooled retinas and purified by chromatography on concanavalin A (ConA)–Sepharose followed by sodium dodecyl sulfate (SDS)–polyacrylamide gel electrophoresis. Figure 2 illustrates the time course of labeling and turnover of rhodopsin along with the standard deviation of two separate measurements of four pooled retinas for each time point. The leucine turnover followed the course expected on the basis of the 7 to 9-day outer segment renewal period, but the palmitate label remained for a prolonged period, reflecting the long-term retention and turnover of fatty acids in phospholipids as well as the probable turnover of the acyl groups bound to rhodopsin (3).

Labeling and Turnover of Rat Rod Outer Segment Lipids

The turnover of lipid components of outer segment membranes was also studied by intraocular injection of 50 μCi [^{3}H]palmitic acid per eye. As Fig. 3 shows, the palmitate was initially incorporated in the dark into phosphatidylcholine but was subsequently transferred to phosphatidylethanolamine. Ac-

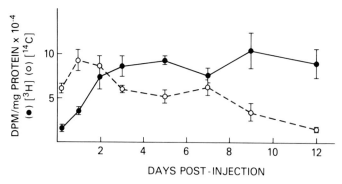

FIG. 2   Time course of rhodopsin following intraocular injection of [^{14}C]leucine (○) and [^{3}H]palmitic acid (●) in rats. Following enucleation, retinas were extracted, and rhodopsin was purified by ConA–Sepharose chromatography and SDS–polyacrylamide electrophoresis. Each point represents the average and standard deviation of two separate measurements of four pooled retinas. [Reprinted with permission from R. S. St. Jules and P. J. O'Brien, *Exp. Eye Res.* **43**, 929 (1986).]

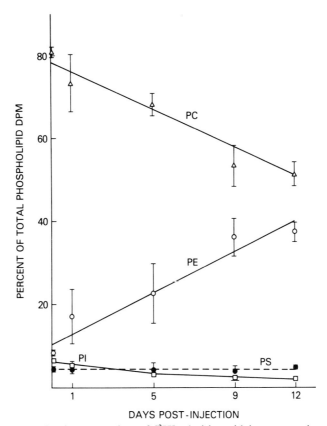

FIG. 3   Intraocular incorporation of [³H]palmitic acid into rat rod outer segment phospholipids in the dark. Each point represents the average of two (2-hr) or four (1-, 5-, 9-, and 12-day) samples ± standard deviation. Each sample contains crude rod outer segments from three retinas. Phospholipids analyzed were phosphatidylcholine (△), phosphatidylethanolamine (○), phosphatidylinositol (□) and phosphatidylserine (●). [Reprinted with permission from M. G. Wetzel and P. J. O'Brien, *Exp. Eye Res.* **43**, 941 (1986).]

ceptable standard deviations were obtained with two or four samples of three retinas each. Rod outer segments were purified by gradient centrifugation before the lipids were extracted and separated by two-dimensional thin-layer chromatography (4).

Labeling of Canine Rhodopsin with Leucine and Palmitic Acid

Using the procedures originally developed by Aguirre (2), miniature poodles were injected intraocularly with a mixture of 20 μCi [¹⁴C] leucine and 200

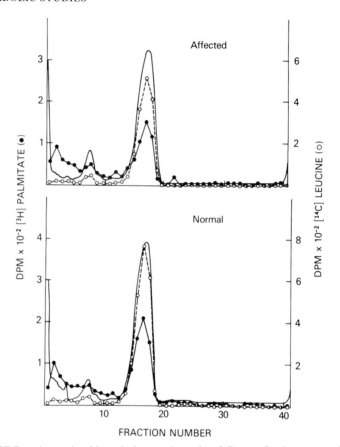

FIG. 4   SDS–polyacrylamide gel electrophoresis of ConA–Sepharose-purified rhodopsin from littermate normal and progressive rod–cone degeneration affected poodles 15 weeks of age injected intraocularly 1 day previously with [^{14}C]leucine and
[^{3}H]palmitic acid. The scan of the Coomassie blue staining pattern is shown as a
solid line with no symbols. The disintegrations per minute (DPM) of [^{14}C]leucine
(○) and [^{3}H]palmitic acid (●) are plotted against the gel fractions. [Reprinted with
permission from M. G. Wetzel, C. Fahlman, P. J. O'Brien, and G. D. Aguirre, *Exp.
Eye Res.* **50**, 89 (1990).]

FIG. 5   Matched sections of the peripheral retina from a normal dog 50 hr after
intraocular injection of 100 μCi [^{3}H]fucose. The bright-field (B) and dark-field (C)
autoradiograms (focus on grains) show label stratified in basal and apical pigment
epithelium (PE), an outer segment layer band (C, arrowhead), external limiting membrane (C, asterisk), and outer and inner plexiform layers (OPL, IPL). The dark-field
autoradiogram (C) best shows the sparse label located over nonnuclear regions of
the outer and inner nuclear layers. Arrows indicate the wall of a blood vessel in the
nerve fiber layer that has an intense accumulation of silver grains. Bar, 40 μm.
[Reprinted with permission from G. Aguirre and P. O'Brien, *Invest. Ophthalmol.
Visual Sci.* **27**, 636 (1986). Photomicrograph courtesy of Gustavo D. Aguirre.]

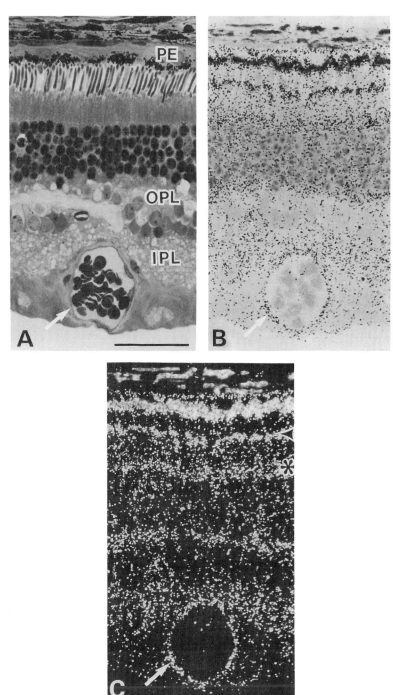

μCi [^{3}H]palmitic acid in a solution of 50% ethanol in physiological saline. One day later the dogs were anesthetized and enucleated in dim red light. The retinas were removed, and rod outer segments were prepared for rhodopsin extraction and purification by chromatography on ConA–Sepharose. Further analysis was carried out by SDS–polyacrylamide gel electrophoresis. Figure 4 shows comparable labeling of rhodopsin with both isotopes in the normal retina as well as the retina of young dogs affected with progressive rod–cone degeneration but prior to the onset of degenerative changes (5). In the same study essentially identical phospholipid labeling patterns were found in the outer segments of normal and diseased dogs using three different fatty acid precursors introduced by intraocular injection. These results were paralleled by *in vitro* incubations of trephine punches of retinas, showing, once again, no differences between the normal and affected retinas. Thus, intraocular injection can be used to compare metabolic processes in the retinas of large as well as small mammals.

Autoradiography of Intraocularly Labeled Retinas

One of the most useful applications of intraocular injection of isotopes is in autoradiography, which requires higher concentrations of isotope than biochemical studies. Figure 5 illustrates the high degree of labeling possible with this method. Here [^{3}H]fucose-labeled rhodopsin is visualized as a sharp band of silver grains which has been used to determine the rate of rod outer segment renewal in dog retinas (6). Note that the other layers of the retina are also well labeled.

A disadvantage in the use of large eyes is the nonuniformity of labeling in various regions of the retina. In one experiment with [^{3}H]palmitic acid, the specific activity of phospholipids in the nasal quadrant was 65% of that in the superior quadrant. Furthermore, the specific activity in the inferior quadrant was only 6% of that in the superior quadrant (5). With that much variation, it is important to sample several areas of the retina to be assured of adequate tissues for autoradiography. Alternatively, the tissue sections could be exposed for varying time periods to assure adequate exposure. Such variability in label distribution emphasizes the point that quantitation based on grain counts of samples from different areas of the retina may be highly inaccurate. Likewise, biochemical measurements, if not on the entire retina, can be made on trephine punches from many locations to avoid misleading data.

References

1. A. I. Goldman and P. J. O'Brien, unpublished observation (1978).
2. N. Buyukmihci and G. D. Aguirre, *Invest. Ophthalmol.* **15**, 579 (1976).
3. R. S. St. Jules and P. J. O'Brien, *Exp. Eye Res.* **43**, 929 (1986).
4. M. G. Wetzel and P. J. O'Brien, *Exp. Eye Res.* **43**, 941 (1986).
5. M. G. Wetzel, C. Fahlman, P. J. O'Brien, and G. D. Aguirre, *Exp. Eye Res.* **50**, 89 (1990).
6. G. Aguirre and P. O'Brien, *Invest. Ophthalmol. Visual Sci.* **27**, 635 (1986).

[5] *In Vitro* Biosynthetic Studies with Isolated Vertebrate Retinas

Steven J. Fliesler

Introduction

In the mid 1950s, Ames and Hastings (1) developed and described an *in vitro* system for studying water and electrolyte balance in neural tissue, using the rabbit retina as a model for the brain. Early on, it was recognized that the isolated neural retina affords an ideal system in which to study a variety of aspects of neuronal biochemistry, physiology, and cell biology. Under appropriate conditions, the retina can be sustained *in vitro* for several hours with preservation of normal cellular architecture and metabolic and electro-physiological competence. The vertebrate retina can be thought of as an "instant tissue slice," being only 0.1–0.3 mm in thickness. Hence, small molecules (e.g., ions, biogenic precursors, and metabolites) can diffuse readily into and out of the tissue. With judicious choice of radiolabeled precursors and pulse–chase protocols, one can label intracellular substrate pools of retinal cells to relatively high specific activities, and subsequently follow precursor–product relationships, intracellular transport of macromolecules, and even assembly and turnover of cellular organelles, using biochemical and cell biological methods.

Perhaps the most significant advantage of the *in vitro* system is that it affords the investigator the ability to manipulate the external environment of the retina at will, rapidly and reproducibly, in a myriad of ways that might be otherwise difficult or impossible to achieve with an intact animal. Obvious environmental variables of physiological significance would include ambient temperature, lighting conditions, atmospheric composition (e.g., aerobic versus anaerobic), and the identities and concentrations of extracellular constituents. Using appropriate pharmacological agents, one can selectively inhibit a particular biosynthetic reaction or pathway and examine the resulting effects on specific cells or cellular processes, without the potential toxicity problems, dilution factors, or tissue accessibility problems (i.e., involving the blood–retina barrier) that may arise when trying to perform similar experiments by systemic administration of the same compounds. Furthermore, the isolated retina is well suited for parallel electrophysiological studies to evaluate the consequences of variations in extracellular composition and ambient conditions.

Methods in Neurosciences, Volume 15

Although intravitreal administration of pharmacological compounds or radiolabeled precursors can circumvent some of the problems inherent to the whole-animal (systemic) approach and may even be the requisite method of choice for some studies (2), certain disadvantages may prevail. For example, some compounds have low solubility in the vitreous body, resulting in precipitation following intravitreal injection. Hence, the actual concentration of the injected compound in the vitreous body becomes uncertain, and the concentration of the compound reaching the retina may be significantly lower than that necessary to produce the desired effect. Other factors leading to variability of intravitreal injections may include the following: differences in exact intravitreal placement of the injected bolus; differences in the extent of backwash of injected material out of the injection site; eye-to-eye differences in vitreal volume; and differential rates of clearance of injected material from the vitreal cavity by retinal uptake versus competing pathways. Incubating isolated retinas in a medium of defined composition and volume obviates these problems. Under appropriate conditions, even relatively water-insoluble compounds can be maintained in incubation media at a well-defined concentration. Also, one can expose isolated retinas to much higher concentrations of radiolabeled precursors or pharmacological agents, and sustain those concentrations for much greater durations, than can be achieved with intravitreal administration of the same compounds.

In the early 1970s, studies concerning visual pigment (rhodopsin) biosynthesis and rod outer segment (ROS) membrane assembly in vertebrate retinal rod cells were greatly facilitated by the further development and utilization of procedures for maintaining vertebrate retinas in short-tem organ culture, primarily employing bovine (3) and frog (*Rana pipiens*) retinas (4). Most subsequent studies concerning metabolism, intracellular transport, and membrane assembly in the retina have employed *in vitro* systems of the same or similar design. In this chapter, the specifications and practical considerations of such systems are described, with particular emphasis on amphibian retinas, and specific examples are given to illustrate the use of isolated retinas for studying the biosynthesis and metabolism of molecules employed in the assembly of ROS membranes.

Methods

Incubation Media: Preparation and Practical Considerations

Ideally, the medium in which isolated retinas are incubated should mimic, as closely as possible, the composition of the interstitial fluid that normally bathes retinal cells in the living animal. In practice, because the interstitial fluid is a complex mixture of constituents (some of which have yet to be defined), a reasonable approach is to use a relatively simple balanced salt solution (e.g., Krebs–Ringer solution) with an ionic composition that approximates that of the interstitial fluid (1). In addition, the medium should contain a biologically compatible buffer and a suitable carbon source. Bicarbonate is most often chosen as the buffer, since it is a physiological constituent and can maintain the pH in the range 7.2–7.4 by utilizing a defined atmosphere containing carbon dioxide (e.g., 95% O_2–5% CO_2 by volume). It is recommended to also include 15–25 mM HEPES [4-(2-hydroxyethyl)-1-piperazineethanesulfonic acid; cell culture grade], preadjusted to pH 7.4, to compensate for variations in pH that occur when the tissue is subjected to conditions where the pCO_2 is not strictly controlled (e.g., during initial dissection, during transfer of tissue from one container to another, and during rinses).

α-D-Glucose (5–10 mM) is usually the carbon source of choice for utilization by neural tissues. However, unlike mammalian retinas (e.g., rat), the isolated frog retina is remarkable in that it does not require an exogenous carbon source to maintain normal tissue levels of ATP over incubation periods of up to 8 hr under normoxic conditions (5). The use of carbon sources that compete with the uptake of radiolabeled precursors should be avoided, so as to attain high specific activities of the intracellular substrate pools. For instance, when employing radiolabeled sugars as biogenic precursors, one should substitute either L-lactate (10–20 mM, preadjusted to pH 7.4), glycerol, or a Krebs cycle intermediate (e.g., pyruvate, fumarate) for glucose. Similarly, inclusion of amino acids in the medium is not recommended when using radiolabeled amino acids as precursors (i.e., during the pulse phase of pulse–chase protocols). However, it is otherwise often desirable to supplement the incubation medium with an amino acid mixture. Typically, casamino acids (an acid hydrolysate of casein; e.g., Amicase, Sigma, St. Louis, MO) are employed at a final concentration of 0.01 mg/ml. The stock solution of casamino acids (e.g., 1 mg/ml) should be filtered (0.45 μm; Millipore, Bedford, MA) prior to use. Alternatively, one may use appropriate dilutions of commercially available, cell culture tested, concentrated stock solutions of amino acids, such as minimal essential medium (MEM) amino acid solution (50× concentrate; Sigma) or MEM nonessential amino acid solution (100× concentrate; Sigma).

Antibiotics generally are not necessary when incubations are performed for up to 4–6 hr, since microbial growth is not generally significant in such short-term cultures. However, when prolonged incubations are being performed (≥6 hr) or when using mammalian retinas, it is advisable to supplement the medium prophylactically with penicillin G (4–8 μg/ml) and streptomycin sulfate (6–12 μg/ml) (3, 6).

Table I provides a convenient guide for the preparation of a simple incubation medium suitable for short-term incubation of amphibian retinas,

TABLE I   Preparation of Amphibian Ringer's–Bicarbonate Medium[a,b]

Reagent stock	Volume to prepare 100 ml medium (ml)	Final concentration	
Distilled water[c]	40	—	
NaCl, 1.0 M	12	120	mM
KCl, 0.1 M	2	2	mM
CaCl$_2$, 0.1 M	2	2	mM
MgSO$_4$, 0.1 M	2	2	mM
KH$_2$PO$_4$, 0.1 M	1.25	1.25	mM
NaHCO$_3$, 0.1 M	25	25	mM
HEPES, 0.5 M, pH 7.4	3	15	mM
MEM amino acids (50×)[d]	2	1×	
Sodium pyruvate, 1.0 M[e]	2	20	mM
D-Glucose, 1.0 M	1	10	mM

[a] See text for contraindications to using amino acids and glucose in medium. Add reagents in the order given.

[b] Antibiotics (penicillin G, final concentration 4–8 μg/ml; streptomycin sulfate, final concentration 6–12 μg/ml) may be added to medium.

[c] Adjust final volume of medium to 100 ml with water, after addition of all other reagents.

[d] Casamino acids (1 mg/ml stock; final concentration 10 μg/ml) may be substituted.

[e] Add to medium in place of glucose, immediately prior to use, after sparging medium with 95% O$_2$–5% CO$_2$.

commonly referred to as either Ringer's–bicarbonate–glucose (RBG) or Ringer's–bicarbonate–pyruvate (RBP) medium. All stock reagents should be at least analytical reagent grade; wherever possible, cell culture grade reagents are preferable. Glass-distilled or reverse-osmosis-purified water should be employed for the preparation of all stock solutions and for adjusting the final volume of the medium. The individual stock solutions should be sterilized by filtration (≤0.45 μm) into autoclaved glass reagent bottles equipped with lined screw caps, and they can be stored at 4°C for several months prior to use. The reagents should be added in the order given, so as to avoid precipitation of salts (particularly calcium phosphate).

It is convenient to make 500 ml stocks of the NaCl and NaHCO$_3$ solutions and 100 ml stocks of the other reagents. A 2× concentrated mixture of the salts and HEPES buffer can be prepared, filtered, and stored at 4°C for several months prior to use, without precipitate formation or other obvious changes in consistency. Carbon sources and amino acids can then be added and the final volume adjusted with water immediately prior to use. Because pyruvate is prone to oxidation, the stock solution of sodium pyruvate (1.0

M) should be aliquoted and stored at $-20°C$; the requisite amount should be thawed and added to the medium immediately prior to use (*after* sparging the medium; see below). This medium is typically 280 (±20) mOsmol/kg; slight hypertonicity tends to result in better preservation of cellular morphology than is obtained with isotonic or hypotonic media, without compromising the metabolic competence of the retina (6).

To assure complete saturation of the medium with the gas (typically 95% O_2–5% CO_2), the medium is sparged on ice for 15–20 min via a gas dispersion tube (Pyrex, 12 × 150 mm, with fritted end; Fisher Scientific, Pittsburgh, PA) that has been autoclaved prior to use. Sparging should be avoided if the medium contains constituents that produce excessive foaming, such as serum or egg ultrafiltrate. Wherever possible, such constituents should be added to the medium only after sparging. The medium is then allowed to equilibrate to the incubation temperature of choice, while maintaining a positive pressure of gas over the medium so as to stabilize the pH in the range 7.2–7.4. Phenol red (e.g., 8 mg/liter; GIBCO/BRL, Grand Island, NY) may be added to the medium to aid monitoring of pH.

The RBG or RBP medium described in Table I can be modified easily to be suitable for incubation of retinas from other species. For example, juvenile to adult *Xenopus laevis* retinas can be maintained with high metabolic activity and good morphological integrity in RBG or RBP that has been supplemented with 5–25% (by volume) Wolf–Quimby amphibian culture medium (GIBCO/ BRL) (7, 7a). Similarly, primate (8), human (9, 10), and canine (11) retinas have been maintained successfully in culture for up to 8 hr in RBG or RBP, where the NaCl concentration has been adjusted to 140 mM and the osmolarity has been adjusted by addition of 2% (w/v) sucrose. Alternatively, one may employ commercially prepared tissue culture media for incubation of retinas, such as RPMI 1640 (GIBCO/BRL), which has been used successfully for short-term incubations of bovine (12) and rat (13) retinas. The osmolality of the medium employed for incubation of mammalian retinas should be in the range 300 ± 20 mOsmol/kg.

For pulse incubations of short duration (e.g., ≤30 min), the minimum recommended incubation volume is as follows: for frog and rat retinas, 1.0 ml per retina; for *Xenopus* retinas, 0.2 ml per retina; for bovine retinas, 2.5 ml per retina. For incubations of longer duration (especially chase incubations), media volumes should be 2–4 times the minimum recommended volume. Retinas can be maintained for many hours to even days in defined culture media if care is taken to change the medium often (e.g., every 4 hr) and if microbial growth is prevented with suitable antibiotics. For example, Basinger and Hoffman (6) have reported successful maintenance of viable and morphologically intact frog retinas using a 4-hr pulse with radiolabeled leucine in RBG, followed by a 32-hr chase in RBG containing amino acids and antibiotics.

Apparatus

The essential components of the incubation apparatus consist of flasks to contain the retinas and incubation medium, a temperature-controlled water bath capable of regulated agitation of the contents of the flasks, and a gas delivery system to distribute the gas mixture to each flask at a defined and controlled rate. Such a system is depicted in Fig. 1.

Although small volume Fernbach flasks (Kimax No. 26502) provide maximum surface area for optimal gas exchange (6), commercially available Erlenmeyer flasks (Pyrex or Kimax; 25- or 50-ml capacity) are quite suitable. The flasks should be thoroughly cleaned and sterilized (autoclaved) prior to use. The volume of the medium in the flasks should be no more than 5 or 10 ml, respectively. Each flask is fitted with a rubber stopper (No. 0 for 25-ml flasks, No. 1 for 50-ml flasks), into which two 14-gauge hypodermic needles (1–1.5 inch length, with blunted ends) are inserted. One needle serves as the inlet port for the gas mixture, while the other is the outlet.

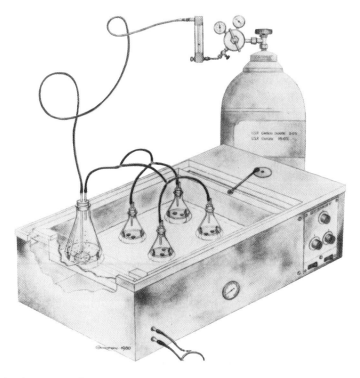

FIG. 1 Apparatus for *in vitro* metabolic studies of retinas. See text for details. [Reproduced with permission from S. F. Basinger and R. T. Hoffman, *in* "Methods in Enzymology" (L. Packer, ed.), Vol. 81, p. 772. Academic Press, New York, 1982.]

A compressed gas cylinder (e.g., H or T cylinder of high purity 95% O_2–5% CO_2) is fitted with a two-stage regulator and an in-line adjustable flow meter (Model 7221, Matheson, Dorsey, MD). The gas is bubbled through a humidifier flask before being introduced to the incubation flasks, so as to prevent evaporation of the medium during the incubation. The humidifier consists of a 250-ml Erlenmeyer flask partially filled with distilled water and fitted with a two-hole rubber stopper. A gas dispersion inlet tube is inserted through one hole (fritted end submerged under the water level in the flask), while a piece of glass tubing is used as the gas outlet. Alternatively, one can use a side-arm flask with a one-hole stopper; in this case, the side arm serves as the gas outlet. The humidifier flask should be set inside the water bath, so as to maintain the temperature of the humidified gas close to that of the incubation temperature. Latex or Tygon tubing (0.25 inch i.d.) is used to connect the flow regulator to the humidifier and the humidifier outlet to the inlet ports of the incubation flasks. A system of tubing and Y connectors is employed to construct a manifold for distribution of gas to multiple flasks. To ensure equal distribution of gas among the flasks, tubing lengths should be equal at each branch point; also, if an odd number of flasks is to be employed when using three or more flasks, a "dummy" flask should be included. Gas flow should be regulated at the rate of 1–2 ft³/hr per flask.

While we typically employ a Dubnoff metabolic incubator (shallow form shaking incubator; GCA/Precision, Chicago, IL), any temperature-controlled shaking water bath equipped to hold Erlenmeyer flasks of the desired capacity will suffice. The water level in the bath should be slightly above that of the medium in the flasks. The water bath should have removable or interchangeable flask clamps capable of securing flasks of the appropriate sizes employed for these incubations. The shaking cycle should be set at about 40 cycles/min; this rate is gentle enough so as to not cause significant mechanical disruption of the tissue, but is vigorous enough to ensure adequate exchange of nutrients and gases between the tissue and medium during the incubation. A temperature-controlled circulator can be coupled to the water bath to provide water temperatures below ambinet room temperature, if necessary.

Incubation Conditions: Temperature, Lighting, and Time

Routinely, amphibian retinas are incubated at 21–23°C, whereas mammalian retinas are incubated at 37°C. Typically, retinas are incubated either in complete darkness or in dim red light (Kodak, Rochester, NY, No. 1A photographic safelight, with 15-W incandescent bulb). Alternatively, normal fluorescent room lighting may be appropriate if one is not concerned about visual pigment "bleaching" or the potential effect of lighting conditions on the particular metabolic pathway being studied. For experiments involving the determination of the effects of light on some cellular process, dark-adapted and light-adapted retinas may be incubated side-by-side in separate flasks in the light, provided the dark-adapted retinas are kept in light-tight flasks (14). This can be accomplished easily by wrapping the flasks to be kept dark in black plastic electrical tape, and by using black tubing for all gas connections.

The duration of the incubation will be determined by the nature of the cellular process under investigation. In the case of rhodopsin biosynthesis and transport to the outer segment, *in vitro* studies with bovine (3), frog (4), and *Xenopus* (7) retinas have demonstrated that 1 hr is sufficient time for *de novo* synthesis and transport of the protein to the outer segment. Hence, pulse labeling of retinas for the purpose of studying these processes should take place over a short duration (e.g., 10–30 min), with a subsequent chase duration of at least 30–60 min. Obviously, longer incubation times (e.g., 4–6 hr) will permit greater accumulation of newly synthesized proteins in outer segments, and may even be required when using rat retinas (13).

Preparation of Intact Amphibian Retinas

The following methods for obtaining intact retinas from amphibian eyes have proved relatively simple and effective. The procedures are generally performed under dim red light, since the adhesional interaction between the neural retina and retinal pigment epithelium (RPE) is reduced in the dark-adapted state, and so as not to bleach the visual pigment. For improved visualization, it is helpful to wear a pair of magnifying loupes (Mark II Magni-Focuser, No. 107-2.75X, Edroy Product Co., Nyack, NY) or to employ a dissecting microscope during some of the procedures. For optimal tissue viability, it is important to remove and hemisect the eyes and transfer the eyecups to oxygenated medium rapidly. If multiple retinas are being harvested, they should be stored in a flask containing ice-chilled oxygenated incubation medium (at least 2 ml per retina) in a covered ice bucket until they are ready for use.

Eyes from adult leopard frogs (*Rana pipiens*) are enucleated with a pair of blunt, curved scissors (No. 86, Miltex Instrument Co., Lake Success, NY). Because the eyes of juvenile to adult *Xenopus laevis* toads are considerably smaller (~1.5–2.5 mm diameter) than those of frogs (~6–9 mm diameter), sharp pointed scissors are utilized for enucleation of *Xenopus* eyes. Holding the eye between the thumb and index finger against some paper toweling on the laboratory bench, the eye is punctured and partially hemisected at the ora serata with sharp, pointed scissors. For frog eyes, we use curved iris scissors (Storz Instruments, St. Louis, MO, E3412), while grasping the cornea with a pair of lightly curved dressing forceps (Storz Instruments, E1410). Placing the blade of the scissors (curve up) behind the lens and cutting circumferentially at the ora serata, the hemisection is completed. The lens and anterior segment are removed in one motion by anterior movement and closure of the scissor blades. For *Xenopus* eyes, we perform the hemisection with a pair of Noyes sharp-pointed iridectomy scissors (Miltex Instrument Co., No. 18-1540), holding the cornea with a pair of fine-tip jeweler's forceps (Miltex Instrument Co., No. 17-305), and removing the lens and anterior segment in a similar manner.

The eyecup is then submerged in oxygenated incubation medium in a 35-mm petri dish. The edge of the sclera is fixated with jeweler's forceps, while the retina–RPE–choroid complex is carefully teased away from the sclera by gentle circumferential traction at the anterior edge with another pair of forceps. As the tissue partially detaches from the eyecup, the optic nerve is exposed posteriorly; by grasping the optic nerve with forceps and pulling the tissue anteriorly, removal of the retina–RPE–choroid from the eyecup is effected. It is imperative to avoid contact with the retina as much as possible during this procedure, so as to minimize gross mechanical disruption of the tissue and loss of photoreceptor outer segments. The RPE–choroid is detached from the neural retina by grasping the edge of the RPE–choroid with one pair of forceps and the edge of the neural retina with the other pair and gently pulling the two layers apart, while keeping the tissue submerged in the medium. The neural retina is then transferred to a flask by carefully grasping the retina by its edge with forceps. For *Xenopus* retinas, we perform transfers with an inverted Pasteur pipette, applying a suction bulb to the tapered end after breaking it off. Retinas are drawn up into the barrel of the pipette in a column of medium; by simply touching the end of the pipette to the surface of the medium in the flask, retinas transfer by gravity from the pipette to the flask. Care must be taken not to draw air bubbles into the pipette during this process, in order to avoid mechanical agitation and outer segment loss. If multiple retinas are being harvested, they should be transferred to and stored in ice-chilled, oxygenated incubation medium in a covered ice bucket until ready for use.

Use of Radiolabeled Precursors

The choice of radiolabeled precursors will depend on the desired products to be radiolabeled and the proposed type of analysis to be employed to assess incorporation of the radiolabel. For instance, [^{35}S]methionine (or TRAN[^{35}S]LABEL, a mixture of radiolabeled methionine and cysteine; ICN Radiochemicals, Irvine, CA) is a suitable precursor for generalized radiolabeling of total cellular proteins, and its incorporation into proteins is readily assayed by techniques such as polyacrylamide gel electrophoresis (PAGE) and autoradiography (or fluorography), or scintillation counting of trichloro-acetic acid (TCA) precipitable material. When using weak β-emitters, such as ^{3}H, fluorography is a desirable alternative to conventional autoradiography. In the latter method, the gel is impregnated with a fluorescent "enhancer" (e.g., Autofluor, National Diagnostics, Mannville, NJ: Amplify, Amersham, Arlington Heights, IL) prior to being dried and exposed to X-ray film. In addition, the use of intensifier screens and exposure temperatures in the range of -70 to $-80°C$ significantly decreases the requisite exposure times for obtaining usable fluorograms.

However, [^{35}S]methionine is a relatively poor choice for subsequent analysis of incorporation by microscopic autoradiography, since the energetics and path length of ^{35}S β-particle emission preclude favorable resolution of radiolabeled proteins in tissue sections by this method. In this case, L-[4,5-^{3}H]leucine would be a more appropriate choice as a radiolabeled precursor. In addition, the amount of radioactivity [i.e., millicuries or disintegrations per minute (dpm)] utilized in a given incubation will be determined, to some degree, by the incubation conditions (e.g., pulse–chase versus continuous labeling protocol), the kind of analysis to be employed for assessing incorporation of the radioisotope into cellular products, the desired time frame for obtaining the analytical results, the specific activity of the isotopic precursor, and (in many intances) the purchase cost of the radioisotope.

For continuous labeling protocols of 1–5 hr in duration, with subsequent analysis of radiolabeled proteins by biochemical methods (e.g., PAGE/fluorography, TCA-precipitable counts), L-[4,5-^{3}H]leucine (specific activity 40–140 Ci/mmol) at levels of 1–10 μCi/ml is suitable, using the higher end of the range for shorter incubation times. Under these conditions, one should obtain usable fluorograms of dried gels by exposure of X-ray film (Kodak, X-OMAT XAR-5 film) in cassettes with intensifier screens for 1–3 weeks at $-80°C$. For pulse–chase protocols involving pulse durations of no longer than 20 min, L-[4,5-^{3}H]leucine levels of 0.1–0.5 mCi/ml should be employed. Similarly, [^{3}H]leucine levels of 0.1–0.5 mCi/ml are ideal for assessing protein synthesis and transport of newly synthesized proteins in cellular compartments by light or electron microscopic autoradiography. Using these levels, exposure times of 3–10 days should provide adequate light microscopic autoradiograms, while electron microscopic autoradiograms will require exposure times of 2–4 months (6). As a rule, the corresponding ^{14}C-labeled amino acid or ^{35}S-labeled amino acids (methionine, cysteine, or mixtures of these) can be used for biochemical experiments at a 10-fold lower level than the ^{3}H-labeled amino acid, with similar results.

The following additional general guidelines for useful ranges of radioisotopic substrates should be considered when studying *de novo* metabolism in vertebrate retinas in short-term organ cultures: D-[2-^{3}H]mannose, 0.1–0.5

mCi/ml (15–30 Ci/mmol), for N-linked oligosaccharide and glycoprotein metabolism; [1,2,3-³H]glycerol, 0.2–0.5 mCi/ml (30–50 Ci/mmol), for glycerophospholipid metabolism; [³H]acetate, 5–15 mCi/ml (5–10 Ci/mmol), for general lipid metabolism; (3R,S)-[5-³H]mevalonic acid, 0.5–5 mCi/ml (3–9 Ci/mmol), for isoprenoid lipid metabolism. In each case, the higher end of the concentration range should be employed when using pulse–chase protocols.

It is often advantageous to employ dual labeling protocols (e.g., ³⁵S- or ¹⁴C-labeled precursors in combination with ³H-labeled compounds) to study two separate metabolic pathways simultaneously in the same tissue. In such cases, it is advisable to utilize a 10- to 20-fold higher concentration (in dpm/ml) of the lower energy radioisotope. Such protocols presume the ability to separate or distinguish the radiolabeled products derived from each of the precursors employed.

Whenever possible, it is desirable to obtain radiolabeled precursors in sterile aqueous solutions, so that they may be added directly to a concentrated stock of incubation medium and the final volume adjusted appropriately with distilled water. Alternatively, if the radioisotopes are provided in an ethanolic or methanolic solution, the organic solvent should be removed by evaporation (e.g., under a gentle stream of nitrogen or argon) or lyophilization prior to use in the incubation medium. In the latter case, the relative volatility of the radiolabeled compound also should be considered.

Use of Inhibitors

It is often desirable to block a specific metabolic pathway and examine the effects of the inhibition on some cellular process. The following levels of metabolic inhibitors have been found to be at least 85% effective in short-term organ cultures of vertebrate retinas (2–6 hr): puromycin or cycloheximide (Sigma), 0.1 mM, for inhibition of protein synthesis; iodoacetic acid (Sigma), 1.0 mM, for inhibition of glycolysis; KCN or NaCN, 0.1 mM, for inhibition of respiration; isobutylmethylxanthine (Sigma), 4 mM, for inhibition of cyclic nucleotide metabolism; tunicamycin (Boehringer-Mannheim, Indianapolis, IN, or Sigma), 20 μg/ml, for inhibition of N-linked oligosaccharide synthesis and protein glycosylation; castanospermine (Boehringer-Mannheim), 0.1 mg/ml, for inhibition of N-linked oligosaccharide posttranslational processing; mevinolin (lovastatin, Merck Sharpe & Dohme, Rahway, NJ), 5 μM, for inhibition of de novo isoprenoid lipid biosynthesis.

Other pharmacological agents that perturb specific cellular functions or processes have been useful in understanding membrane trafficking in retinal cells. Monensin (Sigma) is a Na^+ and H^+ ionophore that perturbs intra-Golgi and post-Golgi vesicular transport (15). It can effectively disrupt membrane traffic at a concentration of 50–100 nM, without significantly inhibiting protein or lipid synthesis in the retina (16, 17). Similarly, brefeldin A (BFA; Epicentre Technologies, Madison, WI) blocks vectorial vesicular transport between the endoplasmic reticulum and the Golgi apparatus and disrupts normal Golgi organization (18). This compound is effective in short-term retina incubations at a concentration of 5 μg/ml, without inhibiting lipid or protein synthesis (19, 20).

For water-soluble compounds, it is desirable to make 100–1000× concentrated stocks of the inhibitors in distilled water or incubation buffer. For compounds that have limited solubility in water or aqueous buffers (e.g., tunicamycin, monensin, brefeldin A), dimethyl sulfoxide (DMSO) is the solvent of choice, but it should not exceed a final concentration of more than 0.2% (v/v) in the incubation medium. Solvents such as ethanol or methanol should be avoided, since they are easily metabolized by the retina and (at certain levels) may be toxic to the retina or appreciably perturb retinal metabolism. Some compounds (e.g., monensin) may require sonication in order to effect complete solubilization in the stock solution.

As a rule, retinas should be "preincubated" with the inhibitors for 30–60 min prior to addition of radiolabeled precursors, in order to permit sufficient time for diffusion of the inhibitors into the cells. This may be particularly important for relatively hydrophobic compounds (e.g., tunicamycin). However, small ionic compounds (e.g., KCN, iodoacetic acid) generally enter cells rapidly and, therefore, do not require preincubation. Companion retinas are incubated in parallel in medium containing an equal volume of the solvent used for solubilization of the inhibitor, as a control. Another desirable side effect of preincubation is the depletion of intracellular substrate pools, which affords higher specific activities and greater labeling efficiencies on addition of radiolabeled precursors.

Initiation and Termination of Incubations

Prior to initiating the incubation, the desired volume of medium is transferred to each flask, and the medium is equilibrated to the appropriate temperature under the desired controlled atmosphere. The incubation is then initiated by transferring retinas to the medium, either with fine-tip jeweler's forceps or with an inverted Pasteur pipette (e.g., for *Xenopus* retinas; see above), followed by brief, gentle swirling of the flasks and reinsertion of the stoppers. Adsorption of storage medium to the reinas can result in variable dilution of the incubation medium; hence, when radioactive precursors are employed, aliquots of the medium should be taken for assay of radioactivity after addition of the retinas.

Following the desired duration of exposure to radiolabeled substrates, the retinas are gently poured out of the flasks into petri dishes or 20-ml polystyrene beakers (diSPo beakers, No. B2718-20, American Scientific Products, McGaw Park, IL) and rapidly rinsed by transfer with jeweler's forceps through three to four serial changes of chilled chase medium (~5–10 ml each). The chase medium should contain a 10^2- to 10^3-fold excess of the nonradioactive form of the precursor. If the incubation protocol requires a subsequent chase phase, the retinas are then transferred to flasks containing temperature-equilibrated chase medium and the incubation continued for the desired duration. At the end of the incubation, the retinas are poured into petri dishes and briefly rinsed by transferring to fresh, temperature-equilibrated medium or balanced salt solution (e.g., Dulbecco's phosphate-buffered saline), prior to subsequent processing.

Preparation of Rod Outer Segment Membranes

In studies concerning the biosynthesis and intracellular transport of ROS membrane precursors, the incubated retinas are processed to obtain a purified ROS membrane fraction for subsequent analysis of incorporated radioactivity. We employ a modification of the discontinuous sucrose density gradient method of Papermaster and Dreyer (21), essentially as described by Fliesler and Basinger (22).

Briefly, incubated retinas are transferred to 17-ml ultracentrifuge tubes (e.g., Ultra-Clear tubes, No. 344061, Beckman Instruments, Fullerton, CA) containing 3–4 ml of ice-chilled, buffered 42% (w/w) sucrose solution (containing 65 mM NaCl, 2 mM MgCl$_2$, 0.15 mM CaCl$_2$, 0.1 mM Na$_2$ EDTA, and 10 mM Tris–acetate, pH 7.4), and ROS are sheared from the neural retinas by vortexing (three to five 10-sec bursts). At this point, one may opt to disintegrate the retinas further by homogenization with a motor-driven or hand-operated Teflon pestle (moderately loose fit) and withdraw aliquots of the retinal homogenate for subsequent analyses. The homogenized retinas are then overlayered with ice-chilled buffered sucrose solutions (containing the same constituents as given above, but without NaCl) having the following volumes and densities: 2 ml of 1.17 g/cm^3, 2 ml of 1.15 g/cm^3, 5 ml of 1.13 g/cm^3, and 3 ml of 1.10 g/cm^3. Following centrifugation (60–90 min at 100,000 g, 4°C), the material that forms a band at the 1.10–1.13 g/cm^3 interface (i.e., ROS membranes) is harvested with a Pasteur pipette, avoiding mixing of the gradient layers or inadvertent contamination with material from the other sucrose density layers. The harvested membranes are transferred to a plastic centrifuge tube, diluted at least 3-fold with ice-chilled hypotonic buffer (10 mM Tris–acetate, pH 7.4, containing 5 mM MgCl$_2$), and collected by centrifugation (20 min at 25,000 g, 4°C). The resulting membrane pellet is usually washed 2–3 more times to remove residual sucrose and soluble constitutents by repeated resuspension in buffer and collection by centrifugation, as described above.

Selected Results

The following examples serve to illustrate the use of isolated vertebrate retinas to study the biosynthesis of ROS membrane precursors and their assembly into ROS membranes, as well as the use of inhibitors to perturb these processes. Details of the analytical methods employed [e.g., measurement of specific activity of TCA-precipitable material, sodium dodecyl sulfate (SDS)-PAGE, fluorography, and light and electron microscopic autoradiography] are given in the original literature cited and references cited therein.

Time Course of Incorporation of [³H]Leucine into Retinal Proteins

A simple and convenient way to evaluate the effect of the chosen *in vitro* conditions on the viability and metabolic competence of retinas (e.g., in the presence versus absence of some pharmacological agent) is to measure the incorporation of a radiolabeled amino acid into retinal proteins as a function of incubation time, comparing the specific activity values obtained in the presence and absence of the pharmacological agent. Figure 2 illustrates an experiment to determine the effect of tunicamycin (TM) on protein synthesis in *Xenopus laevis* retinas *in vitro* over a 6-hr period (7). The incorporation of [³H]leucine was linear for up to 6 hr in the presence and absence of TM, indicative of ongoing protein synthesis over the time course. Although the slopes of the two lines differ by about 20%, suggesting a decreased rate of protein synthesis in the presence of TM, the differences in the specific activity values are not statistically significant until after 2 hr. Hence, pulse–chase protocols employing moderately short exposures to [³H]leucine should yield radiolabeled retinal proteins of comparable specific activities in the presence and absence of TM. Similar results have been obtained with *Rana pipiens* retinas (22).

Polyacrylamide Gel Electrophoresis and Fluorographic Analysis of [³H]Mannose Incorporation into Retinal Glycoproteins

The diversity of radiolabeled proteins that are synthesized during incubation of retinas with radiolabeled precursors can be assessed by subjecting the detergent-solubilized tissue to SDS-PAGE, followed by exposure of the gel

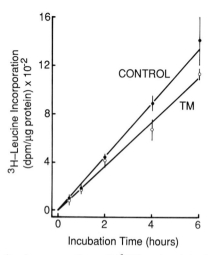

FIG. 2   Time course for incorporation of [³H]leucine into *Xenopus* retina TCA-precipitable material, in the presence and absence of tunicamycin (TM) (7). Incubations were performed at 21°C under an atmosphere of 95% O_2–5% CO_2 and dim red light, using the apparatus shown in Fig. 1. Neural retinas [three retinas per 3 ml of RBP medium, supplemented with 25% (by volume) Wolf–Quimby tissue culture medium per 25-ml flask] were preincubated for 1 hr with or without TM (20 µg/ml; final DMSO concentration 0.2%), then transferred to fresh medium (±TM) containing L-[4,5-³H]leucine (0.1 mCi/ml; initial specific activity 136 Ci/mmol) and the incubations continued. At each time point (0.5, 1, 2, 4, and 6 hr) retinas were retrieved and briefly rinsed with fresh nonradioactive medium, and the retinal proteins were precipitated with ice-cold 10% TCA. The TCA-precipitable material was resolubilized in 1 N NaOH, and aliquots were taken for measurement of protein content and incorporated radioactivity. Note the linearity of incorporation over the 6-hr time course in both the presence and absence of TM, demonstrating continuous protein synthesis and cellular viability under the conditions employed. [Reproduced from S. J. Fliesler, M. E. Rayborn, and J. G. Hollyfield, *J. Cell Biol.* **100**, 574 (1985), by copyright permission of the Rockefeller University Press.

to X-ray film (i.e., autoradiography or fluorography) (7, 7a, 10, 16, 17, 22). Figure 3 shows a Coomassie blue-stained SDS–polyacrylamide gel and corresponding fluorogram obtained from an experiment in which *Xenopus* retinas were incubated with D-[2-³H]mannose in the presence or absence of TM, using a protocol similar to that described above for studying the time course of [³H]leucine incorporation into retinal proteins (7). In this case, retinas were preincubated in the presence or absence of TM (20 µg/ml), then pulse labeled with [³H]mannose (0.5 mCi/ml) for 1 hr (±TM) and chased for 4 hr (±TM) in RBP medium supplemented with 0.1 mM L-leucine, 5 mM α-D-mannose, and 25% (by volume) Wolf–Quimby tissue culture medium. The

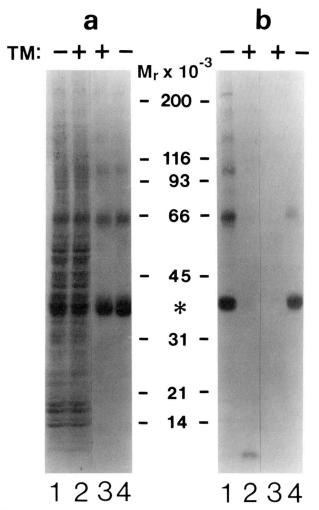

FIG. 3 SDS–polyacrylamide gel electrophoresis and fluorographic analysis of retinal and ROS membrane proteins obtained following a 1-hr pulse–4-hr chase incubation of *Xenopus* retinas with [^{3}H]mannose (0.5 mCi/ml) in the presence (+) or absence (−) of tunicamycin (TM, 20 μg/ml) (7). (a) Coomassie blue-stained gel; (b) fluorogram. Lanes 1 and 2, retina (180 μg protein); lanes 3 and 4, ROS membranes (30 μg protein). Note the simplicity of the staining pattern of ROS membrane proteins compared to that of whole retina, and the simplicity of the corresponding fluorograms. Virtually all of the [^{3}H]mannose incorporation is associated with monomeric opsin (migration position denoted by the asterisk; apparent M_r ∼36,000) and its larger aggregates. Tunicamycin abolishes incorporation of [^{3}H]mannose into retinal glycoproteins under the conditions employed. The migration positions of standard proteins (Bio-Rad, Richmond, CA) of known molecular mass are indicated. See text for details. [Adapted from S. J. Fliesler, M. E. Rayborn, and J. G. Hollyfield, *J. Cell Biol.* **100**, 574 (1985), by copyright permission of the Rockefeller University Press.]

retinas were then homogenized in 42% (w/v) sucrose solution, aliquots were removed for SDS-PAGE analysis, and ROS membranes were prepared from the remaining homogenate by discontinuous sucrose density gradient centrifugation as described above. After resuspension of the ROS membranes, aliquots were taken for SDS-PAGE analysis. The aliquots of retinal homogenate and ROS membranes were solubilized in Laemmli sample buffer and then subjected to one-dimensional SDS-PAGE on a 7.5–15% acrylamide gradient slab gel (10, 16). The gel was stained with Coomassie blue, destained, and subjected to fluorography as previously described (10, 16).

The simplicity of the ROS membrane protein composition is easily appreciated from the Coomassie blue-stained gel (Fig. 3a, lanes 3 and 4), compared with that of total retina (Fig. 3a, lanes 1 and 2). In both whole retina and ROS membranes, opsin (denoted by the asterisk) is the principal constituent, accounting for at least 90% of the protein staining in the ROS samples. The corresponding fluorogram (Fig. 3b) is striking in that, even in whole retina, virtually all of the incorporated radioactivity corresponds to opsin and its higher molecular weight aggregates. In the lanes in which samples were obtained from retinas incubated in the presence of TM (Fig. 3b, lanes 2 and 3), no incorporated radiolabel is observed. This finding is consistent with the expected inhibition of N-linked oligosaccharide biosynthesis caused by TM. Such perturbation of protein glycosylation results in aberrant ROS disk membrane assembly, as evaluated by electron microscopy of TM-treated retinas (7).

Autoradiographic Localization of Radiolabeled Proteins in Incubated Retinas

The distribution of newly synthesized, radiolabeled proteins among the various cellular layers and subcellular compartments of the retina is readily evaluated by microscopic autoradiography. Following incubation of the retina with a suitable radiolabeled precursor (e.g., [³H]leucine), the tissue is fixed, osmicated, serially dehydrated, embedded in plastic, sectioned, and the sections coated with photographic emulsion and exposed for varying lengths of time prior to development of the autoradiograms (7, 7a, 10, 16, 17, 22).

Figure 4 displays both bright-field (Fig. 4a) and dark-field (Fig. 4b) light microscopic autoradiograms obtained from a *Xenopus* retina that had been incubated for 4 hr in RBG containing [³H]leucine (10 μCi/ml), followed by a 1-hr chase in RBG supplemented with 20% (by volume) Wolf–Quimby tissue culture medium. Intense labeling of all retinal cell layers is apparent, indicative of vigorous protein synthetic activity under the conditions em-

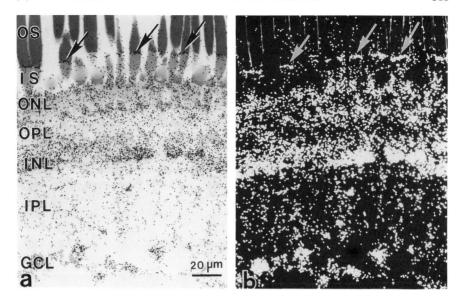

FIG. 4   Bright-field (a) and dark-field (b) light microscopic autoradiograms obtained from a *Xenopus* retina following a 4-hr pulse–1-hr chase incubation with [³H]leucine (10 μCi/ml) in RBG medium supplemented with 20% (by volume) Wolf–Quimby tissue culture medium. Note the intense labeling of all cell layers, indicative of active protein synthesis throughout the retina under the conditions employed. Also note the "bands" of silver grains localized to the inner segment (IS)–outer segment (OS) junctional regions (denoted by arrows), corresponding to the assembly of newly synthesized proteins into nascent disk membranes. Mixed-aldehyde fixation, Epon embedment (1-μm-thick sections), and toluidine blue staining were employed, and the exposure time was 8 days. Consult text and Refs. 16 and 22 for details of methods. Abbreviations: OS, outer segment layer; IS, inner segment layer; ONL, outer nuclear layer; OPL, outer plexiform layer; INL, inner nuclear layer; IPL, inner plexiform layer; GCL, ganglion cell layer.

ployed. The labeling pattern is even more vivid in the dark-field compared to the light-field autoradiogram. A coherent "band" of silver grains (indicated by the arrows) at the base of the outer segment (OS) of each rod cell represents the assembly of newly synthesized proteins into ROS membranes.

For evaluation of incorporation of radiolabeled proteins into discernable ultrastructural elements, autoradiography at the electron microscopic level is required. Figure 5 shows electron micrographic autoradiograms obtained from *Xenopus* retinas that had been incubated in the presence or absence of castanospermine (Cas, an inhibitor of N-linked oligosaccharide posttranslational processing), using [³H]mannose as a radiolabeled precursor (7a).

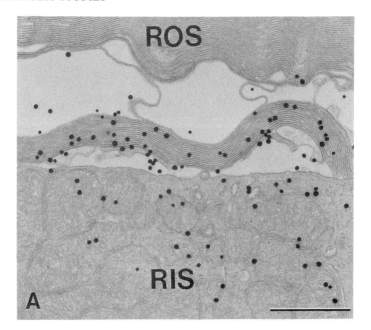

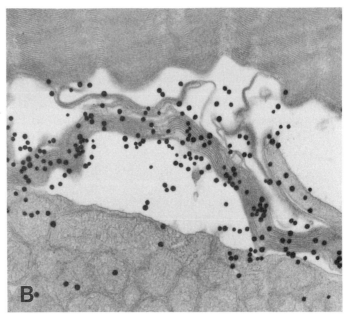

Following a 1-hr preincubation at 22°C in darkness [four retinas per 5 ml of RBP, supplemented with 2 μg/ml casamino acids and 5% (by volume) Wolf–Quimby tissue culture medium, per 25-ml flask] in the presence or absence of Cas (0.1 mg/ml; final DMSO concentration 0.1%), retinas were transferred to fresh medium ($\pm$Cas) containing D-[2-^{3}H]mannose (0.2 mCi/ml; 20 Ci/mmol) and incubated an additional 4 hr under normal fluorescent room lighting. After brief, gentle rinsing, the retinas were fixed and processed for conventional Epon embedment and electron microscopic autoradiography.

The accumulation of silver grains (seen as black dots in Fig. 5) over a discrete group of disk membranes at the base of the ROS in the autoradiograms signifies that newly synthesized glycoproteins were assembled into those membranes during the incubation, and it serves to identify those membranes as newly assembled disks. The greater labeling density of the basal disks in the Cas-treated specimen (Fig. 5B) relative to the disks in the control specimen (Fig. 5A) is consistent with the expected inhibition of N-linked oligosaccharide processing, which would result in a greater than normal incorporation of [^{3}H]mannose into the oligosaccharide chains of the membrane-bound glycoproteins. Examination of the ultrastructural features of the disk membranes in the micrographs of the Cas-treated and control retinas reveals that this particular metabolic perturbation does not result in abnormal disk membrane assembly, unlike the case with tunicamycin (7).

These results were corroborated and extended by biochemical analyses of the retinal and ROS proteins using specific activity measurements of TCA-precipitable material, SDS-PAGE and fluorography, and quantitation of the radioactivity incorporated into opsin by excision and solubilization of the opsin band from the SDS–polyacrylamide gel and subsequent measurement of its radioactivity content by scintillation counting (7a). The apparent molecular mass of opsin was slightly greater (by ~2–3 kDa) and its [^{3}H]mannose content was about 2.3-fold greater in the Cas-treated retinas, compared to

FIG. 5 Electron microscopic autoradiograms of the inner segment–outer segment (RIS, ROS) junctional region of rod cells obtained following a 4-hr incubation of *Xenopus* retinas with D-[2-^{3}H]mannose (0.2 mCi/ml) in the absence (A) or presence (B) of castanospermine (0.1 mg/ml) (7a). See text for details. Note the lamellar appearance and the concentration of silver grains (black dots) over a discrete group of disk membranes at the base of the ROS in both specimens, indicative of incorporation of newly synthesized glycoproteins into ultrastructurally normal nascent disk membranes. The exposure time was 2 months. Bar, 1 μm. [Reproduced with permission from S. J. Fliesler, M. E. Rayborn, and J. G. Hollyfield, *Proc. Natl. Acad. Sci. U.S.A.* **83,** 6435 (1986).]

controls, consistent with "hyperglycosylation" of opsin owing to inhibition of oligosaccharide processing.

Acknowledgments

The author thanks Scott F. Basinger for originally instructing the author in the design, construction, and use of the *in vitro* system described in this chapter, for helpful comments and suggestions during the preparation of the manuscript, and for permission to use Fig. 1 herein. The author also gratefully acknowledges the following colleagues and friends, whose collaborative efforts provided significant contributions to the studies cited herein: Joe G. Hollyfield, Mary E. Rayborn, Scott F. Basinger, Rosemary T. Hoffman, R. Kennedy Keller, Gareth A. Tabor, Mary Lou Mattheke, Eric Holtzman, and Barry S. Winkler. This work was supported, in part, by U.S. Public Health Service Grants EY06045 and EY07361 (National Eye Institute/National Institutes of Health), and by an unrestricted departmental grant from Research to Prevent Blindness, Inc. The author is a Research to Prevent Blindness James S. Adams Scholar.

References

1. A. Ames III and A. B. Hastings, *J. Neurophysiol.* **19,** 201 (1956).
2. P. J. O'Brien, this volume [4].
3. P. J. O'Brien, C. G. Muellenberg, and J. J. Bungenberg de Jong, *Biochemistry* **11,** 64 (1972).
4. S. F. Basinger and M. O. Hall, *Biochemistry* **12,** 1996 (1973).
5. B. S. Winkler and S. J. Fliesler, in preparation (1993).
6. S. F. Basinger and R. T. Hoffman, *in* "Methods in Enzymology" (L. Packer, ed.), Vol. 81, p. 772, Academic Press, New York, 1982.
7. S. J. Fliesler, M. E. Rayborn, and J. G. Hollyfield, *J. Cell Biol.* **100,** 574 (1985).
7a. S. J. Fliesler, M. E. Rayborn, and J. G. Hollyfield, *Proc. Natl. Acad. Sci. U.S.A.* **83,** 6435 (1986).
8. R. J. Ulshafer, C. A. Garcia, and J. G. Hollyfield, *Invest. Opthalmol. Visual Sci.* **19,** 1236 (1980).
9. R. J. Ulshafer and J. G. Hollyfield, *in* "Structure of the Eye" (J. G. Hollyfield, ed.), p. 115. Elsevier/North-Holland, New York, 1982.
10. S. J. Fliesler, G. A. Tabor, and J. G. Hollyfield, *Exp. Eye Res.* **39,** 153 (1984).
11. M. G. Wetzel, C. Fahlman, J. P. Alligood, P. J. O'Brien, and G. D. Aguirre, *Exp. Eye Res.* **48,** 149 (1989).
12. S. J. Fliesler and G. J. Schroepfer, Jr., *J. Neurochem.* **46,** 448 (1986).
13. R. S. St. Jules and P. J. O'Brien, *Exp. Eye Res.* **43,** 929 (1986).
14. R. E. Anderson, M. B. Maude, P. A. Kelleher, M. E. Rayborn, and J. G. Hollyfield, *J. Neurochem.* **41,** 764 (1983).
15. A. M. Tartakoff, *Cell (Cambridge, Mass.)* **32,** 1026 (1983).

16. M. L. Mattheke, S. J. Fliesler, S. F. Basinger, and E. Holtzman, *J. Neurosci.* **4,** 1086 (1984).
17. S. J. Fliesler and S. F. Basinger, *J. Biol. Chem.* **262,** 17516 (1987).
18. J. Lippincott-Schwartz, L. C. Yuan, J. S. Bonifacino, and R. D. Klausner, *Cell (Cambridge, Mass.)* **56,** 801 (1989).
19. S. J. Fliesler and R. K. Keller, *J. Cell Biol.* (*Abstr.*) **109,** 206 (1989).
20. D. Deretic and D. S. Papermaster, *J. Cell Biol.* **113,** 1281 (1991).
21. D. S. Papermaster and W. J. Dreyer, *Biochemistry* **32,** 2438 (1974).
22. S. J. Fliesler and S. F. Basinger, *Proc. Natl. Acad. Sci. U.S.A.* **82,** 1116 (1985).

[6] Isolation of Post-Golgi Membranes Transporting Newly Synthesized Rhodopsin

Dusanka Deretic and David S. Papermaster

Introduction

Retinal photoreceptors are highly polarized cells in which light-sensitive disk membranes and associated proteins involved in visual transduction are organized in a specialized domain, the rod outer segment (ROS). This domain is continually renewed by the addition of new disks at the base (1), followed by circadian or diurnal shedding of the tips of the ROS, which are destroyed by the adjacent pigment epithelial cells (2, 3). In amphibians, disk renewal involves addition of 3 μm^2/min of ROS membranes (4); approximately 85% of these membranes is composed of a single membrane protein, rhodopsin (5). As in other polarized cells, a common biosynthetic machinery is used for the synthesis of the proteins and lipids, which are then sorted to their site of function, the ROS. Synthesis and polarized sorting of a large amount of a relatively simple membrane are unique features of retinal rods that make them excellent candidates for studies of membrane biosynthesis and protein trafficking. Such studies are of interest both for elucidating general mechanisms of attainment and maintenance of cell polarity and for understanding of inherited or acquired retinal degenerations that may involve mutations or injury which impair transport and sorting of newly synthesized molecules in rods.

Newly synthesized rhodopsin is transported to the outer segment on membranous vesicles in a polarized manner (6, 7). Rhodopsin is sorted away from synaptophysin, a synaptic vesicle protein, in the trans-Golgi cisternae of frog rods (8). Isolation of the post-Golgi compartment or the trans-Golgi network (9) of photoreceptor cells along with separation from other biosynthetic membranes is therefore necessary to study sorting of newly synthesized proteins. The post-Golgi compartment represents a very small fraction of the total cell membranes in a retinal homogenate. To isolate it we have modified previously described methods for retinal subcellular fractionation (10, 11). These modifications enable us to isolate and to separate post-Golgi membranes involved in the transport of newly synthesized rhodopsin from other biosynthetic and inner segment compartments (12).

Methods in Neurosciences, Volume 15

Subcellular Fractionation of Retinal Tissue

Isolation of Rod Outer Segments from Frog Retina and Retinal Rehomogenization

Arrival of newly synthesized proteins to the ROS can be used as one criterion for the completion of maturation and accurate sorting of the ROS proteins. Photoreceptor cells offer great advantage for sorting studies, since ROS represent a well-defined compartment, enclosed by the plasma membrane and connected to the rest of the cell via a narrow connecting cilium. ROS are easy to isolate, and several methods for their isolation and purification have been described. In our studies we have focused on the mechanism of rhodopsin transport; therefore, we chose a method designed for ROS membrane protein studies described by Papermaster and Dreyer (13). Moderate shear forces are employed for ROS removal, so that isolated ROS are relatively free of contamination and retinal tissue is not extensively damaged. After separation from the reminder of the retina by flotation of ROS on high-density sucrose, the crude ROS are recovered and rehomogenized. The ROS disk membranes are then purified on a step sucrose gradient which includes divalent cations to shift contaminating membranes away from the ROS membranes to a higher buoyant density. This preparation yields purified ROS disk membranes.

Biosynthetic compartments from photoreceptor cell inner segments are isolated from the reminder of the retina by rehomogenization of the retinal pellet in 0.25 M sucrose under conditions of slightly greater shear. As a consequence of retinal anatomy, this homogenization preferentially releases photoreceptor inner segment membranes, while the rest of the retina remains relatively unbroken in large fragments. Retinal fragments and nuclei are then sedimented at low speed after addition of EDTA to disrupt divalent cation cross-linking of unrelated membranes and to inhibit Ca^{2+}-sensitive proteases. The resulting pellet contains approximately 85% of the retinal tissue but less than 10% of the newly synthesized rhodopsin (10). The supernatant after this centrifugation, therefore, contains photoreceptor organelles involved in the biosynthesis of the ROS proteins, which can be further separated according to their buoyant density.

Choice of Shallow Linear Sucrose Density Gradient for Retinal Subcellular Fractionation

Conditions for retinal subcellular fractionation on step sucrose gradients were previously described (10, 11). Although useful separations were achieved using this fractionation procedure, considerable heterogeneity persisted after gradient separation, owing to the similar buoyant densities of the fragments of the cell membranes. We found that fractionation of the membranes on a shallow linear density gradient that is divided into 14 to 15 fractions results in improved separation.

This approach has its foundation in earlier studies of membrane trafficking in other cells. Studies of endocytosis in hepatocytes by Dunn and Hubbard (14), employed 1.11–1.25 or 1.06–1.20 g/ml linear sucrose gradients overlying a 1.22 g/ml cushion, which enabled them to separate endosomes (1.08–1.13 g/ml) from the trans-Golgi membranes (1.11–1.16 g/ml), plasma membrane (1.14–1.17 g/ml), and lysosomes (1.18–1.25 g/ml). Similar gradients were also used for the study of the biogenesis of the hepatocyte plasma membrane (15). The density of endoplasmic reticulum (ER) membranes in sucrose is approximately 1.19 g/ml (16). We use a linear 1.06–1.20 g/ml sucrose gradient with a 1.22 g/ml cushion in order to follow movement of newly synthesized, [^{35}S]methionine-labeled rhodopsin from the ER to the Golgi and subsequently to post-Golgi membranes in retinal photoreceptors. The retinal subcellular fractionation procedure is schematically outlined in Fig. 1.

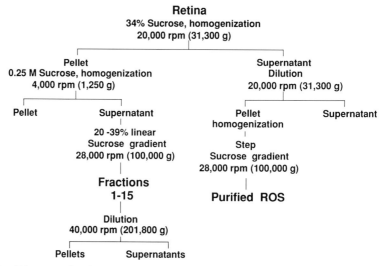

FIG. 1   Diagram of retinal subcellular fractionation. ROS are sheared from the retina and floated on 34% sucrose. The retinal pellet is rehomogenized in 0.25 M sucrose, retinal fragments and nuclei are removed by low-speed centrifugation, and the supernatant is further fractionated on a linear 20–39% sucrose gradient. Crude ROS are rehomogenized and purified on a step sucrose gradient.

Methods

Stock Solutions

> 1 M NaCl: 5.84 g NaCl to 100 ml with water
> 0.1 M MgCl$_2$: 2.03 g MgCl$_2$·6H$_2$O to 100 ml with water
> 1 M Tris–acetate, pH 7.4: 30 g Tris base, pH adjusted to 7.4 with acetic acid, to 250 ml with water
> 0.2 M EDTA: 3.72 g EDTA (disodium salt dihydrate) to 50 ml with water
> Stock 42% (w/w) sucrose solution: 151.5 g sucrose/350 g solution in water [η (refractive index), 1.4036; ρ (density), 1.1870 g/ml at 20°C]
> Stock 49% (w/w) sucrose solution: 150 g sucrose/300 g solution in water (η, 1.4179; ρ, 1.2241 g/ml at 20°C)

The weight of sucrose is calculated for Sigma (St. Louis, MO) S-9378 sucrose, which contains a small amount of water. All sucrose concentrations are formulated on a weight per weight basis so that solutions are simply and accurately prepared on a top-loading balance. Sucrose solutions are prepared on the day before the experiment. It is critical to check the refractive index of stock sucrose solutions before proceeding.

> Protease inhibitor stock solutions (1000×):
> 10 mg/ml antipain (10 μg/ml final)
> 1 mg/ml (2 mM) leupeptin (2 μM final)
> 10 mg/ml [100,000 kallikrein inhibitory units (KIU)/ml] aprotinin (100 KIU/ml final)

Protease inhibitors are purchased from Sigma. Stock solutions are kept frozen and are added on the day of experiment. The volume added to the sucrose solutions is a sum of equal volumes of each protease inhibitor.

Sucrose Solutions

Component	Homogenizing media		Step gradient solutions			Linear gradient solutions	
	34% Sucrose (η = 1.3833)[a]	0.25 M Sucrose (8.5%, η = 1.3453)	1.10 g/ml Sucrose (24%, η = 1.3710)	1.11 g/ml Sucrose (25%, η = 1.3730)	1.13 g/ml Sucrose (30%, η = 1.3811)	20% Sucrose (η = 1.3635)	39% Sucrose (η = 1.3980)
Stock 42% sucrose	191 g	10.2 g	31.2 g	34.2 g	40.1 g	—	—
Stock 49% sucrose	—	—	—	—	—	41.7 g	81.3g
1 M NaCl	13 ml	2.5 ml	—	—	—	—	—

(continued)

Sucrose Solutions (*continued*)

Component	Homogenizing media		Step gradient solutions			Linear gradient solutions	
	34% Sucrose (η = 1.3833)[a]	0.25 M Sucrose (8.5%, η = 1.3453)	1.10 g/ml Sucrose (24%, η = 1.3710)	1.11 g/ml Sucrose (25%, η = 1.3730)	1.13 g/ml Sucrose (30%, η = 1.3811)	20% Sucrose (η = 1.3635)	39% Sucrose (η = 1.3980)
0.1 M MgCl$_2$	0.4 ml	0.5 ml	0.05 ml	0.05 ml	0.05 ml	0.1 ml	0.1 ml
1 M Tris–acetate	1 ml	0.5 ml	0.05 ml	0.05 ml	0.05 ml	0.1 ml	0.1 ml
Water to weight	229.31 g	49.95 g	55.0 g	55.5 g	56.5 g	99.7 g	99.7 g
Protease inhibitors	0.69 ml	0.05 ml	—	—	—	0.3 ml	0.3 ml
	230 g	50 g	55.0 g	55.5 g	56.5 g	100 g	100 g

[a] Refractive indexes are measured at 20°C.

Medium for [35S]Methionine Incorporation

The incubation medium is prepared using the MEM Select-Amine Kit (GIBCO Laboratories, Grand Island, NY). To prepare 1 liter of the medium, each vial of amino acids and vitamins from the kit is reconstituted in 10 ml sterile water and 5.5 ml of each solution is combined to give the final concentration as described by Wolf and Quimby (17). Methionine is omitted and added only to the chase medium. Salts are dissolved in approximately 300 ml of water to give the following final concentrations according to Greenberger and Besharse (18):

> 64 m*M* NaCl (3740 mg/liter)
> 1 m*M* MgCl$_2$ (203 mg/liter MgCl$_2$·6H$_2$O)
> 35 m*M* NaHCO$_3$ (2940 mg/liter)
> 2 m*M* KCl (150 mg/liter)
> 1.8 m*M* CaCl$_2$ (18 μl of 100 m*M* solution)
> 4.4 m*M* Glucose (800 mg/liter)

The pH of the solution is adjusted to 7.5, and the solution is filter sterilized and added to the mixture of amino acids and vitamins. The final volume is adjusted to 1 liter with sterile water, divided in half, and 2.25 ml of the methionine solution is added to one half (chase medium).

Equipment

> Red safelights (Kodak, Rochester, NY, 1A filter and 15-W bulb).
> Dissection tools (large forceps, two small forceps, fine scissors, blades), guillotine

Erlenmeyer flasks (25 ml) with stoppers, connected to the 95% O_2–5% CO_2 (by volume) tank

Orbital shaker (Lab Line) or a water bath with orbital shaker

Syringes (10 and 3 ml) and needles (15, 18, and 26 gauge)

8 × 50 ml Angle rotor (Beckman Instruments Inc., Palo Alto, CA, JA-20), 15-ml polycarbonate tubes and adapters

SW 40 rotor (Beckman) and 13.5-ml ultraclear tubes

Motor-driven loose-fitting Teflon–glass homogenizer (Thomas Scientific, Swedesboro, NJ, Tissue Grinder, size AA)

Pipettes, automatic pipettors, and tips

Gradient maker (Hoefer, San Francisco, CA)

Büchler Auto Densi-Flow IIC fractionator (Büchler Instruments, Fort Lee, NJ)

Fraction collector (Gilson, Middleton, WI)

Procedure

Frogs, *Rana berlandieri* (100–250 g, Rana Co., Brownsville, TX), are maintained at 20°C under dim white light in a 12-hr light/dark cycle and fed live crickets. Because frog rhodopsin synthesis is maximal in the afternoon (D. Deretic and D. S. Papermaster, unpublished observation, 1989) the light cycle is shifted to lights on at 12 midnight, lights off at 12 noon, for several weeks before use of the frogs. Frogs are dark adapted for 2 hr (from 8 to 10 AM) to facilitate retinal isolation, and retinal disections are started 2 hr before the time of light offset (10 AM). All experiments are conducted under dim red light.

Frogs are sacrificed by decapitation using a small animal guillotine (Harvard Apparatus, Millis, MA), and retinas are isolated as decribed (11). Seven retinas are incubated per 15 ml of oxygenated medium in 25-ml Erlenmeyer flasks on the orbital shaker at a constant room temperature of 20°C (if such a room is not available, a water bath with an orbital shaker can be used). [^{35}S]Methionine (1000 Ci/mmol, New England Nuclear, Boston, MA) is added to a final concentration of 25 μCi per retina, and retinas are incubated for varying time periods of incorporation and chase. After isotope incorporation, retinas are briefly rinsed in a petri dish with 34% ice-cold sucrose homogenizing medium and transferred to a polycarbonate tube with fresh medium on ice (0.3 ml per retina).

The ROS are sheared from the retina by five passes through a 15-gauge trochar by gentle aspiration with a 10-ml syringe. The homogenate is deposited in the polycarbonate tube and is overlaid with 1 ml of 1.10 g/ml sucrose gradient solution and centrifuged at 20,000 rpm for 20 min at 4°C in a JA 20 rotor. The ROS are collected from the 1.10–34% sucrose interface, diluted with 1 volume of 10 mM Tris–acetate, pH 7.4, and centrifuged at 20,000 rpm at 4°C for 20 min (JA 20 rotor). The resulting crude ROS pellet is resuspended in 0.15–0.5 ml of 1.10 g/ml sucrose gradient solution per retina and homogenized by several passes through a 26-gauge needle. The ROS suspension is overlaid on a step sucrose gradient prepared by underlayering from the bottom of a 13.5 ml SW 40 tube as follows: 3 ml of 1.11, 5 ml of 1.13, and 2 ml of 1.15 g/ml (34% sucrose) solution. Gradients are centrifuged at 28,000 rpm in an SW 40 rotor in an L8 ultracentrifuge (Beckman) for 30 min at 4°C. The ROS layer is collected from the 1.11–1.13 interface with an 18-gauge needle on a 10-ml syringe, diluted with 2 volumes of 10 mM Tris–acetate, pH 7.4, pelleted at 20,000 rpm in a JA 20 rotor at 4°C for 20 min, and resuspended in the same buffer. This yields a preparation of purified ROS disk membranes.

The retinal pellet obtained after removal of crude ROS and excess 34% sucrose homogenizing medium is rehomogenized in 0.25 M sucrose homogenizing medium (0.2 ml/retina) with five passes of a loose-fitting Teflon–glass homogenizer (1 ml maximal volume) driven by a GT21 motor controller (G. K. Heller Corp., Floral Park, New York) at setting 3, in the cold room in an ice bucket under dim red light. Homogenized aliquots are collected into a 13-ml polycarbonate tube, 0.2 M EDTA is added to a final concentration of 2 mM and mixed thoroughly, and the homogenate is centrifuged at 4000 rpm at 4°C for 4 min in a JA 20 rotor. The supernatant is collected, and 3 ml of supernatant is overlaid on 10 ml of a linear 20–39% sucrose density gradient which is prepared as follows: a 0.5 ml cushion of 49% sucrose is prepared in the 13.5-ml ultraclear tube for the SW 40 rotor; 5.25 ml of 39% sucrose is pipetted into the first chamber and 5.25 ml of 20% sucrose into the second chamber of the gradient maker that is connected to a Büchler fractionator, which deposits a linear gradient on the underlying cushion. Gradients are centrifuged at 100,000 g_{av} (28,000 rpm) at 4°C, for 13 hr in an SW 40 rotor in an L8 ultracentrifuge. Fractions (0.9 ml) are collected from the top of the gradient using the Büchler fractionator and a fraction collector. As the more dense fractions (11–14) are collected, the fractionator occasionally fails to advance sufficiently. This can be managed by manually advancing the sampling needle slowly into the gradient. A small aliquot of each fraction is used to measure the refractive index and to determine galactosyltransferase activity according to Bartles et al. (15).

Retinal subcellular fractions are diluted with 10 mM Tris–acetate, pH 7.4, and membranes are pelleted by centrifugation at 40,000 rpm for 40 min in an SW 40 rotor. Pellets are resuspended in 5 μl/retina of the same buffer and aliquoted for determination of protein concentration, radioactivity, for analysis by sodium dodecyl sulfate–polyacrylamide gel electrophoresis (SDS-PAGE) and for electron microscopic (EM) analysis. Samples are resuspended in Optifluor (Packard Instrument Co., Meriden, CT) and radioactivity is determined in a Beckman LS7000 scintillation counter. Protein samples are solubilized in 50% hexyl-β-D-glucopyranoside (final concentration 8%), and protein concentrations are determined using the Bradford protein assay modified for membrane proteins (19). Membranes from different retinal fractions are solubilized and separated on 10% polyacrylamide gels in the presence of SDS (20). Gels are either impregnated with 1 M sodium salicylate, dried, and autoradiographed or blotted onto Immobilon P membranes (Millipore Corp., Bedford, MA) (21) for autoradiography and/or Western blotting analysis. Supernatants containing soluble proteins are stored frozen; proteins are precipitated with 20% trichloroacetic acid (TCA) and analyzed by the same methods.

Use of Linear Sucrose Density Gradients for Studies of Photoreceptor Membrane Biosynthesis and Intracellular Transport

The kinetics of transport of newly synthesized proteins in frog retinal rods *in vivo* was established by early EM autoradiographic studies (1, 5). This transport is relatively slow in frogs, as newly synthesized membrane proteins arrive at the ROS after approximately 2 hr following the isotope injection. Movement of newly synthesized, [^{35}S]methionine-labeled rhodopsin through the subcellular compartments of the inner segments of retinal rods can be followed by pulse–chase experiments in which isotope incorporation and chase times are chosen to parallel the kinetics observed *in vivo*. An example of one such experiment is shown in Fig. 2A. After a short period of isotope incorporation (30 min) radiolabeled membrane proteins with the highest specific activity are found in the fraction with a density that corresponds to that of ER membranes (fractions 14–15). Longer incubation (90 min) results in the distribution of radiolabeled proteins into the lighter gradient fractions (fractions 7–12). When 90 min of incorporation is followed by a 2-hr chase, a very low buoyant density fraction (fraction 5, 1.09 g/ml) becomes highly labeled. The pattern of isotope incorporation into newly synthesized rhodopsin parallels the distribution of total radiolabeled protein since rhodopsin is the major radiolabeled protein in all of the retinal subcellular fractions. Radiolabeled rhodopsin is also recovered from the isolated ROS disk membranes after a 2-hr chase but is barely detectable after 90 min of incorporation.

The composition of the separated subcellular compartments can be studied by quantitation of the markers for the membranes of interest. Figure 2B shows the distribution of the trans-Golgi membranes (1.12–1.16 g/ml, as determined by galactosyltransferase activity), and Fig. 2C shows the distribution of plasma membranes (1.13–1.16 g/ml, as determined immunochemically by the Na^+,K^+-ATPase content) and synaptic vesicles (1.10–1.15 g/ml, as determined immunochemically by the synaptophysin content). A small fraction of ROS membranes (~3%) remain with the retina and distribute

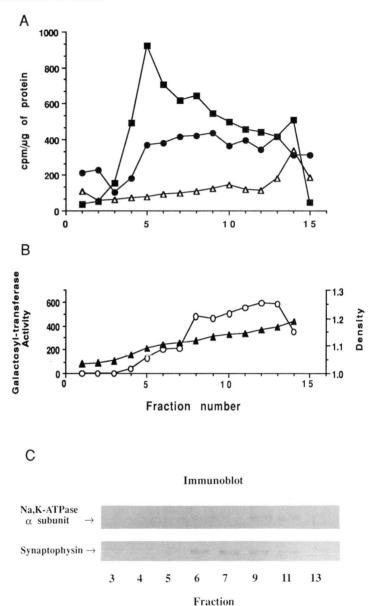

FIG. 2   (A) The distribution of radiolabeled retinal membrane proteins separated on linear sucrose density gradients changes as newly synthesized proteins move through the biosynthetic subcellular compartments. The highest specific activity shifts from the fractions with greater buoyant density after 30 (△) or 90 min (●) of isotope incorporation to a fraction of very low buoyant density after a 2-hr chase (■). (B)

in the linear gradient at their usual density (fractions 7 and 8, 1.12–1.13 g/ml). The distribution of galactosyltransferase activity resembles the distribution of radiolabeled proteins after 90 min of isotope incorporation, suggesting that at this time the majority of newly synthesized membrane proteins are processed in the Golgi apparatus. The subcellular fraction (fraction 5) that accumulates newly synthesized rhodopsin after it has passed through the Golgi has a buoyant density in sucrose (1.09 g/ml) that is different from all of the other organelles. The kinetics of appearance of newly synthesized rhodopsin in this low buoyant density fraction suggests that it contains post-Golgi membranes. Additional criteria used to assign the origin of this fraction include the orientation of rhodopsin in the membranes and inhibition of delivery of radiolabeled rhodopsin by the fungal antibiotic brefeldin A (BFA) [see Deretic and Papermaster (12) for more details].

Post-Golgi membranes are well separated from other biosynthetic membranes by our retinal subcellular fractionation procedure. Further purification of subcellular organelles can be achieved by modifying the densities of the linear sucrose gradient, by subsequent sedimentation on a second sucrose gradient, by use of a gradient made from a different medium, or by immunoisolation using antibodies that have been conjugated to a solid support as we describe below.

Immunoisolation of Membranes by Monoclonal Antibodies to the Carboxy-Terminal Domain of Rhodopsin Bound to Methacrylate Beads

We use immunoisolation, as originally described by Burger and co-workers (22) for synaptic vesicle isolation, for further purification of post-Golgi membranes that are specifically involved in rhodopsin transport. Methacrylate beads are coated either with a monoclonal antibody to the cytoplasmic (C-terminal) domain of rhodopsin or with a nonspecific immunoglobulin (IgG)

The distribution of trans-Golgi membranes determined by galactosyltransferase activity (○) resembles the distribution of radiolabeled proteins after 90 min of isotope incorporation. The density of each fraction (▲) is highly reproducible. (C) Membranes containing synaptophysin and Na^+,K^+-ATPase, as determined by immunoblotting, are found in more dense fractions and are separated from the low buoyant density subcellular fraction that accumulates newly synthesized proteins with kinetics expected from the post-Golgi membranes. [Modified from D. Deretic and D. S. Papermaster, *J. Cell Biol.* **113**, 1281 (1991), by copyright permission of the Rockefeller University Press.]

of the same subclass as a control. Immunobeads are blocked to prevent nonspecific binding and incubated with the retinal subcellular fraction enriched in the post-Golgi membranes (fraction 5). Morphological and biochemical analysis shows that more than 85% of the radiolabeled membranes from the membrane pellet of this sucrose gradient fraction are immunoisolated with the specific monoclonal antibody, whereas only 10% of the radiolabeled proteins are absorbed by the beads coated with the control IgG. Thus, the membranes in fraction 5 are significantly purified post-Golgi membranes even before application of the immunoisolation procedure. Immunoisolated membranes are a suitable starting material for further studies of the molecule(s) involved in the polarized sorting of newly synthesized rhodopsin.

Procedure

Preparation of Immunobeads

Purified monoclonal antibody and control IgG are dialyzed against water. The antibody concentration should be 2–6 mg/ml; if the concentration is lower, antibody is concentrated by ultrafiltration or by spinning in a Centricon concentrator (Amicon, Danvers, MA). Eupergit C1Z methacrylate beads (150 mg; 1 μm diameter, manufactured by Röhm Pharma, Weiterstadt, Germany, distributed by Accurate Chemical and Scientific Co., Westbury, NY) are washed once with water and incubated with 1 mg of antibody or control IgG of the same subclass at a final concentration of 0.5 mg/ml. The suspension is incubated in an end-over-end rotator (Labindustries Inc., Berkeley, CA) at controlled temperature of 20°C (in a room with controlled temperature or a thermostat), until approximately 50% of the antibody is coupled (45 min to 1 hr). Beads are pelleted by a 15-sec spin in an Eppendorf microcentrifuge and incubated for 12 hr at 20°C with 3 ml of 1 M glycine, pH 6.5, to block remaining binding sites. The antibody concentration in the remaining supernatant is measured in order to estimate the amount of antibody coupled to the beads. The final concentration of bound antibody or IgG is usually about 7 μg/mg of beads. Immunobeads are washed by six alternate washes in 150 mM NaCl containing 100 mM Tris-HCl, pH 8, or 100 mM sodium acetate, pH 4.5, respectively. Immunobeads are stored in 150 mM NaCl, 20 mM Tris-HCl, pH 7.2 at 4°C, for several weeks without loss of activity.

Immunoisolation

Immunobeads are blocked for 1 hr at room temperature with 5% nonfat dry milk and 1% bovine serum albumin (BSA) in phosphate-buffered saline (PBS) in order to reduce nonspecific binding, then washed and resuspended in PBS. The coated immunobeads (2.5 mg in 50 μl) are incubated in an end-over-end rotator for 2 hr at 4°C with the sucrose gradient fraction containing radiolabeled post-Golgi membranes (20 μg in ~150–200 μl, equivalent to fraction 5 membranes pooled from four retinas). After several washes with 0.25 M sucrose homogenizing buffer, each sample is divided in two portions and one-half of the immunobeads, with bound membranes, is resuspended in 150 mM NaCl, 10 mM Tris, pH 7.4, containing 2% SDS and protease inhibitors (as in homogenizing medium) and analyzed by SDS-PAGE. The other half is fixed and processed for EM analysis.

Conclusion

Retinal subcellular fractionation on sucrose density gradients combined with immunoisolation provides a useful system for studies of photoreceptor membrane biosynthesis and post-Golgi transport of newly synthesized rhodopsin. Membranes of the biosynthetic compartments of the frog rod inner segment are separated based on their biophysical and immunological properties. This yields purified and enriched starting materials that can be used to study components of the transport membranes. Some of these components, by interacting with the target membranes, may generate the capacity for polarized sorting. Further development and application of this method may lead to sufficient purification of biosynthetic membranes so that they can be used for *in vitro* reconstitution of photoreceptor membrane synthesis and transport.

References

1. R. W. Young and B. Droz, *J. Cell Biol.* **39,** 169 (1968).
2. M. M. LaVail, *Science* **194,** 1071 (1976).
3. S. Basinger, R. Hoffman, and M. Matthew, *Science* **194,** 1074 (1976).
4. J. C. Besharse, *in* "The Retina: A Model for Cell Biological Studies" (R. Adler and D. Farber, eds.), p. 297. Academic Press, New York, 1986.
5. M. O. Hall, D. Bok, and A. D. E. Bacharach, *J. Mol. Biol.* **45,** 397 (1969).
6. D. S. Papermaster, B. G. Schneider, and J. C. Besharse, *Invest. Ophthalmol. Visual. Sci.* **26,** 1386 (1985).
7. D. S. Papermaster, B. G. Schneider, D. Defoe, and J. C. Besharse, *J. Histochem. Cytochem.* **34,** 5 (1986).
8. R. Schmied and E. Holtzman, *J. Neurobiol.* **20,** 115 (1989).
9. G. Griffiths and K. Simons, *Science* **234,** 438 (1986).
10. D. S. Papermaster, C. A. Converse, and J. Siu, *Biochemistry* **14,** 1343 (1975).
11. D. S. Papermaster, *in* "Methods in Enzymology" (S. Fleischer and B. Fleischer, eds.), Vol. 96, p. 609. Academic Press, New York, 1983.
12. D. Deretic and D. S. Papermaster, *J. Cell. Biol.* **113,** 1281 (1991).

13. D. S. Papermaster and W. J. Dreyer, *Biochemistry* **13,** 2438 (1974).
14. W. A. Dunn and A. L. Hubbard, *J. Cell Biol.* **98,** 2148 (1984).
15. J. R. Bartles, H. M. Feracci, B. Stieger, and A. L. Hubbard, *J. Cell Biol.* **105,** 1241 (1987).
16. W. E. Balch, W. G. Dunphy, W. A. Braell, and J. E. Rothman, *Cell (Cambridge, Mass.)* **39,** 405 (1984).
17. K. Wolf and M. C. Quimby, *Science* **144,** 1578 (1964).
18. L. M. Greenberger and J. C. Besharse, *Invest. Ophthalmol. Visual Sci.* **24,** 1456 (1983).
19. B. O. Fanger, *Anal. Biochem.* **162,** 11 (1987).
20. U. K. Laemmli, *Nature (London)* **227,** 680 (1970).
21. P. Matsudaira, *J. Biol. Chem.* **262,** 10035 (1987).
22. P. M. Burger, E. Mehl, P. L. Cameron, P. R. Maycox, M. Baumert, F. Lottspeich, P. DeCamilli, and R. Jahn, *Neuron* **3,** 715 (1989).

Section III

Photoreceptor Membrane and Protein Preparation and Characterization

[7] Preparing Rod Outer Segment Membranes, Regenerating Rhodopsin, and Determining Rhodopsin Concentration

J. Hugh McDowell

Introduction

Rhodopsin is a member of a receptor family that expresses its activity through interaction with a G protein. Bovine rhodopsin serves as an excellent model for G-protein-linked receptors because it is available in large quantities and is easily prepared in a highly pure form. Disk membranes prepared from bovine rod outer segments have been estimated to have over 95% of their protein present as rhodopsin (1). Bovine rod outer segments can be prepared that contain most of the components involved in visual transduction and can be used to study reactions of the visual cycle. Alternatively, disk membranes can be prepared that contain essentially only rhodopsin (and phospholipids), and these are convenient for studying properties of rhodopsin in its native environment or for reconstituting with other components of the visual cycle or other G-protein-linked receptor systems (2). The aim of this chapter is to provide simple and rapid techniques for the preparation of rod outer segments from bovine retinas as well as to indicate similar approaches for other species. Methods are presented for measuring the amount of rhodopsin present and for reconstituting rhodopsin from opsin.

Rod Outer Segment Preparation

Rod cell outer segments (ROS) are easy to prepare owing to their unusually low density compared to other retinal cells and cell organelles. Most techniques rely on modifications of the discontinuous sucrose density gradient procedure described by Papermaster and Dreyer (3). This procedure and variations of it yield outer segments containing variable amounts of the soluble ROS proteins. Continuous density gradients using sucrose or other materials (4, 5) have also been used to isolate ROS, and the procedure of Schnetkamp *et al.* has been estimated to retain 3 or 4 times as much of the soluble ROS proteins as a normal discontinuous gradient technique (6). We use discontinuous gradients because we find them easier and faster to pre-

Methods in Neurosciences, Volume 15

pare, and we obtain a good yield of rhodopsin from either fresh or frozen retinas (0.5–0.8 mg/retina) with acceptable levels of soluble ROS proteins for most other purposes. A further advantage of our procedure is that it can be performed entirely by the use of a refrigerated centrifuge and does not require an ultracentrifuge.

Solutions

Solution A: 0.1 M potassium phosphate buffer, pH 7.0, containing 1 mM MgCl$_2$, 0.5 mM dithiothreitol (DTT) [or dithioerythritol (DTE)], and 0.1 mM EDTA

Solution B: 50% (w/v) sucrose in 0.1 M potassium phosphate buffer, pH 7.0, containing 1 mM MgCl$_2$, 0.5 mM DTT (or DTE), and 0.1 mM EDTA

Solution C: 45% (w/v) sucrose in 0.1 M potassium phosphate buffer, pH 7.0, containing 1 mM MgCl$_2$, 0.5 mM DTT (or DTE), and 0.1 mM EDTA

Sucrose density gradient solutions:
d = 1.105, 102 ml of B diluted to 200 ml with A
d = 1.115, 108.5 ml of B diluted to 200 ml with A
d = 1.135, 129 ml of B diluted to 200 ml with A
d = 1.15, 192.5 ml of B diluted to 200 ml with A

The density of each gradient solution is checked at 4°C with a hydrometer and adjusted if necessary to ensure reproducible gradients.

Procedure

All procedures are performed in the dark and at 4°C. Thawed retinas (200) (Jim and Wanda Lawson, Lincoln, NE) are mixed with 180 ml of 45% sucrose (solution C) in a capped flask and shaken vigorously by hand for about 3 min. Centrifuge in a fixed-angle rotor for 5 min at 3000 g (Beckman JA20 rotor at 5000 rpm). The supernatant is filtered through four single layers of gauze into a 1-liter graduated cylinder. Dilute 1:1 with buffer (solution A) and then centrifuge 7 min at 4400 g (Beckman JA20 rotor at 6,000 rpm). Remove the supernatant and discard. Resuspend each pellet in about 1 ml of sucrose solution (d = 1.105) and wash each tube with an additional 1 ml, combining all the suspended pellets and washes.

Prepare six gradients by overlayering 18 ml of d = 1.135 with 17 ml of d = 1.115 sucrose. Keep cold and mark the interfaces between the solutions as well as the top of the $d = 1.115$ layer. Layer the suspended pellets on top of the gradients, distributing the suspension among the gradients. Ensure that the weights of the tubes to be placed opposite one another in the centrifuge rotor are equal (adjusting the liquid levels to the same height visually is usually sufficient). Centrifuge in a swinging bucket rotor for 1 hr at 27,000 g (Beckman JS13 rotor at 13,000 rpm) and allow the centrifuge to decelerate with no brake. The gradients are viewed under dim red light while the ROS are collected from the marked 1.115–1.135 interface using a syringe fitted with a long cannula. Often most of the gradient is cloudy, but the ROS are generally found in a thick band at the interface. After determining the rhodopsin content of the ROS as described later, the ROS are diluted 1:1 with buffer (solution A) and centrifuged at 39,000 g (Beckman JA20 rotor at 18,000 rpm), and the pellets are stored at $-70°C$, preferably under an inert atmosphere such as argon or nitrogen.

Preparation of Rod Outer Segments from Other Species

For most species, it is clearly not feasible to prepare ROS at the scale described above. Scaling down the procedure has been successful for preparation of ROS from many species. Sucrose solutions of the same densities are used as described, and the procedure is shortened to minimize handling loses.

Procedure

Retinas are homogenized in about 6 ml of $d = 1.115$ sucrose in buffer A. Layer 3 ml of the homogenized retinas on top of a gradient of 3 ml of $d = 1.15$, 4 ml of $d = 1.135$, and 4 ml of $d = 1.115$ in a 15-ml centrifuge tube. After marking the interfaces on the side of the tube and adjusting the level of liquid in opposing tubes to the same height, the gradients are centrifuged at 27,000 g (Beckman JS13 rotor at 13,000 rpm) for 1 hr at 4°C. Although the majority of ROS generally migrate to the 1.115–1.135 interface, we have found varying amounts of rhodopsin at other places in the gradient; thus, all areas should be collected and examined for the presence of rhodopsin. Turbid material from each interface is collected, diluted 3-fold with buffer A, and centrifuged at 12,100 g (Beckman JA20 rotor at 10,000 rpm) for 30 min. The collected ROS can then be suspended in an appropriate amount of buffer A or other buffer, and the rhodopsin concentration can be measured.

Although the above procedure has worked well for most species, the procedure must be modified for some species. For rats and mice, the entire contents of the eye excluding only the lens is used instead of retinas. Alligators and horses have retinas that are very difficult to separate from the vitreous body. For these, the retina and vitreous body are collected together and the volume measured. Sufficient 80% (w/v) sucrose in buffer A is added to yield a final concentration of 45% sucrose. After the mixture is shaken, the procedure for the large-scale bovine ROS preparation above is followed.

Measuring the Concentration of Rhodopsin

The concentration of rhodopsin can easily be determined from its light-sensitive OD_{498} using the procedure of Wald and Brown (7). This procedure is problematic only when there is a relatively high concentration of free retinal. The rhodopsin in a sample is solubilized in a detergent that frees all the rhodopsin but does not denature it. Selection of the detergent depends to some extent on the species of interest since rhodopsins vary in stability (8). We use Ammonyx-LO, which is primarily lauryldimethylamine oxide (provided as a generous gift from the Onyx Chemical Company, Jersey City, NJ, as a 30% w/v solution).

A suspension of ROS is mixed with no less than an equal volume of a 2% solution of Ammonyx-LO in 0.1 M NH_2OH, 67 mM sodium phosphate, 1 mM $MgCl_2$, 0.1 mM EDTA, 1 mM DTE, pH 7.0. The final rhodopsin concentration should be 0.3–1 mg/ml. Hydroxylamine is present to promote complete bleaching on exposure to light and to shift the spectrum of the all-*trans*-retinal produced on bleaching to shorter wavelengths, preventing its

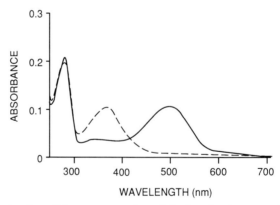

FIG. 1   Determination of the concentration of rhodopsin. A suspension of rod outer segments (100 μl) was solubilized in detergent (900 μl) as described in the text. The spectrum was determined before (——) and after (– – –) bleaching for 5 min on a light box. The ΔOD_{498} measured was 0.0970, which gives a concentration of 23.9 μM rhodopsin in the original suspension.

interference with the absorbance at 498 nm. The solubilized sample is centrifuged at 39,000 g (Beckman JA20 rotor at 18,000 rpm) for 20 min, and the absorbance at 498 nm is measured. The sample is bleached for 5 min either on a light box or using a flood lamp at a distance of about 30 cm. The bleached sample is checked for turbidity and centrifuged if necessary. The absorbance at 498 nm is again measured, and the ΔOD_{498} along with appropriate dilution factors are used to calculate the initial rhodopsin concentration, where the molar extinction coefficient is 40,600 M^{-1} (7). Figure 1 shows spectra from a typical measurement of rhodopsin concentration.

For samples having a large excess of retinal, such as samples that are partially denatured or contain an unknown amount of opsin, the background from the changes in retinal oxime ΔOD_{498} on exposure to light can still interfere with the determination of rhodopsin. This interference can be minimized by reducing the retinal to retinol using $NaBH_4$. A freshly prepared solution of 10 mg/ml $NaBH_4$ in water is added to the membrane sample (not a solubilized sample) to a final concentration of 1.3 mg/ml. The sample is then incubated at room temperature for 1 hr before solubilizing and following the procedure above. This reduces the interference of a large excess of retinal but does not completely eliminate it. Figure 2 shows a typical measurement of rhodopsin following this procedure with a 3-fold molar excess of 11-*cis*-retinal over the original opsin concentration.

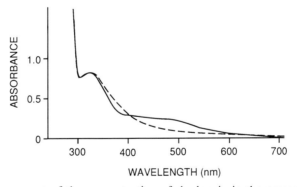

FIG. 2   Measurement of the concentration of rhodopsin in the presence of a large excess of 11-*cis*-retinal. ROS disk membranes were bleached, then (as part of a study on the thermal stability of opsin) denatured at 56°C for 1 min. To determine the amount of regenerable opsin present, 2% bovine serum albumin and a 3-fold molar excess of 11-*cis*-retinal over the original opsin concentration was added. The excess retinal was reduced by adding $NaBH_4$ and the suspension solubilized with an equal volume of detergent-containing buffer, as described in the text. The spectrum was determined before (———) and after (– – –) bleaching. The ΔOD_{498} measured was 0.0985, which gives a concentration of 4.85 μM regenerable opsin in the original suspension. (In this sample, 73% of the opsin was irreversibly denatured.)

Regeneration of Rhodopsin

In vivo, rhodopsin is regenerated after bleaching as a normal part of the visual cycle (9). *In vitro*, however, 11-*cis*-retinal must be added after bleaching. Addition of a 3-fold molar excess of 11-*cis*-retinal over rhodopsin followed by incubation in the dark overnight is generally sufficient to regenerate all the opsin present. The 11-*cis*-retinal (which may be requested from the National Eye Institute, Bethesda, MD) is added most often as an ethanol solution, with care taken to ensure that the final ethanol concentration is well below 1% (v/v). We examined the rate of regeneration of rhodopsin in bovine disk membrane suspensions prepared by the procedure of Smith *et al.* (10) using a 10-fold molar excess of 11-*cis*-retinal. Previous reports indicated that this procedure should yield apparent first-order kinetics (11); however, we observed somewhat variable results owing to changes in the turbidity of the suspension. The kinetic data often showed a rapid regeneration that took minutes and accounted for about 70–80% of the total amount regenerated, and this was followed by a very slow regeneration that took hours to reach completion. We concluded that the retinal was not evenly distributed among the disk membranes and that, once incorporated into the disk membranes, retinal was not easily transferred to another disk membrane owing to its low water solubility (12). To overcome this problem, 2% (w/v) bovine serum albumin (BSA) was added to provide a means of transporting retinal among the disk membranes. Changes in turbidity were also markedly reduced in the presence of BSA. Under these conditions, first-order kinetics were observed as shown in Fig. 3.*

Procedure

Bleached ROS are suspended in buffer [e.g., 0.1 M potassium phosphate buffer, pH 7.0, containing 1 mM MgCl$_2$, 0.5 mM DTT (or DTE), and 0.1 mM EDTA] to 1 mg/ml. In the dark, 11-*cis*-retinal is dissolved in ethanol at

---

* The apparent rate constant for regeneration is the second-order rate constant for the reaction multiplied by the concentration of 11-*cis*-retinal:

$$\text{Opsin} + 11\text{-}cis\text{-retinal} \xrightarrow{k} \text{rhodopsin}$$

$$d[\text{rhodopsin}]/dt = k[11\text{-}cis\text{-retinal}][\text{opsin}]$$

At high retinal concentrations, the regeneration follows pseudo-first-order kinetics where $k_{app} = k[11\text{-}cis\text{-retinal}]$.

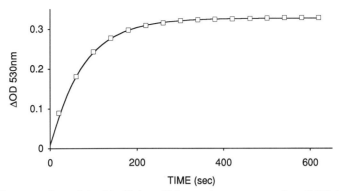

FIG. 3   Regeneration of rhodopsin in a disk membrane suspension. ROS disk membranes were suspended to 0.3 mg/ml in 0.1 M potassium phosphate buffer, pH 7.0,
containing 1 mM MgCl$_2$, 0.5 mM DTT, 0.1 mM EDTA, and 2% (w/v) bovine serum
albumin. The suspension was bleached for 3 hr at room temperature with orange
light ($t_{1/2}$ for bleaching was about 1 min under these conditions). The bleached suspension was placed in a themostated cuvette at 25°C, and a 10-fold molar excess of 11-
cis-retinal in ethanol was added and quickly mixed. The final ethanol concentration
was 0.2% (w/v). The increase in OD$_{530}$ was measured at 40-sec intervals for 10 min
using a Hewlett Packard 8452A diode array spectrophotometer. The OD$_{530}$ was used
instead of OD$_{498}$ to avoid interference caused by absorbance of the excess free retinal
present. The line drawn is a least-squares fit of the data to first-order kinetics.

10 mg/ml. Add 2 μl of retinal for every milliliter of ROS suspension, which
yields approximately a 3-fold molar excess of 11-cis-retinal. For complete
regeneration, incubate at 4°C overnight under an inert atmosphere such as
nitrogen or argon. For experiments that require rapid, complete regeneration,
2% BSA must be included in the buffer and more 11-cis-retinal should be
added. For example, the conditions in Fig. 3 gave a $t_{1/2}$ of regeneration of
about 1 min, so that the regeneration was essentially complete in about
10 min.

Summary

Simple procedures have been presented for the preparation of bovine rod
outer segments, determination of the concentration of rhodopsin, and regeneration of rhodopsin. These procedures only require access to a refrigerated
centrifuge and a spectrophotometer in a dark room. They lend themselves
well to modifications to fit existing equipment or desired experimental protocols.

Acknowledgments

Research was supported by Grants EY 06225 and EY 06226 from the National Institutes of Health and an unrestricted departmental award from Research to Prevent Blindness. The technical assistance of Joseph P. Nawrocki is gratefully acknowledged.

References

1. W. Krebs and H. Kühn, *Exp. Eye. Res.* **25,** 511 (1977).
2. R. S. Molday and L. L. Molday, this Volume [8].
3. D. S. Papermaster and W. J. Dreyer, *Biochemistry* **13,** 2438 (1974).
4. P. P. M. Schnetkamp, A. A. Klompmakers, and F. J. M. Daemen, *Biochim. Biophys. Acta* **552,** 379 (1979).
5. R. S. Molday and L. L. Molday, *J. Cell Biol.* **105,** 2589 (1987).
6. S. W. Hall and H. Kühn, *Eur. J. Biochem.* **161,** 551 (1986).
7. G. Wald and P. K. Brown, *J. Gen. Physiol.* **37,** 189 (1953).
8. S.-L. Fong, A. T. C. Tsin, C. D. B. Bridges, and G. I. Liou, *in* "Methods in Enzymology" (L. Packer, ed.), Vol. 81, p. 133. Academic Press, New York, 1982.
9. R. R. Rando, *J. Bioenerg. Biomembr.* **23,** 133 (1991).
10. H. G. Smith, G. W. Stubbs, and B. J. Litman, *Exp. Eye Res.* **20,** 211 (1975).
11. H. Matsumoto, K. Horiuchi, and T. Yoshizawa, *Biochim. Biophys. Acta* **501,** 257 (1978).
12. E. Z. Szuts and F. I. Harosi, *Arch. Biochem. Biophys.* **287,** 297 (1991).

[8]   Isolation and Characterization of Rod Outer Segment Disk and Plasma Membranes

Robert S. Molday and Laurie L. Molday

Introduction

The outer segment of the rod photoreceptor cell consists of an ordered stack of over 1000 closed disks surrounded by a separate plasma membrane. Each disk consists of a continuous membrane in which two closely spaced lamellar membrane domains are joined by a hairpin loop domain referred to as the rim region. The disk membrane encloses a lumen compartment generally referred to as the intradiskal space. Except at the base of the rod outer segment (ROS), the plasma membrane lipid bilayer is physically separated from the disk membrane lipid bilayer. At the proximal or basal region, where new membrane is added as part of the ROS renewal process, open disklike structures are observed which appear to evaginate from the ciliary plasma membrane (1). The membrane of these disklike structures appears to be continuous with the ROS plasma membrane. The highly organized ROS structure is maintained by a network of fibrous cytoskeletal elements that link the rim regions of adjacent disks to one another and the rim region of the disks to the plasma membrane (2, 3).

An important step in the analysis of the molecular structure, function, and morphogenesis of ROS is the development of preparative procedures to purify intact ROS from retinal tissue extracts, separate the soluble or cytosolic fraction from the ROS membrane, and isolate the disk and plasma membranes. In this chapter, methods to purify and fractionate ROS are described, and recent studies on the compositional analysis of defined ROS fractions are briefly reviewed.

Purification of Intact Rod Outer Segments

General Considerations

A number of methods have been developed to isolate ROS from rod-dominant retinas and, in particular, from bovine and frog retinas. Early methods (4, 5) have been refined to increase the yield and purity of ROS (6) and to obtain intact, sealed ROS structures (7–9). These procedures take advantage of the

Methods in Neurosciences, Volume 15
Copyright © 1993 by Academic Press, Inc. All rights of reproduction in any form reserved.

fragile nature of the ciliary connection between the outer and inner segment of the rod cell, the stability of the ROS in isotonic or hypertonic solution, and the relatively low buoyant density of the outer segment. Generally, freshly dissected retinas in sucrose solution are shaken or gently homogenized to break off the ROS from the rest of the photoreceptor cell at the cilium, and a crude ROS suspension is then obtained after removal of retinal tissue. ROS are further purified by either discontinuous or continuous sucrose gradient density centrifugation to remove contaminating subcellular organelles. Continuous sucrose gradients have been particularly effective in separating sealed ROS from unsealed or fragmented ROS (7, 10). Sealed ROS that band at a greater bouyant density than fragmented ROS consist largely of stacks of disks surrounded by a plasma membrane. Intact ROS are preferentially obtained if freshly dissected retinas are used as the starting material and if care is taken to maintain the ROS in sucrose solution (~20%, w/v, sucrose). Although sucrose gradients have been most widely used, other gradients such as Ficoll–sucrose (9) have also produced relatively pure, intact ROS. For frog ROS preparations, Percoll gradient centrifugation has been particularly effective in the isolation of intact ROS (11, 12).

Purification Method

Rod outer segments are typically isolated under dim red light from the retinas of 80 freshly dissected bovine eyes (10, 13). The retinas are placed in a 125-ml Erlenmeyer flask containing 30 ml of homogenizing buffer (20%, w/v, sucrose, 20 mM Tris–acetate, pH 7.2, 2 mM $MgCl_2$, 10 mM glucose, and 5 mM taurine). The retina suspension is gently shaken for about 1 min and subsequently filtered through either cheesecloth or a fine Teflon screen to remove the bulk retina tissue. The crude ROS suspension is then layered on six 24-ml 25–60% (w/v) continuous sucrose gradients containing 20 mM Tris–acetate, pH 7.2, 10 mM glucose, and 5 mM taurine and centrifuged at 25,000 rpm (75,000 g) for 45 min at 4°C in a Beckman SW-27 swinging bucket rotor. A small upper band at a density of 1.13 g/ml is composed of broken ROS and disk membranes. The major pink band having a density of about 1.14 g/ml constitutes the intact, sealed ROS. Directly below this band is a diffuse, white band composed of other subcellular organelles and a sharp red band containing red blood cells. The dark pellet is composed largely of pigment granules from retinal pigment epithelial cells and some unbroken cells. When previously frozen retinas are used in place of freshly dissected retinas, the lower ROS band is diminished and the upper ROS band is increased such that the amount of sealed and unsealed ROS is roughly equal.

For studies requiring sealed ROS, the lower ROS band is carefully collected using a syringe with a wide-bore needle and mixed with homogenizing buffer to yield a final volume of about 100–150 ml. The ROS are then centrifuged at 8000 rpm (7710 g) for 10 min in a Sorvall SS-34 rotor, and the pellet is resuspended in 4 ml of homogenizing buffer. Typically, 40–50 mg of sealed ROS are obtained from 80 freshly dissected bovine retinas. A typical sodium dodecyl sulfate (SDS)–polyacrylamide gel pattern of ROS proteins under reducing conditions is shown in Fig. 1. The ROS preparation can be frozen in homogenizing buffer for storage, although the sealed property of the ROS is generally compromised. This preparative procedure can be scaled down

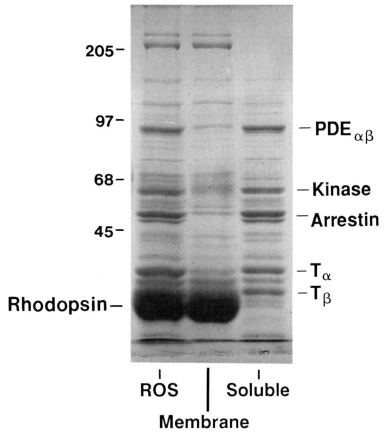

FIG. 1 SDS–polyacrylamide gel electrophoresis of intact purified ROS, the ROS membrane fraction, and the ROS soluble fraction. Following purification on continuous sucrose gradient, intact ROS were lysed in 10 mM Tris buffer, pH 7.2, and the ROS membranes separated from the soluble fraction by centrifugation. Lanes were loaded with 15–30 μg protein, and the gels were stained with Coomassie blue. PDE, Phosphodiesterase; Kinase, rhodopsin kinase; T, transducin.

for the isolation of ROS from other rod-dominant species such as rat, pig, and human.

Separation of Rod Outer Segments into Soluble and Membrane Fractions

General Considerations

As first reported by Godchaux and Zimmerman (7) and subsequently by Kühn (14), ROS can be readily separated into a soluble and membrane fraction by hypotonic lysis of unbleached ROS followed by centrifugation. Under these conditions, soluble proteins and proteins weakly associated with the membrane, including transducin, phosphodiesterase, arrestin, and rhodopsin kinase, appear in the supernatant. Differential extraction of some proteins can be achieved by altering the state of bleaching of the ROS, changing the ionic strength of the solution, and including nucleotides such as GTP (14). Integral membrane proteins such as rhodopsin, the 220-kDa rim protein, peripherin/rds, the cGMP-gated channel, and the $Na^+/Ca^{2+} - K^+$ exchanger are found in the pellet. Additional nonintegral, membrane-associated proteins can be extracted from the membrane fraction with chelating agents and high ionic strength buffers. In particular, the calcium-binding protein calmodulin can be extracted by washing the membranes with EGTA (15), and glyceraldehyde-3-phosphate dehydrogenase can be extracted with physiological saline buffer (16). Figure 1 shows a typical SDS–polyacrylamide gel pattern of proteins present in intact ROS and in the membrane and soluble fractions obtained after hypotonic lysis of unbleached ROS.

Osmotically active ROS membranes can also be isolated by hypotonic lysis of ROS in distilled water followed by flotation on 5% Ficoll according to the method of Smith et al. (17). These membrane vesicles consist of both disk membrane and plasma membrane vesicles in a ratio similar to that found in ROS, namely, 20:1 (see Fig. 5).

Fractionation Method

Generally, 1 ml of sealed ROS (6–8 mg protein) in homogenizing buffer is centrifuged in a Sorvall SS-34 rotor at 8000 rpm (7710 g) for 10 min. The supernatant is carefully removed, and the pellet is resuspended in 2 ml of 1 mM Tris or 1 mM HEPES buffer, pH 7.2, at 4°C. After 1 hr at 4°C, the ROS suspension is centrifuged at 12,000 rpm (17,300 g) for 30 min, and the supernatant is retained as the soluble fraction. The supernatant is centrifuged

again at high speed [>17,000 rpm (>34,800 g) for 30 min] to remove residual
membrane. The membrane pellet from the initial centrifugation is washed
twice with 1 mM Tris or HEPES buffer to remove remaining soluble proteins,
and the final pellet is resuspended in 2 ml of buffer. If the membrane is to
be stored frozen, it is desirable to resuspend the ROS in homogenizing buffer
or a related buffer containing sucrose.

Additional membrane-associated proteins can be extracted from the ROS
membranes by washing the membranes with 150 mM NaCl and 2 mM EDTA.
The extraction is routinely monitored by SDS–polyacrylamide gel electrophoresis of the supernatant and membrane fractions. When unbleached ROS
membranes are used, transducin subunits (37 and 39 kDa), phosphodiesterase
subunits (often appearing as a doublet at 89–90 kDa), and arrestin (52 kDa)
are readily visible in the soluble fraction (Fig. 1). Rhodopsin appears as the
major band at 36–38 kDa in the membrane fraction, but is absent in the soluble
fraction. The ROS and ROS membrane fractions are also characterized by
several proteins in the range of 220–250 kDa when SDS–polyacrylamide gels
are loaded with over 30 μg protein per lane.

Separation of Rod Outer Segment Disk and Plasma Membranes

General Considerations

Over the years there has been considerable debate concerning the molecular
composition of ROS disk and plasma membranes. The view that disk and
plasma membranes are similar, if not identical, in composition has developed
from morphological and immunocytochemical analysis of the outer segment
and from functional studies. Electron microscopic studies have suggested
that disk and plasma membranes arise from the same newly formed membrane at the base of the ROS. This membrane appears as an evagination of
the ciliary membrane (1). Immunocytochemical studies using both monoclonal and polyclonal antirhodopsin antibodies have shown that rhodopsin
is present in high concentrations in both disk and plasma membranes (18,
19). At a functional level, several studies have reported that disk membranes,
as well as the plasma membranes, contain cGMP-gated cation channel activity (20–22) and Na$^+$/Ca^{2+} exchange activity (23). The purity of the disk
membranes used in these studies, however, was not confirmed, and the
possibility that fusion occurred between disk and plasma membranes was
not addressed. Although these studies suggest that the two membranes are
similar, other studies indicate that differences in protein composition exist
between the disk and plasma membranes. Several proteins that have been
shown to be present in the plasma membrane by lactoperoxidase-catalyzed

radioiodination are absent in the disk membranes (24, 25). Neuraminidase-sensitive ricin-binding glycoproteins present in ROS plasma membranes also have been shown to be absent in disk membranes (13, 26).

To resolve the question of whether disk and plasma membranes are similar, it is necessary to isolate ROS plasma membranes and disk membranes for biochemical analysis of the protein and lipid compositions. Development of such methods, however, has been impeded by (1) the relatively low amount of the plasma membrane (5–6%) relative to disk membranes in ROS; (2) the lack of suitable disk membrane- and plasma membrane-specific markers for monitoring the stages of membrane fractionation; (3) the similarity in physical properties of the disk and plasma membranes; and (4) the presence of cytoskeletal proteins that link the rim regions of the disks to the plasma membrane.

An affinity density perturbation method employing ricin–gold particles has been developed to overcome many of these problems (13). Generally, this procedure first involves the treatment of intact ROS with neuraminidase to remove sialic acid residues and expose galactose residues on ROS plasma membrane-specific sialoglycoproteins. These include glycoproteins with apparent subunit molecular masses of 230 and 110 kDa (13, 26). The 230-kDa protein has been identified as the $Na^+/Ca^{2+} - K^+$ exchanger (27). The exposed galactose residues are then labeled with ricin–gold particles that serve both as electron-dense markers to identify the plasma membrane by electron microscopy and as agents to increase the density of the plasma membrane for density gradient separation. Other galactose-specific lectins such as peanut agglutinin that also bind to neuraminidase-treated ROS (28) can, in principle, be used in place of ricin.

The extent and specificity of binding of the ricin–gold particles to ROS plasma membranes can be visualized by transmission electron microscopy (Fig. 2). After removing excess ricin–gold reagent by repeated washing, the labeled ROS are lysed in hypotonic buffer to produce fragmented ROS in which unlabeled disks are still attached to the ricin–gold-labeled plasma membrane (Fig. 2). The disks are then dissociated from the plasma membrane by either mild trypsin treatment or prolonged exposure to hypotonic buffer. The former method is more efficient in dissociating intact disks from plasma membrane vesicles (Fig. 3) and ultimately produces highly purified disk and plasma membranes. However, it has the disadvantage that proteins of interest may undergo limited proteolysis in the presence of trypsin. Sucrose gradient centrifugation is finally used to separate unlabeled disk membranes from the more dense ricin–gold-labeled plasma membranes.

Typically, from 24 mg of trypsinized ROS membrane protein, 1.6 mg of ROS plasma membrane protein can be obtained as a red pellet with a plasma membrane purity greater than 75%, and 15 mg of disk protein can be isolated

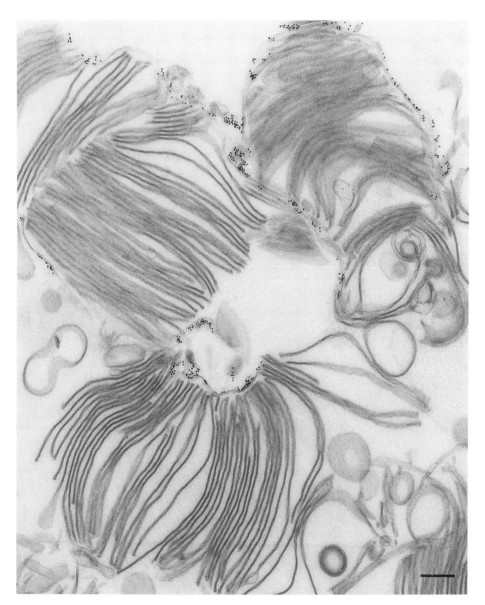

FIG. 2 Electron micrograph of neuraminidase-treated, ricin–gold–dextran-labeled ROS hypotonically lysed in 10 mM Tris buffer, pH 7.2. Note that the gold particles (diameter ~9 nm) are bound to the extracellular surface of the partially inverted plasma membrane and that the unlabeled disks are still attached to the cytoplasmic surface (13, 26). Bar, 0.2 μm.

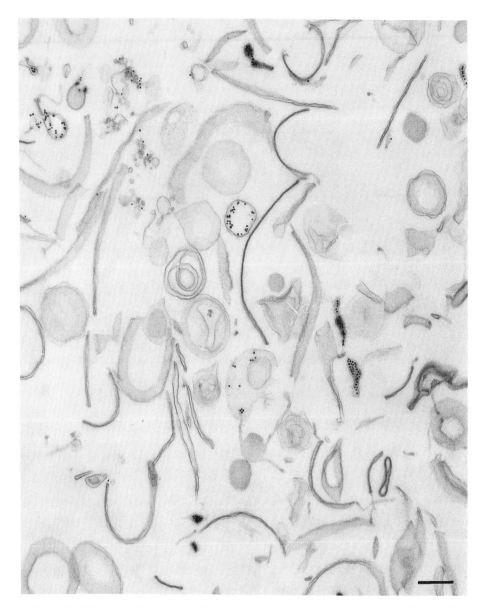

Fɪɢ. 3   Electron micrograph of ricin–gold–dextran-labeled bovine ROS that had been lysed in hypotonic buffer and treated with trypsin. Note that the gold-labeled plasma membranes are dissociated from the unlabeled disk membranes. Disk membranes appear either as flattened disk structures or as vesicles (13). Bar, 0.2 μm.

with a plasma membrane contamination of less than 0.025%. Mild trypsin treatment appears to digest the cytoskeletal matrix that links adjacent disks and the disks to the plasma membrane. Electron microscopic analysis indicates that the disks maintain their unique flattened morphology (10, 13) (Figs. 3 and 4A). The plasma membrane pellet exhibits an intense red color from the bound gold particles. Electron microscopic analysis indicates that most membrane vesicles are labeled with gold particles, with many of the vesicles attaining an inverted orientation with the gold particles bound to the inner surface of the vesicles (Fig. 4B).

In preparations in which hypotonic buffer is used in place of trypsin, all disks are not completely dissociated from the plasma membrane. Electron microscopic analysis indicates that many rim regions of the disks are still associated with fragmented plasma membrane (13). Accordingly, the enriched plasma membrane fraction obtained by dissociation in hypotonic buffer without trypsin is only about 25% pure, and the disk membrane fraction has a plasma membrane contamination of about 0.1%. The extent of contamination of the disks with plasma membrane in these preparations, however, will depend on the extent of the ricin–gold–dextran labeling of the plasma membrane and the size of the gold particles. These parameters affect the extent to which the density of the plasma membrane is increased relative to the unlabeled disk membranes.

SDS–polyacrylamide gel electrophoresis and Western blotting are typically used to assess the purity of the membrane fractions. Generally, disk membranes have a relatively simple protein pattern, with rhodopsin as the major protein and the 220-kDa rim glycoprotein as another characteristic band in nontrypsin-treated preparations. The 220-kDa protein is digested to a 120-kDa fragment in trypsin-treated preparations. The plasma membrane fraction has a more complex pattern, with numerous bands between 20 and 250 kDa. Rhodopsin still appears as a dominant protein. If membrane fractionation is carried out in low ionic strength buffer ($\sim$10 mM), a band at 38 kDa just above rhodopsin also appears as a prominent protein. This protein identified as the glyceraldehyde-3-phosphate dehydrogenase subunit, can be removed by washing the membrane with physiological buffer (16). Several other proteins have been identified as constituents of the plasma membrane, including the 63-kDa cGMP-gated channel subunit (29), 240-kDa channel-associated protein (30), ricin-binding proteins (25), $Na^+/Ca^{2+} - K^+$ exchanger (27), and a GLUT-1 glucose transporter (31). Western blotting or solid-phase competition immunoassays of these proteins can be used to assess the purity of the plasma membrane and disk membranes. This is shown in Fig. 5 for the cGMP-gated channel. An antichannel monoclonal antibody PMc 1D1 (29) is shown to label the channel in ROS membranes,

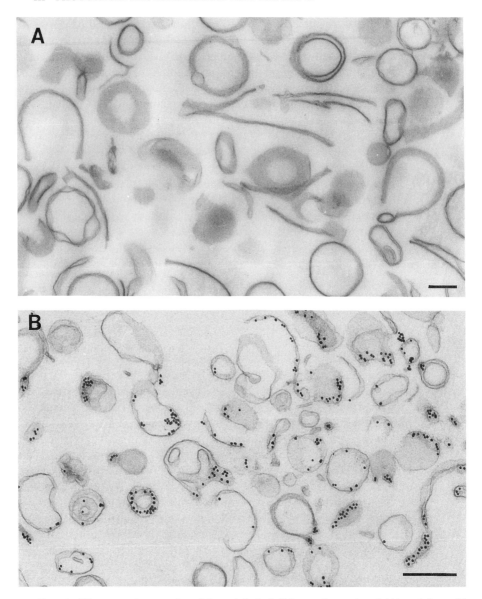

FIG. 4   Electron micrographs of the unlabeled disk membrane band (A) and the gold-labeled plasma membrane pellet (B) obtained after fractionation of trypsin-treated, ricin–gold–dextran-labeled ROS by sucrose density gradient centrifugation (13). Bars, 0.2 μm.

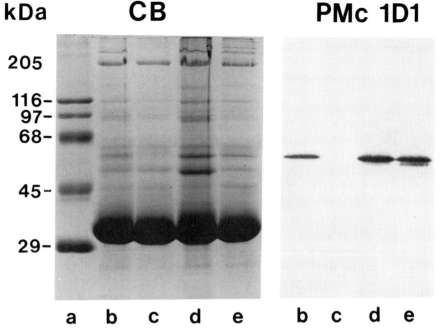

FIG. 5   SDS–polyacrylamide gels and Western blots of bovine ROS membrane preparations. Lane a, molecular weight standards; lanes b, ROS membranes prepared from
hypotonically lysed ROS; lanes c, ROS disk membrane fraction from nontrypsin
preparations; lanes d, ROS plasma membrane enriched fraction from nontrypsin
preparations; lanes e, ROS membrane vesicles prepared by hypotonic lysis of ROS
followed by flotation on Ficoll. The SDS–polyacrylamide gels were either stained
with Coomassie blue (CB) or transferred to Immobilon membranes and labeled with
anti-cGMP-grated channel monoclonal antibody (PMc 1D1). Note that all ROS membrane fractions except disk membranes (lane c) contain detectable amounts of channel. Approximately 30 μg of ROS membrane protein was loaded on each lane.

ROS membrane vesicles isolated by flotation on Ficoll, and plasma membranes, but not in purified disk membranes.

Ricin–Gold–Dextran Affinity Perturbation Method

Isolated, unbleached bovine ROS (30–40 mg protein) in homogenizing buffer
are treated with 0.1 units of *Arthrobacter ureafaciens* neuraminidase (Boehringer-Mannheim, Indianapolis, IN) at 4°C in the dark for at least 2 hr. The
neuraminidase-treated ROS are then washed by centrifugation [8000 rpm

(7710 g) for 10 min] in a Sorvall SS-34 rotor in 10 ml homogenizing buffer to remove the excess neuraminidase, and the pellet is resuspended in 4 ml of homogenizing buffer. Two milliliters of ricin–gold–dextran (gold diameter 10–15 nm; absorbance of about 4 at a wavelength of 520 nm) is added to the ROS suspension, and the mixture is gently agitated for at least 2 hr. The ROS suspension is then diluted with 20 ml of homogenizing buffer and washed twice by centrifugation at 5000 rpm (3020 g) for 5 min in a Sorvall SS-34 rotor. After removal of the unbound ricin–gold–dextran, the ROS are further washed 3 times to remove sucrose and lysed in 10 mM Tris buffer, pH 7.2, for 1 hr at 4°C. The ROS membranes are then washed by centrifugation at 12,000 rpm (17,300 g) for 15 min in 10 mM Tris buffer, pH 7.2, containing 1 mM EDTA to remove the soluble proteins.

The plasma membrane can be dissociated from the disk membranes by either prolonged treatment with low ionic strength buffer or by mild digestion with trypsin. In the former procedure the ROS membrane pellet is resuspended in 8 ml of 1 mM Tris buffer, pH 7.2, and maintained at 4°C in this buffer for 14–16 hr. In the trypsin procedure the ROS membrane pellet is resuspended in 4 ml of 20 mM Tris buffer, pH 7.2, containing 0.2 μg/ml of trypsin treated with N-tosyl-L-phenylalanine chloromethyl ketone (TCPK). After 30 min at 4°C the digestion reaction is stopped by the addition of 4 μg of soybean trypsin inhibitor. Under these conditions many of the high molecular mass proteins are digested, but rhodopsin, which contains a trypsin-sensitive 9-amino acid C-terminal segment, is not digested unless higher trypsin concentrations are used. The trypsinized ROS membranes are then washed twice with 20 mM Tris buffer, pH 7.2, by centrifugation at 15,000 rpm (27,000 g) for 30 min in a Sorvall SS-34 rotor. The final pellet is resuspended in 4 ml of the same buffer.

The dissociated ROS membranes are fractionated into disk and plasma membranes by sucrose density gradient centrifugation using a Beckman SW-41 rotor. Typically, the ROS membranes (20–30 mg protein) are layered on four gradients consisting of 1 ml of 60% (w/v) sucrose in 20 mM Tris buffer, pH 7.2, and 9 ml of a 15–50% (w/v) sucrose gradient in the same buffer. Centrifugation is carried out at 35,000 rpm (208,000 g) for 3 hr at 4°C. The gold-labeled plasma membrane fraction is generally obtained as a red pellet for trypsin-treated preparations or as a pellet or a band at the interface of the 50–60% sucrose layer for nontrypsin-treated preparations. The density of the enriched plasma membrane for nontrypsinized preparations is lower than that for the trypsinized sample owing to the contaminating, unlabeled disks still associated with the plasma membrane. The disk membranes for both preparations are found as a band having a density of about 1.13 g/ml. In general the band for trypsinized preparations is significantly larger as a result of the increased amount of dissociated disks. The disk band of each gradient is collected with a syringe, diluted with 3 volumes of 20 mM Tris buffer, pH 7.2, and centrifuged at 15,000 rpm (27,000 g) for 30 min in a Sorvall SS-34 rotor. The disk pellet is then resuspended in about 2 ml of buffer to obtain a protein concentration of 6–8 mg/ml. The plasma membrane fraction is washed in the same buffer and resuspended in 0.5–1 ml. Generally, the samples are exposed to light after the sucrose gradient centrifugation. The fractions are analyzed by SDS–polyacrylamide gel electrophoresis (13) (Fig. 5).

In this isolation procedure, ricin–gold–dextran conjugates have been widely used. These reagents have been prepared by coupling ricin I (ricin 120) or ricin II (ricin 60) to glutaraldehyde-activated dextran as previously described (32). However, commercially available ricin–gold conjugates can be used in place of the ricin–gold–dextran conjugates. Generally, gold particles having a diameter of about 10–15 nm are best, but larger gold particles have also been used.

Related Methods

Related affinity density perturbation methods have also been developed. In one related procedure, a monoclonal antibody, PMe 2D9, which binds to an extracellular domain of the 230-KDa ricin-binding protein of ROS plasma membranes has been directly conjugated to gold–dextran particles and used in place of the ricin–gold–dextran reagent to isolate disk and plasma membranes. The two methods are identical except that the ROS do not have to be treated with neuraminidase when the PMe 2D9 antibody is used since the antibody binds to the surface of ROS which have not been treated with neuraminidase (D. Reid and R. S. Molday, 1991, unpublished results).

Ricin bound to Sepharose particles has been used to separate disk and plasma membranes for lipid analysis (33). In this procedure ricin–Sepharose particles are used to bind neuraminidase-treated ROS. After washing the Sepharose to remove unbound ROS, hypotonic lysis of the ROS is carried out, and the disk and plasma membranes are dissociated by trypsin or low ionic strength buffer as indicated above. The membranes are then separated by differential centrifugation. Potential advantages of this method are the relative ease of separating the plasma membrane-bound Sepharose particles from the free disks by low-speed centrifugation and the ability to dissociate the plasma membrane from the ricin–Sepharose particles by competition with 1 M galactose. Detailed description of the methods, including the extent of disk and plasma membrane recovery and SDS–polyacrylamide gel electrophoresis analysis of the proteins in these fractions, however, has not yet been reported.

Finally, several reports have used concanavalin A–polystyrene or concanavalin A–Sepharose particles to bind ROS and effect separation by differential centrifugation (34, 35).

Characterization of Rod Outer Segment Disk and Plasma Membranes

Protein Composition

The development of methods to fractionate ROS into a soluble fraction and disk and plasma membrane fractions has contributed toward our analysis of ROS proteins and their role in ROS structure, morphogenesis, and function. The soluble fraction is operationally defined as proteins that do not require detergents for solubilization. This fraction includes proteins that are contained within the cytoplasmic compartment of ROS and proteins that are weakly associated with the disk or plasma membrane by (1) interaction with integral membrane proteins, (2) noncovalent association to the surface of the lipid bilayer, or (3) weak interaction with the lipid bilayer by way of covalently bound lipid molecules. In the latter case, for example, it has recently been shown that the C terminus of the transducin γ subunit and the PDE α subunit are posttranslationally modified by carboxymethylation and prenylation (36–38). These functional groups have been suggested to enhance the association of the proteins with the disk membrane.

Many of the proteins contained within the soluble fraction have been identified and characterized, and in many cases their sequences have been determined by cDNA analysis. Such proteins include enzymes of the visual cascade system (transducin, phosphodiesterase, arrestin protein, phosphatase 2A, rhodopsin kinase), calcium-binding proteins (recoverin and calmodulin), and metabolic enzymes (glycolytic enzymes, pentose shunt enzymes, creatine kinase, nucleotide kinases, etc.). A partial listing of soluble and weakly associated ROS proteins is presented in Table I (39–69).

Membrane proteins are operationally defined as proteins which require detergents for solubilization. In most cases these proteins span the lipid bilayer one or more times. Hydrophobic stretches of 19–26 amino acids are considered as the putative transmembrane segments. Rhodopsin is the most well characterized of the integral membrane proteins of ROS and has been shown to contain seven hydrophobic segments that serve as membrane-spanning regions (49, 50). Some membrane proteins that are firmly anchored to the bilayer by covalently bound lipids may require detergent for solubilization, and therefore are operationally classified as membrane proteins.

ROS membrane proteins can be divided into proteins that are predominantly, if not exclusively, found in the ROS plasma membrane and proteins

TABLE I   Rod Outer Segment Proteins

Protein	M_r^a	Selected references
Soluble and membrane-associated proteins		
Phosphodiesterase		39, 40
α subunit	88,000	
β subunit	84,000	
γ subunit	11,000	
Protein kinase C	85,000	41
Rhodopsin kinase	68,000	42, 43
Arrestin (48K protein or S-antigen)	48,000	44, 45
Creatine kinase	43,000	46
Transducin		14, 47, 48
α subunit	39,000	
β subunit	37,000	
γ subunit	8,000	
Pyrophosphatase	44,000	51
Glyceraldehyde-3-phosphate-dehydrogenase	38,000	16
Phosducin (33K protein)	33,000	52, 53
Recoverin	26,000 (23,000)	54, 55
Calmodulin	20,000 (16,500)	15, 56
Phosphatase 2A	38,000	57
Other proteins		
Glycolytic enzymes		31
Nucleotide diphosphokinase		58, 59
Pentose shunt enzymes		60
Guanylate kinase		58, 59
Tubulin	58,000	64
Disk membrane proteins		
Rim protein[b]	220,000	40
Rhodopsin	38,000	6, 10, 13, 49, 50, 61
Peripherin/rds[b]	35,000 (39,000)	10, 62
ROM-1[b]	33,000 (37,000)	63
Retinol dehydrogenase[c]	37,000	73
Plasma membrane proteins		
cGMP-gated channel-associated protein	240,000	30
$Na^+/K^+/Ca^{2+}$ exchanger	230,000 (130,000)	27, 65
Ricin-binding sialoglycoprotein	160,000	26
Ricin-binding sialoglycoprotein	110,000	13, 26
cGMP-gated channel	63,000 (79,600)	29, 66, 67
GLUT-1 glucose transporter	50,000	31
Rhodopsin	38,000	13, 34
Guanylate cyclase[c]	112,000	68, 69

[a] Subunit M_r values were determined by SDS–polyacrylamide gel electrophoresis from bovine ROS (values may vary depending on electrophoresis conditions and the gel system employed); values in parentheses were estimated from sequence analysis when they deviate significantly from M_r estimated by SDS–polyacrylamide gel electrophoresis.
[b] Localized to the rim region of disks.
[c] Localization has not yet been established.

localized in the disk membrane (13). To date only rhodopsin has been conclusively shown to be present in similar quantities in both the disk and plasma membrane (13, 34). Proteins that have been localized to the plasma membrane by immunochemical analysis are absent or present in extremely low amounts in the disk membrane preparations. For example, the cGMP-gated channel has been shown by both Western blotting and immunocytochemical studies to be predominantly present in the ROS plasma membrane (29). More sensitive solid-phase radioimmune competition assays have further shown that the channel protein can be detected in purified disk fractions, but in amounts that are 200-fold lower than that in the plasma membrane (70). It is not clear if the small quantity of channel in the disk fraction represents channel protein that is inherently present in the disk membranes (i.e., is not sorted to the plasma membrane), or if this represents a residual contamination of the disk membrane fraction by plasma membrane. Other proteins including the 240-kDa channel-associated protein, the $Na^+/Ca^{2+} - K^+$ exchanger, ricin-binding proteins, and the GLUT-1 glucose transporter have also been shown to be localized to the plasma membrane.

A number of disk membrane proteins have also been identified and partially characterized. Rhodopsin is by far the most abundant disk membrane protein, accounting for about 90% of the total disk membrane protein. Rhodopsin is preferentially localized along the lamellar region of the disk membrane, as shown by immunogold labeling studies (10). Other disk membrane proteins that have been identified include the high molecular mass (220 kDa) rim protein (71), peripherin/rds (10), and rom-1 (63, 72). Immunocytochemical studies indicate that these proteins, in contrast to rhodopsin, are localized along the rim region of the disks. Recently, retinol dehydrogenase has been isolated from ROS (73). This protein has yet to be localized, but on the basis of its function to reduce the all-*trans*-retinal group released from rhodopsin, one may speculate that this enzyme is likely to be present in both the disk membrane and plasma membrane in close proximity to rhodopsin. Guanylate cyclase has also been purified (68, 69), but its localization within the ROS has not yet been determined by immunocytochemical methods. A listing of disk and plasma membrane proteins is given in Table I.

Lipid Composition

The lipid composition of ROS from several species has been extensively investigated (74). More recently, studies have been directed toward defining the lipid composition of isolated disk and plasma membranes. Boesze-Battaglia and Albert (75) have reported that the ROS plasma membrane is high in C14:0 (20%) saturated fatty acid and 18:2 (9%) and 18:3 (8%) unsaturated fatty acids, and low in C22 : 6 docosahexaenoic acid (5%). In contrast, disk membranes are characterized by a high docosahexaenoic acid content (35%), a relatively high saturated C18 : 0 content (19%), and a low content of C14 : 0 (1.4%), C18 : 2 (1.1%), and C18 : 3 (1.1%) fatty acids. The cholesterol content between the plasma membrane and disk membrane is also significantly different, with the plasma membrane containing a relatively high cholesterol to phospholipid ratio of 0.4 compared to disk membranes with a ratio of 0.11 (75). The differences in lipid composition between the disk membrane and plasma membrane indicate that specific sorting mechanisms occur for lipids as well as proteins.

Functional Studies

ROS disk and plasma membrane preparations have also been used for functional studies. In particular cGMP-gated channel activity and Na^+/Ca^{2+} exchange activities have been measured by solubilizing the disk membrane or plasma membrane fractions in CHAPS detergent and reconstituting the proteins in liposomes containing calcium for measurements of cGMP-dependent or Na^+-dependent calcium efflux (27, 29). Such studies have confirmed that essentially all the activity of these ion transporters resides in the plasma membrane. The ability of rhodopsin to activate phosphodiesterase by way of transducin has also been studied in plasma membrane and disk membrane preparations (76). Results indicate that rhodopsin contained in the plasma membrane does not effectively activate the cascade system compared with rhodopsin in disk membranes. The inability of plasma membrane rhodopsin to activate transducin has been attributed to the high cholesterol content of the ROS plasma membrane.

Conclusions

Preparations of highly purified ROS disk and plasma membranes have been developed based on the specific binding of lectin or antibody reagents to the surface of isolated ROS, dissociation of the disks from the plasma membrane by hypotonic lysis or mild trypsin digestion, and separation of labeled plasma membrane from the unlabeled disk membranes by differential density centrifugation. Analyses of the disk and plasma membranes indicate that the protein compositions of these membranes are different. With the exception of rhodopsin, membrane proteins that have been identified and partially characterized to date are preferentially localized in either the disk membrane or the plasma membrane. Significant differences in the lipid composition of disk and plasma membranes have also been found. These studies lead to the conclusion that highly selective protein and lipid sorting mechanisms occur within the ROS to direct specific proteins and lipids to either the disk or plasma membrane. The molecular mechanism for this sorting process, however, remains to be determined. Isolated disk and plasma membrane preparations in conjunction with soluble protein preparations should prove highly useful for further analyses of the structure, function, and morphogenesis of ROS.

Acknowledgments

The work from our laboratory described in this chapter was supported by grants from the National Institutes of Health (EY 02422), the Medical Research Council of Canada, and the RP Eye Research Foundation of Canada.

References

1. R. H. Steinberg, S. K. Fisher, and D. H. Anderson, *J. Comp. Neurol.* **190,** 501 (1980).
2. J. Usukura and E. Yamada, *Biomed. Res.* **36,** 389 (1981).
3. D. J. Roof and J. Heuser, *J. Cell Biol.* **95,** 487 (1982).
4. F. D. Collins, R. M. Love, and R. A. Morton, *Biochem J.* **51,** 292 (1952).
5. D. G. McConnell, *J. Cell Biol.* **27,** 459 (1965).
6. D. S. Papermaster and W. J. Dreyer, *Biochemistry* **13,** 2438 (1974).
7. W. Godchaux and W. F. Zimmerman, *Exp. Eye Res.* **28,** 483 (1979).
8. W. Krebs and H. Kühn, *Exp. Eye Res.* **25,** 511 (1977).
9. P. P. M. Schnetkamp, A. A. Klompmakers, and F. J. M. Daemen, *Biochim. Biophys. Acta* **552,** 379 (1979).
10. R. S. Molday, D. Hicks, and L. L. Molday, *Invest. Ophthalmol. Visual Sci.* **28,** 50 (1987).
11. M. S. Biernbaum and M. D. Bownds, *J. Gen. Physiol.* **85,** 83 (1985).
12. H. E. Hamm and M. D. Bownds, *Biochemistry* **24,** 4512 (1985).
13. R. S. Molday and L. L. Molday, *J. Cell Biol.* **105,** 2589 (1987).
14. H. Kühn, *Nature (London)* **250,** 588 (1980).
15. S. Nagao, S. Yamazaki, and M. W. Bitensky, *Biochemistry* **26,** 1659 (1987).
16. S.-C. Hsu and R. S. Molday, *J. Biol. Chem.* **265,** 13308 (1990).
17. H. G. Smith, G. W. Stubbs, and B. J. Litman, *Exp. Eye Res.* **20,** 211 (1975).
18. D. Hicks and R. S. Molday, *Exp. Eye Res.* **42,** 55 (1986).
19. I. Nir and D. S. Papermaster, *Invest. Ophthalmol. Visual Sci.* **24,** 868 (1983).
20. A. Caretta, A. Cavaggioni, and T. Sorbi, *J. Physiol. (London)* **295,** 171 (1979).
21. K.-W. Koch and U. B. Kaupp, *J. Biol. Chem.* **260,** 6788 (1985).
22. K. Puckett and S. M. Goldin, *Biochemistry* **25,** 1739 (1986).

23. P. P. M. Schnetkamp, *J. Physiol.* **373,** (1986).

24. V. M. Clark and M. O. Hall, *Exp. Eye Res.* **34,** 847 (1982).

25. P. L. Witt and M. D. Bownds, *Biochemistry* **26,** 1769 (1987).

26. L. L. Molday and R. S. Molday, *Biochim. Biophys. Acta* **897,** 335 (1987).

27. D. M. Reid, U. Friedel, R. S. Molday, and N. J. Cook, *Biochemistry* **29,** 1601 (1990).

28. A. S. Polans and M. D. Burton, *Invest. Opthalmol. Visual Sci.* **29,** 1523 (1988).

29. N. J. Cook, L. L. Molday, D. Reid, U. B. Kaupp, and R. S. Molday, *J. Biol. Chem.* **264,** 6996 (1989).

30. L. L. Molday, N. J. Cook, U. B. Kaupp, and R. S. Molday, *J. Biol. Chem.* **265,** 18690 (1990).

31. S.-C. Hsu and R. S. Molday, *J. Biol. Chem.* **266,** 21745 (1991).

32. R. S. Molday and D. W. Laird, *in* "Immuno-gold Labeling in Cell Biology" (A. J. Verkleij and J. L. M. Leunissen, eds.), pp. 29. CRC Press, Boca Raton, Florida, 1989.

33. K. Boesze-Battaglia and A. D. Albert, *Exp. Eye Res.* **49,** 699 (1989).

34. K. M. P. Kamps, W. J. De Grip, and F. J. M. Daemen, *Biochim. Biophys. Acta* **687,** 296 (1982).

35. D. Matesic and P. A. Liebman, *Nature (London)* **326,** 600 (1987).

36. Y. Fukada, T. Takao, H. Ohguro, T. Yoshizawa, T. Akino, and Y. Shimonishi, *Nature (London)* **346,** 658 (1990).

37. R. K. Lai, D. Perez-Sala, F. J. Canada, and R. R. Rando, *Proc. Natl. Acad. Sci. U.S.A.* **87,** 7673 (1990).

38. O. C. Ong, I. M. Ota, S. Clarke, and B. K.-K. Fung, *Proc. Natl. Acad. Sci. U.S.A.* **86,** (1989).

39. W. Baehr, M. J. Devlin, and M. L. Applebury, *J. Biol. Chem.* **254,** 11669 (1979).

40. J. B. Hurley, *Annu. Rev. Physiol.* **49,** 793 (1987).

41. G. Wolbring and N. J. Cook, *Eur. J. Biochem.* **201,** 601 (1991).

42. H. Kühn, *Biochemistry* **17,** 4389 (1978).

43. K. Palczewski, J. H. McDowell, and P. A. Hargrave, *J. Biol. Chem.* **263,** 14067 (1988).

44. H. Kühn, *Prog. Retinal Res.* **3,** 124 (1984).

45. U. Wilden, E. Wust, I. Weyand, and H. Kühn, *FEBS Lett.* **207,** 292 (1986).

46. T. Wallimann, G. Wegmann, H. Moser, R. Huber, and H. M. Eppenberger, *Proc. Natl. Acad. Sci. U.S.A.* **83,** 3816 (1986).

47. W. Baehr, E. A. Morita, R. J. Swanson, and M. L. Applebury, *J. Biol. Chem.* **253,** 6452 (1982).

48. B. K.-K. Fung, *J. Biol. Chem.* **258,** 10495 (1983).

49. P. A. Hargrave, *Prog. Retinal Res.* **1,** 1 (1982).

50. Y. A. Ovchinnikov, *FEBS Lett.* **148,** 179 (1982).

51. Z. Yang and T. G. Wenzel, *Invest. Ophthalmol. Visual Sci.* **314** (Suppl. Abstr.), 1064 (1990).

52. R. H. Lee, B. S. Lieberman, and R. N. Lolley, *Biochemistry* **26,** 3983 (1987).

53. R. H. Lee, J. P. Whelan, R. N. Lolley, and J. F. McGinnis, *Exp. Eye Res.* **46,** 829 (1988).

54. A. M. Dizhoor, S. Ray, S. Kumar, G. Niemi, M. Spencer, D. Brolley, K. A. Walsh, P. P. Philipov, J. B. Hurley, and L. Stryer, *Science* **251,** 915 (1991).
55. H.-G. Lambrecht and K.-W. Koch, *EMBO J.* **10,** 793 (1991).
56. R. E. Kohnken, J. G. Chafouleas, D. M. Eadie, A. R. Means, and D. G. McConnell, *J. Biol. Chem.* **256,** 12517 (1981).
57. K. Palczewski, P. A. Hargrave, J. H. McDowell, and T. S. Ingebritsen, *Biochemistry* **28,** 415 (1989).
58. S. J. Berger, G. W. DeVries, J. G. Carter, D. W. Schulz, P. N. Passonneau, O. H. Lowry, and J. A. Ferendelli, *J. Biol. Chem.* **255,** 3128 (1980).
59. P. P. M. Schnetkamp and F. J. M. Daemen, *Biochim. Biophys. Acta* **672,** 307 (1981).
60. S. Futterman, A. Hendrickson, P. E. Bishop, M. H. Tollins, and E. Vacano, *J. Neurochem.* **17,** 149 (1970).
61. R. S. Molday, *Prog. Retinal Res.* **8,** 173 (1988).
62. G. Connell and R. S. Molday, *Biochemistry* **29,** 4691 (1990).
63. R. A. Bascom, S. Manara, L. Collins, R. S. Molday, V. I. Kalnins, and R. R. McInnes, *Neuron* **8,** 1171 (1992).
64. D. F. Matesic, N. J. Philip, J. M. Murray, and P. A. Liebman, *J. Cell Sci.* **103,** 157 (1992).
65. N. J. Cook and U. B. Kaupp, *J. Biol. Chem.* **263,** 11382 (1988).
66. N. J. Cook, W. Hanke, and U. B. Kaupp, *Proc. Natl. Acad. Sci. U.S.A.* **84,** 585 (1987).
67. U. B. Kaupp, T. Niidome, T. Tanabe, S. Terada, W. Bonigk, W. Stuhmer, N. J. Cook, K. Kangawa, H. Matsuo, T. Hirose, T. Miyata, and S. Numa, *Nature (London)* **342,** 762 (1989).
68. K.-W. Koch, *J. Biol. Chem.* **266,** 8634 (1991).
69. F. Hayashi and A. Yamazaki, *Proc. Natl. Acad. Sci. U.S.A.* **88,** 4746 (1991).
70. R. S. Molday, D. M. Reid, G. Connell, and L. L. Molday, *in* ''Signal Transduction in Photoreceptor Cells'' (P. A. Hargrave, K. P. Hofmann, and U. B. Kaupp, eds.) pp. 180. Springer-Verlag, Berlin, 1992.
71. D. S. Papermaster, B. G. Schneider, M. A. Zorn, and J. P. Kraehenbuhl, *J. Cell Biol.* **78,** 415 (1978).
72. R. A. Bascom, G. Connell, J. Garcia-Heras, L. Collins, D. Ledbetter, R. Molday, V. Kalnins, and R. McInnes, *Am. J. Hum. Genet. Abstr.* **47,** 392 (1990).
73. S. Ishiguro, Y. Suzuki, M. Tamai, and K. Mizuno, *J. Biol. Chem.* **266,** 15520 (1991).
74. S. J. Fliesler and R. E. Anderson, *Prog. Lipid Res.* **22,** 79 (1983).
75. K. Boesze-Battaglia and A. Albert, *Exp. Eye Res.* **49,** 699 (1989).
76. K. Boesze-Battaglia and A. Albert, *J. Biol. Chem.* **265,** 20727 (1990).

[9]   Immunological Measurement of Rhodopsin

Grazyna Adamus

Introduction

Many different types of assays have been used to detect rhodopsin in ocular tissue (1–8). All immunochemical techniques are based on the interaction of an antibody with an antigen (i.e., rhodopsin). The affinity of an antibody is an important factor in determining its usefulness. High-affinity antibodies are required in immunoassays, molecular biology, and immunocytochemistry, although low-affinity antibodies are useful for immunoaffinity purification. The development of a large number of specific antirhodopsin monoclonal antibodies (MAbs) has allowed the determination of rhodopsin using immunochemical techniques. Application of monospecific, high-activity antipeptide serum is also beneficial. However, the reactivity of antipeptide serum, in many cases, depends on selection of the appropriate peptide. Although most peptides will elicit an antibody response [that is measured in an enzyme-linked immunosorbent assay (ELISA)], the antipeptide antibody may not react with the native protein. Other sera raised against rhodopsin contain many different types of antibodies that are specific for many different epitopes, and the use of the mixed population of antibodies may create a variety of different problems in immunochemical techniques. Table I summarizes the usefulness of monoclonal antibodies versus serum in immunological measurement of rhodopsin.

Assay Methods for Rhodopsin

Specificity of the method is one of the primary considerations, especially when measuring rhodopsin in tissue extracts or homogenates. There are several methods that are used for rhodopsin determination. Competition ELISA and immunostaining of blotted rhodopsin onto membrane are the most popular.

Sample Preparation

A wide variety of rhodopsin-containing samples can be used in the assay: rod outer segments, disk membranes, purified rhodopsin, retina extracts, or

TABLE I   Application of Polyclonal versus Monoclonal
Antibodies in Immunochemical Methods

Method	Serum (polyclonal antibody)	Monoclonal antibody	Mixture of monoclonal antibodies
Immunoblotting	Good	Very good[a]	Excellent
ELISA			
Labeled antibody	Poor	Excellent	NA[b]
Labeled antigen	Very good	Very good	NA
Cell/tissue immunostaining	Good	Very good[a]	Excellent
Gene expression	Very good	Poor	Excellent
Immunoaffinity purification	Poor	Excellent	NA

[a] Depends on antibody specificity.
[b] NA, Not applicable.

pineal extracts. To obtain a membrane fraction enriched in rhodopsin, retinal (or pineal) tissue is homogenized in 10 mM phosphate buffer, pH 7.4, containing 0.9% NaCl (phosphate-buffered saline, PBS) and 0.25 M sucrose at 4°C. The suspension is centrifuged for 30 min at 20,000 g and 4°C. The pellet, which contains rhodopsin, is washed with the same buffer followed by centrifugation. The pellet is resuspended in PBS containing 2% octyl glucoside and incubated for 30 min at room temperature. Supernatant containing rhodopsin is obtained by subsequent centrifugation under the same conditions. The pellet is washed once more with the same buffer, and the two supernatants are pooled for rhodopsin determination.

Rhodopsin can also be prepared by direct solubilization of retinal proteins in mild detergent (2% octyl glucoside) assisted by probe sonication (3 times, 20 sec each). The supernatant containing rhodopsin is collected by centrifugation (30 min, 20,000 g, 4°C) and used in ELISA or Western blotting. This method is recommended when only small amounts of tissue are available.

Coating of Microtiter Plates with Rhodopsin

Ninety-six-well polyvinyl chloride microtiter plates (Falcon, No. 3912, Becton Dickinson, Oxnard, CA) are coated with 1 μg purified rhodopsin [obtained by concanavalin A affinity chromatography (9)] in 100 μl of 0.1 M Tris-HCl, pH 9. The plates are incubated overnight at room temperature and next washed 2 times with the same buffer. It is recommended to prepare a large number of plates for the assay in order to increase the reproducibility of the test. After washing, plates are air-dried, covered with Parafilm, and can be stored in an airtight container or Zip-Loc bags for several weeks.

Enzyme-Linked Immunosorbent Assay

Prior to ELISA, plates are incubated with 200 μl of 1% (w/v) bovine serum albumin (BSA) in 10 mM phosphate buffer, pH 7.2, containing 0.9% NaCl (PBS) in order to block free binding sites. One hundred microliters of serial 2-fold dilutions of antibody (culture supernatant, ascites fluid, serum, or purified antibody) is added to the well. Following 1 hr of incubation, the microplate is washed 5 times with deionized water and rabbit anti-mouse immunoglobulin G (IgG, heavy and light chain; Zymed, No. 61-6500) is added. After 1 hr of incubation, wells are washed again, and 100 μl of protein-A–peroxidase conjugate (Zymed, No. 10-1023) is added to each well. The color reaction is developed by adding 200 μl of peroxidase substrate: o-phenylenediamine (8 mg/10 ml) and hydrogen peroxide (8 μl/10 ml) in 0.1 M citrate–phosphate buffer, pH 5.0. The enzymatic reaction is terminated after 15 min of incubation by adding 25 μl of 2 M H$_2$SO$_4$ and then measured at 490 nm using an ELISA reader. A typical titration curve is shown in Fig. 1.

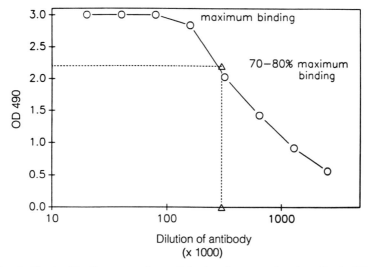

FIG. 1   Antibody titration curve for antirhodopsin monoclonal antibody K16-155C (in ascites fluid) by ELISA. Microtiter wells were coated with 1 μg rhodopsin and incubated with 2-fold serial dilutions of MAb. Color development of the peroxidase reaction at 490 nm is plotted versus antibody dilution. The antibody dilution that gives 70–80% of the maximum binding of rhodopsin is selected for the competition assay.

Competition Assay Using Anti-bovine Rhodopsin Monoclonal Antibodies

Antibody is titered in the ELISA using rhodopsin-coated plates in order to select the minimum dilution of antibody which gives between 70 and 80% of the maximum binding of antigen (see Fig. 1). That amount of antibody is preincubated for 1 hr with a solution containing various amounts of rhodopsin (standard curve), or protein extract containing rhodopsin, in a total volume of 200 μl. The competitor concentration is in the range from 1 mg/ml to 100 pg/ml, obtained by 10-fold dilutions in PBS containing 0.1% octyl glucoside. Then the antigen–antibody mixture is divided in two portions, 100 μl each, transferred to rhodopsin-coated wells, and the standard test is performed.

Two controls are prepared for each experiment: a positive control (C_{Ab}), which contains no competitor, and a negative control (C_N), which contains no antibody. All samples are tested in duplicate. The percentage of specific binding is calculated from the following formula:

$$\% \text{ bound} = \frac{\text{mean OD}_{490} \text{ rhodopsin samples} - \text{mean OD}_{490} \text{ C}_N}{\text{mean OD}_{490} \text{ C}_{Ab} - \text{mean OD}_{490} \text{ C}_N} \times 100\%$$

The percentage of binding is plotted against the amount of rhodopsin required to cause a given competition. The linearity of the assay is determined (Fig. 2). Then the test is repeated. This time, the antibody is preincubated for 1 hr with 2-fold serial dilutions of rhodopsin (for standard curve), or protein extract containing rhodopsin, in a total value of 200 μl. The rhodopsin concentration is chosen over the range of the linear part of the previous competition curve (Fig. 2). The amount of rhodopsin present in the sample tested is calculated from the rhodopsin standard curve.

This protocol provides an assay with a sensitivity of 10 ng rhodopsin per sample, depending on the affinity of the antibody used. This is lower than the reported detection limit of a spectrophotometric assay. The rhodopsin concentration should be adjusted to keep optical density readings in the linear range of the assay. Because the assay conditions may vary from laboratory to laboratory, it is advisable to titer an antibody using the same batch of rhodopsin-coated plates that will be used for routine assay.

Interpretation of the results obtained from the competition assay requires caution, especially for negative results. Most monoclonal antibodies and antisera available have been prepared against bovine rhodopsin. Detection of rhodopsin in extracts prepared from different species requires a knowledge of the cross-reactivity of various anti-bovine rhodopsin antibodies with different rhodopsins. For this purpose, Table II summarizes cross-reactivities

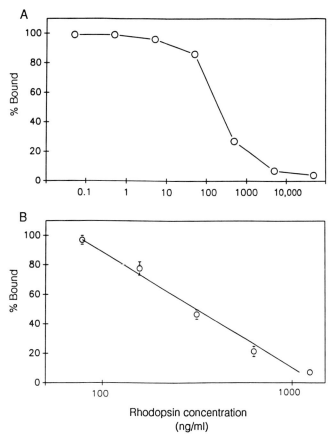

FIG. 2   Competition ELISA using antirhodopsin MAb K16-155C and purified rhodopsin-coated microtiter plates. The percentage of antigen bound is plotted against
the competitor (rhodopsin) concentration on a log scale. (A) The standard curve is
constructed by preincubation of a series of 10-fold dilutions of rhodopsin (100 pg/
ml to 10 μg/ml) with the same final dilution of antibody that gave 70–80% of maximum
binding in the titration assay. (B) Standard curve for rhodopsin determination. The
concentration of rhodopsin in the linear part of the previous competition curve is
chosen. Then, 2-fold dilutions of rhodopsin are preincubated with the same dilution
of MAb. Bars represent the standard deviation of four independent experiments.

of selected, frequently used monoclonal antibodies (6, 10). Although bovine
rhodopsin is used as a standard in most assays, use of rhodopsin from the
same species is recommended. When purified rhodopsin from the desired
animal is not available, bovine rhodopsin may be used as long as it is
cross-reactive.

TABLE II   Cross-Reactivity of Anti-bovine Rhodopsin
Monoclonal Antibodies with Rhodopsin from
Different Species

Source of rhodopsin	Monoclonal antibody				
	R2-12N[a]	B6-30N[a]	K16-155C[a]	G26C[a]	1D4[b]
Bovine	+	+	+	+	+
Human	+	+	+	+	+
Monkey	+	+	+	+	ND[c]
Rabbit	+	−/+	+	+	+
Pig	+	+	+	+	+
Sheep	+	+	+	+	+
Mouse	+	+	+	+	+
Rat	+	+	+	+	+
Guinea pig	+	−	+	+	ND
Dog	+	+	ND	+	+
Cat	ND	ND	ND	ND	+
Alligator	+	−	+	−	ND
Frog	+	+	+	−	+
Fish	+	+/−	+	+	+/−
Snake	+	+	+	+	ND
Chicken	−	−	+	+	ND

[a] MAbs R2-12N and B6-30N are specific for the amino terminus (6), and MAbs K16-155C and G26C are specific for the carboxyl terminus (6; G. Adamus, 1992, unpublished data).
[b] MAb 1D4 is specific for the carboxyl terminus (1, 10; R. Molday, 1992, personal communication).
[c] ND, Not determined.

Immunostaining of Blotted Rhodopsin

Western blotting and dot blotting are convenient methods for immunodetection of rhodopsin immobilized on a solid support. In Western blotting (11), rhodopsin samples are subjected to gel electrophoresis, then electrophoretically transferred onto a membrane. In dot blotting (12), the rhodopsin sample is applied directly to the membrane. Polyvinylidene fluoride (PVDF) membrane is recommended for Western blotting, although nitrocellulose can be employed when the hydrophobic properties of PVDF interfere with direct loading in dot blotting. Rhodopsin subjected to dot blotting retains a conformation close to native, whereas by Western blotting rhodopsin will be mostly denatured. Depending on the procedure used, antibodies with particular characteristics may be required; for example, for Western blotting, antibody that recognizes denatured rhodopsin is needed. Regardless of the blotting method employed, the subsequent immunodetection procedure is identical.

PVDF membrane containing blotted rhodopsin is immersed for 10 sec in 100% methanol and washed with water for 5 min. The membrane is then transferred to the blocking solution (5% normal goat serum, 1% BSA, 0.01% Tween 20 in PBS) to prevent nonspecific binding. A nitrocellulose membrane is placed directly in the blotting solution. After 1 hr of incubation at room temperature, diluted primary antibody is added. For preliminary optimization, the antirhodopsin antibody dilution is chosen using the following general rule: for hybridoma culture supernatant, undiluted to 1:100; for ascites fluid, 1:1000 to 1:100,000; for serum, 1:500 to 1:10,000; and for purified antibody, 0.1 to 2 μg/ml. Higher or lower dilutions may be required with some antibodies. The following procedure is given for detection of rhodopsin using mouse monoclonal antibody.

The membrane is incubated with monoclonal antibody diluted with 1% BSA in PBS for 1 hr at room temperature with agitation. Then the membrane is washed with 0.01% Tween in PBS to remove unbound primary antibody 4 times for 10 min followed by 1 hr of incubation with biotinylated rabbit anti-mouse IgG (secondary antibody; Zymed, No. 61-6540) diluted 1:5000 with PBS containing 1% BSA and 0.01% Tween 20. The membrane is washed again as previously and treated with 1:2000 diluted alkaline phosphatase conjugated with streptavidin (Zymed, No. 42-4322) for 1 hr. After extensive washing, the phosphatase substrate is added: BCIP (5-bromo-4-chloro-3-indolyl phosphate) and NBT (nitro blue tetrazolium) to enhance the signal (Zymed, No. 00-2209).

A positive control contains a sample of bovine rhodopsin. For a negative control primary antibody is omitted or a nonspecific antibody can be substituted. This procedure gives a sensitivity of detection of 10–50 ng rhodopsin, depending on affinity of the antibody used. Other secondary reagents can be used such as peroxidase–Ig, peroxidase–protein A, protein A–gold, phosphatase–Ig, avidin–Ig. However, sensitivity of the method will vary.

Detection of Phosphorylated Forms of Rhodopsin

Fractions containing phosphorylated species of rhodopsin separated by chromatofocusing (13) are subjected to isoelectric focusing in the dark on a 1-mm-thick polyacrylamide gel slab using a pH gradient of 3–7 (Pharmalyte from Pharmacia, Piscataway, NJ). Samples containing 10 μg protein are loaded onto the gel containing 10 mM dodecyl β-maltoside (or 1% octyl glucoside). Isoelectric focusing is performed using a flat-bed Pharmacia apparatus at constant power (25 W for 2 hr at 10°C). After focusing, the pH gradient of the gel is measured by a flat electrode (Bio-Rad, Richmond, CA), and the gel is fixed in 5% sulfosalicylic acid and 10% trichloroacetic acid

pH

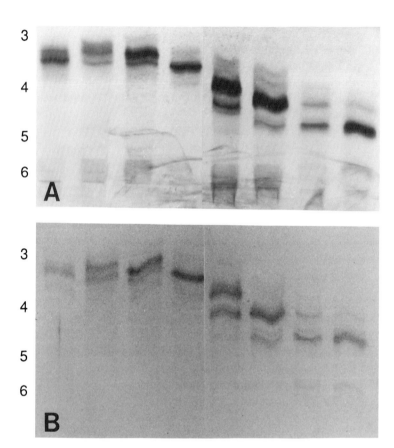

FIG. 3   Effect of monoclonal antibodies with different specificities on immunodetection of rhodopsin and phosphorhodopsin, as demonstrated by analysis of fractions obtained during phosphorhodopsin chromatofocusing and isoelectric focusing. (A) Visualization of proteins in the gel by Coommasie Brilliant Blue staining. (B) Immunostaining of blotted proteins with MAb A5-3N specific for the amino terminus reveals all phosphorylated forms present. (C) Immunostaining of phosphorhodopsin in a similar experiment with MAb A11-82P specific for highly phosphorylated rhodopsin reveals only highly phosphorylated forms.

(1 hr), followed by 10% acetic acid and 30% methanol (30 min), and stained for proteins with 0.25% Coomassie Brilliant Blue.

For immunostaining, unfixed, unstained proteins are blotted to nitrocellulose for 30 min. The membrane is washed 3 times with 0.01% Tween 20 in

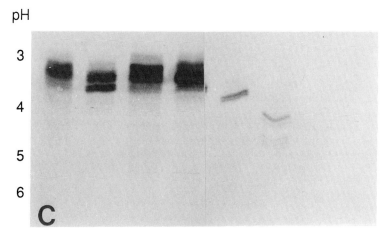

Fig. 3 *(continued)*

PBS, followed by blocking with 1% BSA in PBS (1 hr). Then antiphosphorho-
dopsin monoclonal antibody A11-82P (1:100 diluted culture supernatant) is
added for 1 hr of incubation. The membrane is washed again 4 times with
0.01% Tween 20 in PBS and incubated with phosphatase-conjugated mouse
IgG for 1 hr. The phosphatase substrate is added to develop the color reaction
(Zymed, No. 00-0229). There is only one antibody available that specifically
recognizes phosphorhodopsin. Monoclonal antibody A11-82P (7) binds only
to highly phosphorylated rhodopsin and can be used in Western blotting
as well as in competition ELISA. To detect all phosphorylated species of
rhodopsin, antibody specific for the amino terminus is recommended (Fig. 3).

The immunochemical assays provide an adequately high sensitivity for
most purposes. We have found ELISA and immunostaining of transferred
proteins to be specific and convenient methods for measuring rhodopsin in
a wide variety of samples.

References

1. R. S. Molday, *Prog. Retinal Res.* **8,** 173 (1989).
2. W. J. De Grip, *Prog. Retinal Res.* **4,** 137 (1985).
3. J. J. Schalken and W. J. De Grip, *Exp. Eye Res.* **43,** 431 (1986).
4. J. J. Plantner, H. L. Barbour, and E. L. Kean, *Curr. Eye Res.* **7,** 1125 (1988).
5. R. J. Peterson, P. A. Hargrave, J. H. McDowell, and R. W. Jackson, *Vision Res.* **23,** 267 (1983).
6. G. Adamus, Z. S. Zam, A. Arendt, K. Palczewski, J. H. McDowell, and P. A. Hargrave, *Vision Res.* **31,** 17 (1991).
7. G. Adamus, Z. S. Zam, J. H. McDowell, G. P. Shaw, and P. A. Hargrave, *Hybridoma* **7,** 237 (1988).

8. D. S. Papermaster, *in* "Methods in Enzymology" (L. Packer, ed.), Vol. 81, p. 240. Academic Press, New York, 1982.

9. B. J. Litman, *in* "Methods in Enzymology" (L. Packer, ed.), Vol. 81, p. 150. Academic Press, New York, 1982.

10. D. MacKenzie, A. Arendt, P. Hargrave, J. H. McDowell, and R. S. Molday, *Biochemistry* **23,** 6544 (1984).

11. H. Towbin, T. Staehelin, and J. Gordon, *Proc. Natl. Acad. Sci. U.S.A.* **76,** 4350 (1979).

12. R. Hawkes, *in* "Methods in Enzymology" (J. J. Langone and H. V. Vunakis, eds.), Vol. 121, p. 484. Academic Press, Orlando, Florida, 1986.

13. V. Y. Arshavsky, M. P. Antoch, and P. P. Philippov, *Bioorgan. Membr.* **3,** 1197 (1986).

[10] Preparation and Characterization of Chicken Rod and Cone Pigments

Tôru Yoshizawa and Yoshitaka Fukada

Introduction

Many vertebrates have several types of cones, each of which has a visual pigment with a distinctive absorption maximum. Humans have three types of cone cells, namely, red-, green- and blue-sensitive cones that contain the visual pigments human red, green, and blue, respectively. The integration of the photoresponses from each cone finally generates the sensation of color in the visual cortex. The photoresponse from cones is wider in dynamic range and faster in generation than that of rods. It is of interest to determine how the same light stimulus elicits different responses among the cells. The first step to this study is to isolate physiologically active cone visual pigments, the chemical stability of which is remarkably lower than that of the rod pigment rhodopsin.

One of the best materials to study the cone cell machinery is chicken retina, which shows a relatively high ratio of cone to rod cells in comparison to other animals. Unlike the human retina, the chicken retina contains four kinds of cone pigments, chicken red, green, blue, and violet, in addition to rhodopsin. Since the pioneering work on chicken red by Wald (1), who termed the pigment iodopsin,* only digitonin has been used as a detergent to solubilize cone pigments, because the use of other detergents causes denaturation of the cone pigments. Although digitonin is generally a good detergent for solubilizing visual pigments in stable form, it is difficult to remove digitonin from the extract by dialysis or other means. In addition, digitonin forms a large micelle, which may hinder protein–protein interactions essential for signal transduction. Thus, we focused our study on extracting cone pigments using a detergent other than digitonin (2).

3-[(3-Cholamidopropyl)dimethylammonio]-1-propanesulfonate (CHAPS) has a higher critical micellar concentration (CMC) value (0.49%) and a lower micelle molecular weight (6150, Ref. 3) than digitonin (0.09%, Ref. 4, and

---

* The term "iodopsin" is a specific name for the chicken red-sensitive cone pigment (11). Because there are no specific terms for other cone pigments, it would be better to use a name derived from both the animal species and the color characterizing the spectral sensitivity of the pigment. In this chapter, we designate the chicken red-sensitive cone pigment chicken red instead of iodopsin.

Methods in Neurosciences, Volume 15

70,000, Ref. 3), and it is easily removed by dialysis. Here we describe a novel method (2) to extract rod and cone visual pigments in stable form from chicken retina using CHAPS in the presence of phosphatidylcholine (PC). The absorption maxima of the pigments purified by subsequent column chromatography (Fig. 1) in the CHAPS–PC system were in good agreement with those determined microspectrophotometrically compared to those reported in digitonin, suggesting that the conformations of pigments in the CHAPS–PC system may be closer to the native conformations than those in digitonin. It should be emphasized that isolated chicken red, on absorption of light, can activate the rod G protein transducin (5) and can be phosphorylated by rhodopsin kinase (6). Because these two reactions are thought to be key events in the on- and off-processes, respectively, of light signal transduction in photoreceptor cells, the CHAPS–PC system provides not only photochem-

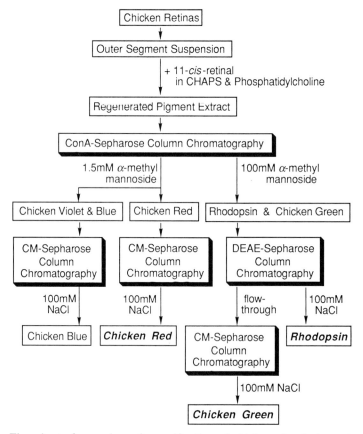

FIG. 1   Flowchart of procedures for purification of chicken visual pigments. Highly purified visual pigments are shown in bold italic type.

ically but also biochemically active cone visual pigments, which will permit us to elucidate the molecular mechanism that elicits the physiological difference between rods and cones (7).

Overview of Procedures

Detergents and Lipids

Because chicken red is the predominant cone pigment in chicken retina, stabilities of chicken red and its apoprotein, R-photopsin,* were examined in detail to determine the best conditions for its extraction and purification. Afterward, it was confirmed that these conditions also stabilized other cone pigments.

In addition to digitonin, many detergents have been tested [cetyltrimethylammonium bromide, Emulphogene BC-720, Triton X-100, cholate, deoxycholate, Ammonyx-LO (Refs. 8, 9), octyl glucoside, and CHAPS (Ref. 2)], among which only CHAPS gave satisfactory results. At higher concentrations of CHAPS (above 1% w/v), however, no chicken red was regenerated when 11-*cis*-retinal was added to extracts of bleached chicken outer segment membranes containing R-photopsin. In extracts with 0.75% CHAPS, a part of the R-photopsin regenerated to form chicken red, but it gradually decomposed in the dark. Moreover, the regenerated chicken red was completely denatured over the course of concanavalin A (ConA)–Sepharose column chromatography, probably owing to removal of endogenous lipids. This observation led us to include PC (1.0 mg/ml) in the buffer for extraction (0.75% CHAPS in buffer P; see below), resulting in significant stabilization of chicken red and other pigments after extraction. Addition of PC at a concentration higher than 1.0 mg/ml to the extraction buffer (0.75% CHAPS in buffer P) prevented effective solubilization of visual pigments. The efficiency of solubilization was also decreased by lowering the CHAPS concentration below 0.75% in the extraction buffer.

Concentration of Detergent during Purification Procedures

To find the optimal concentration of CHAPS during the long purification procedures, the effect of the CHAPS concentration on the stability of R-

---

* The opsin moiety of chicken red, which is responsible for photopic vision, is called photopsin. We use "photopsin" prefixed by the initial letter of the color characterizing the spectral sensitivity of a cone pigment for expression of the opsin moiety. For example, R-photopsin means the opsin moiety of the red-sensitive cone pigment.

photopsin after extraction was studied. The ability of R-photopsin to bind 11-*cis*-retinal (regenerability) gradually decreased after extraction with a mixture of 0.75% CHAPS and 1.0 mg/ml PC. For instance, more than 80% of the regenerability was lost by incubating the extract for 12 hr at 20°C. However, the loss of regenerability was reduced (to ~50% during the same incubation) by diluting the extract with buffer P to lower the CHAPS concentration below 0.6% (0.5–0.6%). As this range of CHAPS concentration is close to the CMC value (0.49%, Ref. 3), the higher concentration of CHAPS (0.6%) was employed to prevent aggregation of pigments. Thus, all the buffers used for further purification procedures contain 0.6% CHAPS and 0.8 mg/ml PC (CHAPS–PC buffer). Partial denaturation of the protein in this buffer was further minimized as described below.

Light Condition

The thermal stabilities of chicken red, rhodopsin, and their opsin moieties were compared. It was clearly shown that chicken red is more stable than R-photopsin at 4°C; that is, only a small amount (less than 10%) of chicken red was thermally bleached during incubation for 300 hr at 4°C, whereas more than 90% of R-photopsin lost its regenerability within 108 hr at 4°C. Similar results were obtained for rhodopsin. It is evident that the pigments are far more stable than their opsin moieties, so purification procedures should be performed under the safe lights after the pigments are regenerated by the addition of 11-*cis*-retinal.

Stabilization by Glycerol

As shown in Fig. 2, the addition of 20% (w/v) of glycerol to the CHAPS–PC buffer effectively stabilized both rod and cone pigments. In Fig. 2B, only a small effect of glycerol on a mixture of rhodopsin and chicken green was observed. This result does not indicate that chicken green is more stable than the other cone pigments, because this fraction contains rhodopsin predominantly. A little degradation without glycerol (Fig. 2B, triangles) may reflect the denaturation of chicken green. In fact, the stabilities of the other three kinds of cone pigments were noticeably improved by addition of 20% (w/v) glycerol (Fig. 2A,C,D). However, it should be emphasized that deletion of glycerol in the elution buffer for the ConA column chromatography resulted in better separation of each visual pigment. Thus, glycerol should be added to the sample after the ConA column chromatography step.

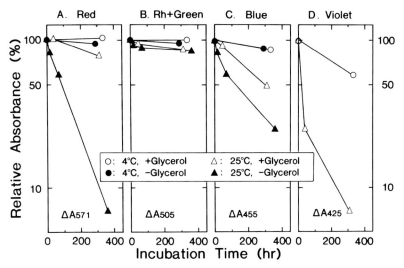

FIG. 2   Effect of glycerol on the thermal stability of chicken visual pigments. A mixture of chicken visual pigments (in buffer A-140) was divided into two portions, one of which was mixed with an equal volume of buffer A-140 containing 40% (w/v) glycerol to give a final concentration of glycerol of 20% (w/v). Another portion was mixed with an equal volume of buffer A-140 without glycerol. They were further divided into two portions, respectively. The four portions were then incubated at either 25 or 4°C. At the appropriate time, an aliquot (0.4 ml) was transferred from each portion to an optical cell to measure the absorbance of each pigment remaining in the sample by the partial bleaching method. The relative absorbance near the maximum (A, 571 nm for chicken red; B, 505 nm for a mixture of chicken rhodopsin and green; C, 455 nm for chicken blue; D, 425 nm for chicken violet) is plotted versus the incubation time. [Reprinted with permission from T. Okano, Y. Fukada, I. D. Artamonov, and T. Yoshizawa, *Biochemistry* **28,** 8848 (1989). Copyright 1989 American Chemical Society.]

Experimental Procedures

Spectrophotometric Measurements

Samples

All the cone pigments except for chicken green are stable in the presence of 10 mM hydroxylamine (hydroxylamine hydrochloride is adjusted to pH 6.6 with NaOH) at 4°C. Only chicken green is bleached, very slowly. The amount of bleached chicken green is less than 6% during the spectrophotometric measurement (3–4 hr). Therefore, all the spectrophotometric measurements can be performed in the presence of 10 mM hydroxylamine at 4°C.

Equipment

The sample in an optical cell (volume, 0.4 ml; width, 2 mm; light path, 1 cm) is kept at a constant temperature (usually 4°C). Moisture on the cell surface is removed by a stream of nitrogen gas. The sample is irradiated in the sample compartment of the spectrophotometer with a 1-kW tungsten–halogen lamp (Rikagaku Seiki Co. Ltd., Tokyo, Japan). A glass optical cell filled with distilled water (light path, 5 cm) is placed between the light source and a filter (see below) to remove heat from the irradiation light.

Partial Bleaching

When a sample contains several kinds of visual pigments, the amount of each pigment can be estimated by a partial bleaching method. A sample is first irradiated with long-wavelength light by which only the visual pigment with the longest absorption maximum could be bleached. After completion of bleaching of this pigment, the wavelength of irradiating light is shifted to shorter wavelengths. The sample is then reirradiated, until the second pigment is completely bleached. Such bleaching is repeated successively until all the pigments in the sample are bleached (see Figs. 4 and 6). In each irradiation, we use the following combinations of cutoff filter (Toshiba Co. Ltd, Tokyo, Japan) and irradiation time: VR68 (>660 nm, deep red light) for 40 min for bleaching of chicken red; VR61 (>590 nm, red light) for 20 min for both chicken green and rhodopsin; VO54 (>520 nm, orange light) for 10 min for chicken blue; and VY50 (>480 nm, yellow light) for 5 min for chicken violet. After bleaching of chicken red by irradiation with the deep red light for 40 min, another irradiation (>660 nm, 40 min) is repeated to confirm the absence of chicken red in the sample. Such irradiation for confirmation is carried out for each pigment.

Hydroxylamine Bleaching

Because chicken green and rhodopsin show spectral curves similar to one another, the amount of each pigment cannot be estimated by the partial bleaching method described above. For instance, a fraction eluted from the ConA–Sepharose column with 100 mM α-methyl-D-mannoside is a mixture of the two pigments (see below). In such a case, the sample is mixed with hydroxylamine at a final concentration of 10 mM, and then the sample is kept in the dark at 23°C. Because chicken rhodopsin is stable in the presence of hydroxylamine, only chicken green is progressively bleached by the incubation. After chicken green is bleached completely, the amount of rhodopsin (or other pigments) can be estimated by the partial bleaching method. The absorption maximum of the difference spectrum between chicken green and its retinal oxime is located at 508 nm, whereas that between rhodopsin and its retinal oxime is at 503 nm (see Figs. 6 and 7).

Buffers

The pH of all buffers is adjusted to 6.6 at 4°C with 5 N NaOH. Buffers should be used within a few days.

> Buffer P (for preparation): 50 mM N-2-hydroxyethylpiperazine-N'-2-ethanesulfonic acid (HEPES), 140 mM NaCl, 1 mM dithiothreitol (DTT), 0.1 mM phenylmethylsulfonyl fluoride (PMSF), 50 kallikrein inhibitor units/ml aprotinin, and 4 μg/ml leupeptin
>
> Buffer E (for extraction): 50 mM HEPES, 0.75% CHAPS, 1.0 mg/ml L-α-phosphatidylcholine (PC) from fresh egg yolk (type XI-E from Sigma, St. Louis, MO; dissolved in chloroform), 140 mM NaCl, 1 mM MnCl$_2$, 1 mM CaCl$_2$, 1 mM DTT, 0.1 mM PMSF, 50 kallikrein inhibitor units/ml aprotinin, and 4 μg/ml leupeptin

To prepare buffer E, remove chloroform from the commercial PC solution with a gentle stream of nitrogen gas at the bottom of a flask. To 1 g of PC in the flask, add 200 ml of water and 7.5 g CHAPS, and dissolve the PC completely by stirring under reduced pressure. Bring the solution to a total volume of 1 liter in water and filter it through a 0.45-μm nitrocellulose membrane by the use of a vacuum filtration unit. After cooling to 4°C, add the other reagents and adjust the pH to 6.6 with 5 N NaOH. The following buffers can be prepared similarly.

> Buffer A-140 (for affinity column): 50 mM HEPES, 0.6% CHAPS, 0.8 mg/ml PC, 140 mM NaCl, 1 mM MnCl$_2$, 1 mM CaCl$_2$, 1 mM DTT, 0.1 mM PMSF, 50 kallikrein inhibitor units/ml aprotinin, and 4 μg/ml leupeptin
>
> Buffer A-10 (for affinity column): The composition is the same as Buffer A-140 except the NaCl concentration is 10 instead of 140 mM
>
> Buffer D-20 (for DEAE- and CM-Sepharose columns): 50 mM HEPES, 0.6% CHAPS, 0.8 mg/ml PC, 20% (w/v) glycerol, 1 mM DTT, 0.1 mM PMSF, 50 kallikrein inhibitor units/ml aprotinin, and 4 μg/ml leupeptin

Isolation of Chicken Retinas

The following procedures are performed at 4°C under red light (>640 nm), which partially bleaches chicken red. After regeneration of chicken red by the addition of 11-*cis*-retinal (see below), manipulations should be carried out under dim red light (>680 nm) to prevent photobleaching of all pigments.

Chicken heads are brought to the laboratory in a light-tight ice box within a few hours after death. Eyelids and connecting tissue are carefully cut off from an eyeball with scissors, and the isolated eyeball is dissected equatorially. After cutting off the pecten, the eyecup is kept in buffer P until the retina detaches spontaneously. The retinas are collected in a tube, pelleted by centrifugation at 16,000 g for 10 min, and stored at $-80°C$ until use.

Isolation of Outer Segments

Frozen retinas in centrifugation tubes are thawed and vigorously shaken for 1 min in buffer P containing 40% (w/v) sucrose (~0.5 ml per retina) in order to detach rod and cone outer segments from retinas. After centrifugation at 20,000 g for 30 min, the supernatant with some floating material is saved. The pellet is mixed with the sucrose solution, followed by centrifugation, and the supernatant is saved. This step is repeated once more. All supernatants thus collected are mixed and then diluted with an equal volume of buffer P, followed by centrifugation at 20,000 g for 40 min to pellet the outer segments. The outer segments are homogenized in buffer P (0.3–0.5 ml per retina) with a Teflon homogenizer (10 strokes). The homogenate is centrifuged (20,000 g, 40 min), and the supernatant is discarded. To remove oil droplets as much as possible, this washing is repeated (at least 5 times) until the supernatant becomes colorless.

Extraction of Outer Segment Proteins

Subsequent operations should be carried out under dim red light (>680 nm) to prevent photobleaching of chicken red. To the outer segment pellet is added buffer E (0.25–0.30 ml per retina) supplemented with a small molar excess of 11-*cis*-retinal (0.03 $\Delta OD \cdot ml^*$ per retina) over the amount of R-photopsin in the pellet, and the sample is homogenized with a Teflon homogenizer (30 strokes) for extraction of the visual pigments. The homogenate is kept in the dark for 30 min to regenerate chicken red, then centrifuged (110,000 g, 40 min). The resultant supernatant is saved (the first extract), and the pellet is again subjected to the same extraction procedure (without

---

* As a measure of the amount of a visual pigment, we use the unit $\Delta OD \cdot ml$, which is the maximal optical density (ΔOD) of the difference spectrum between the pigment and its photoproduct or thermally denatured product (retinal oxime plus opsin) multiplied by the volume (ml). In the case of retinal, ΔOD is the maximal optical density of the absolute absorption spectrum.

addition of 11-*cis*-retinal) to obtain the second extract, which was mixed with the first one. More than 90% of visual pigments will be recovered in the mixture. Then buffer P (1 volume) supplemented with 5 mM of $MnCl_2$ and $CaCl_2$ is added to the supernatant (4 volumes) to decrease the concentration of CHAPS to 0.6%. The diluted preparation is termed the CHAPS–PC extract. Usually 0.03–0.04 ΔOD·ml of rhodopsin, 0.02–0.03 ΔOD·ml of chicken red, and less than 0.01 ΔOD·ml of the other cone pigments are extracted from one retina.

ConA–Sepharose Affinity Column Chromatography

The bed volume of the ConA–Sepharose column (0.25–1.0 ml per 10 retinas) depends on the amount of starting material (usually 500–2000 retinas); approximately 0.7–2.0 ΔOD·ml of visual pigment can be adsorbed to 1 ml of ConA–Sepharose. A ConA–Sepharose column (16 mm in diameter) washed in advance with 10 bed volumes of 1 M NaCl is equilibrated with 5 bed volumes of buffer A-140 at a flow rate of 14 ml/hr. The CHAPS–PC extract is loaded on the column and washed with 6 bed volumes of buffer A-140 and 2 bed volumes of buffer A-10 to remove unbound material including oil droplet components. The bound proteins are then eluted with 1.5, 5, and 100 mM α-methyl-D-mannoside (α-methyl mannoside) in buffer A-10 (e.g., 130 ml, 90 ml, and 70 ml, respectively in Fig. 3). Throughout the procedures (sample loading, washing, and elution), the flow rate is fixed at 8 ml/hr. After washing the column, the absorbance of the eluate is continuously recorded at 280 nm by using a UV-monitoring flow cell. An elution profile of the visual pigments is shown in Fig. 3. Glycerol is added at a final concentration of 20% (w/v) to each fraction (20–25 ml) recovered from the column.

Comments

Do not monitor the flow-through fraction during sample loading. Otherwise, some hydrophobic material having UV absorbance (probably oil droplet components) in the flow-through fraction strongly adheres to the inner surface of the UV-monitoring cell, and will consequently damage it.

Buffer A-140 (containing 140 mM NaCl) supplemented with α-methyl mannoside had been used as an elution buffer in our previous experiment (see Ref. 2). In our current method, however, the concentration of NaCl in the elution buffer is lowered to 10 mM (i.e., buffer A-10). Consequently, the fractions recovered from the ConA–Sepharose column can be subjected directly to the next purification step, DEAE- and CM-Sepharose column chromatography. This modification does not significantly affect the elution profile of visual pigments from the ConA–Sepharose column.

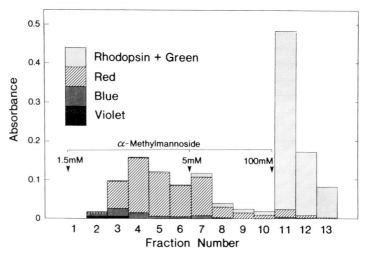

FIG. 3   Elution profile of chicken visual pigments from the ConA–Sepharose column. The CHAPS–PC extract from 546 retinas was subjected to ConA–Sepharose column chromatography. Visual pigments adsorbed to the column (16 × 270 mm) were eluted by increasing the concentration (as shown by arrowheads) of α-methyl mannoside in the elution buffer (buffer A-140). Partial bleaching of each fraction (22 ml) was used to estimate the amount of each visual pigment. The amount of each pigment except for chicken violet was expressed as absorbance at the maximum of the difference absorption spectrum (505 nm for a sum of rhodopsin and chicken green, 571 nm for chicken red, and 455 nm for chicken blue). The amount of chicken violet was calculated from the difference absorbance at 425 nm multiplied by 1.19 for correction of the absorbance. [Reprinted with permission from T. Okano, Y. Fukada, I. D. Artamonov, and T. Yoshizawa, *Biochemistry* **28,** 8848 (1989). Copyright 1989 American Chemical Society.]

Chicken Violet and Blue

Fraction 1 (Fig. 3) has a large amount of UV-absorbing materials without visual pigments. Chicken violet and blue are contained in fraction 2, in which the relative content of chicken violet (38%) is the highest among all fractions. The difference absorption maximum of chicken violet is estimated to be 425 nm by means of partial bleaching of this fraction (Fig. 4A). Fraction 3 displays a peak in the elution of chicken blue, whose difference absorption maximum is determined to be 455 nm by partial bleaching (Fig. 4B).

Chicken Red

The relative content of chicken red significantly increases in fractions 4–6 (Fig. 3), indicating that chicken red binds to the column with higher affinity than chicken violet and blue. Chicken red with the highest purity is recovered in the later fractions. For instance, fraction 5 is composed of more than 92% of chicken red, 2% of a mixture of rhodopsin and chicken green, and 6% of chicken blue (Fig. 4C). The content of chicken red in the corresponding fractions in several experiments ranged from 90 to 96%. The total recovery of chicken red from the ConA column was 86%. A gel electrophoretic analysis of fraction 5 displayed three bands of 36, 70, and 110 kDa (2), which would correspond to chicken red monomer, dimer, and trimer, respectively.

Chicken Green and Rhodopsin

Before the elution of chicken green and rhodopsin, the concentration of α-methyl mannoside is increased to 5 mM in buffer A-10 (an elution buffer), with which a large amount of chicken red remaining in the column is eluted. When about 90% of the chicken red loaded onto the column is recovered, the concentration of α-methyl mannoside in buffer A-10 is increased to 100 mM for elution of chicken green and rhodopsin (fractions 11–13 in Fig. 3). Contamination with a small amount of chicken red in these fractions cannot be avoided, because prolonged elution with 5 mM α-methyl mannoside leads to elution of chicken green and rhodopsin. The three late fractions (fractions 11–13) are mixed together for further purification (see below). The mixture is composed of 1.54 $\Delta OD \cdot ml$ of chicken green and 14.7 $\Delta OD \cdot ml$ of rhodopsin with a little contamination (0.64 $\Delta OD \cdot ml$) of chicken red. The total recovery of the mixture of rhodopsin and chicken green from the ConA column is 87%.

The fractions thus recovered from the ConA column are mixed with glycerol to give a final concentration of 20% (w/v).

DEAE-Sepharose Column Chromatography

The DEAE-Sepharose column bed volume depends on the amount of starting material (~1 ml per 10 retinas). The DEAE-Sepharose column, washed in advance with 5 bed volumes of 1 M NaCl and 10 bed volumes of distilled water, is equilibrated with 5 bed volumes of buffer D-20 at a flow rate of 60 ml/hr. All the fractions (containing chicken green and rhodopsin) eluting with 100 mM α-methyl mannoside from the ConA column (fractions 11–13 in Fig. 3; supplemented with glycerol) are combined and loaded onto the preequilibrated DEAE-Sepharose column (16 mm in diameter) at a flow rate of 14 ml/hr. The column is subsequently washed with 2 bed volumes of buffer D-20. Chicken green does not bind to the column, so it is recovered in the flow-through and washing fractions. Then rhodopsin adsorbed to the column is eluted with buffer D-20 supplemented with 100 mM NaCl. Throughout the chromatography, the eluate from the column is monitored continuously by measuring the absorbance at 280 nm.

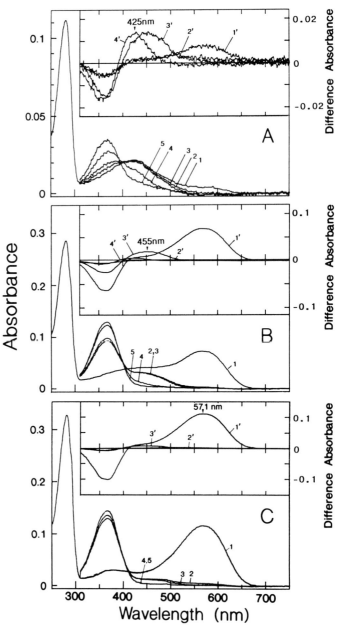

FIG. 4   Determinations of difference absorption maxima of chicken violet (A), blue (B), and red (C) by the partial bleaching method. Spectral changes by the partial bleaching of typical fractions (fractions 2, 3, and 5 in Fig. 3) eluted from the

Comments

In the previous experiment (2), the fractions containing chicken green and rhodopsin were concentrated to 10–20 ml prior to the DEAE-Sepharose column chromatography. Under such conditions, the two pigments were eluted from the column as shown in Fig. 5. However, subsequent column chromatography on CM-Sepharose (see below), which can concentrate chicken green, enabled us to omit the troublesome step of sample concentration prior to the DEAE column chromatography.

Chicken Green

Chicken green passes through the DEAE-Sepharose column without adsorption and is recovered in the first peak (Fig. 5). Some portion of chicken green elutes with retardation, as revealed by a long tail after the first fraction (25–155 ml). The yield of chicken green (shaded part of the first peak in Fig. 5) is 0.92 ΔOD·ml, corresponding to 60% recovery of the chicken green applied to the column. In the tailing part, 0.12 ΔOD·ml (8%) of chicken green is recovered. Thus, the total recovery of chicken green is 68%.

Rhodopsin

After washing the column with 2 bed volumes of buffer D-20, rhodopsin bound to the column is eluted by increasing the concentration of NaCl to 100 mM in buffer D-20. This fraction (shaded part of the second peak in Fig. 5) contains 10.2 ΔOD·ml of rhodopsin, corresponding to 69% of rhodopsin

---

ConA–Sepharose column are shown. Curve 1 shows the absorption spectrum of the fraction before irradiation. Curves 2, 3, 4, and 5 are the spectra after sequential irradiations with deep red light (>660 nm, for 80 min), red light (>590 nm, for 40 min), orange light (>520 nm, for 20 min), and yellow light (>480 nm, for 10 min), respectively. (*Insets*) Difference spectra calculated from those before and after the sequential irradiations. Curve 1′, curve 1 − curve 2 (chicken red); curve 2′, curve 2 − curve 3 (a mixture of rhodopsin and chicken green); curve 3′, curve 3 − curve 4 (chicken blue); and curve 4′, curve 4 − curve 5 (chicken violet). Fraction 2 was composed of 19% chicken red, 10% of a mixture of rhodopsin and chicken green, 33% chicken blue, and 38% chicken violet. Fraction 3 was composed of 71% chicken red, 2% of a mixture of rhodopsin and chicken green, 20% chicken blue, and 7% chicken violet. Fraction 5 was composed of 92% chicken red, 2% of a mixture of rhodopsin and chicken green, and 6% chicken blue. Because fraction 5 contained no chicken violet, curve 4′ is not shown in (C). [Reprinted with permission from T. Okano, Y. Fukada, I. D. Artamonov, and T. Yoshizawa, *Biochemistry* **28**, 8848 (1989). Copyright 1989 American Chemical Society.]

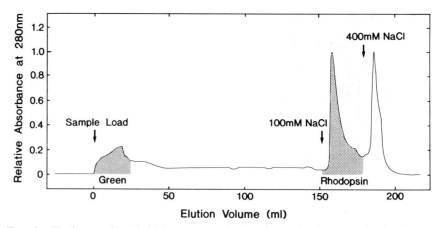

FIG. 5 Elution profile of chicken green, rhodopsin, and other proteins by DEAE-Sepharose anion-exchange column chromatography. A mixture of chicken green and rhodopsin (fractions 11–13 in Fig. 3, supplemented with glycerol) was concentrated and desalted with buffer D-20 by use of an Amicon (Danvers, MA) ultrafiltration cell (Model 8050) fitted with a YM30 membrane filter. Then the sample (22 ml) was loaded onto the DEAE-Sepharose column (16 × 300 mm). The column was washed with 120 ml of buffer D-20, followed by successive elution with 100 and 400 mM NaCl dissolved in buffer D-20. [Reprinted with permission from T. Okano, Y. Fukada, I. D. Artamonov, and T. Yoshizawa, *Biochemistry* **28,** 8848 (1989). Copyright 1989 American Chemical Society.]

applied to the column. The ratio between absorbances at 280 and 503 nm is 2.0 (Fig. 6B). The molecular weight of rhodopsin is estimated to be 37 kDa by gel electrophoresis (2). No visual pigment is detected in the third peak fraction eluted by buffer D-20 containing 400 mM NaCl.

CM-Sepharose Column Chromatography

As judged from the amino acid sequences (10), all the cone pigments are expected to have positive charges at pH 6.6, while rhodopsin has a negative charge. Thus, it is possible to purify and/or concentrate cone pigments such as chicken red, green, and blue by a cation exchanger such as CM-Sepharose.

The CM-Sepharose column bed volume depends on the volume of a loading sample rather than the amount of visual pigment; the bed volume should be greater than 1/20 volume of the loading sample. Otherwise, cone visual pigments, once adsorbed to the column, partly elute during the loading procedure. A CM-Sepharose column (16 mm in diameter) is washed with 5 bed volumes of 1 M NaCl and 10 bed volumes of distilled water, then

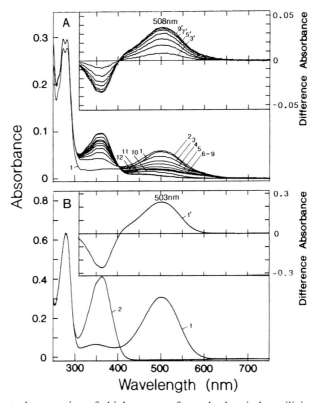

FIG. 6   Spectral separation of chicken green from rhodopsin by utilizing differential susceptibility to hydroxylamine. (A) Curve 1 is an absolute absorption spectrum of the chicken green fraction (shaded part of the first peak in Fig. 5). Immediately after adding 4 μl of 1 M hydroxylamine (pH 6.6) to 0.4 ml of the sample at 4°C, it was brought to 23°C (curve 2), and then the spectrum was recorded every hour until no change was observed (curves 3–9). (*Inset*) Difference spectra before and after the incubation with hydroxylamine (curve n', curve 2 − curve n, with n = 3, 5, 7, 9). All difference spectra showed an absorption maximum at 508 nm and formed an isosbestic point at 404 nm. These observations indicate that only chicken green was bleached by the incubation with 10 mM hydroxylamine at 23°C for 7 hr. The pigments still remaining were then successively bleached by deep red light (>660 nm, for 80 min: curve 10), red light (>590 nm, for 40 min: curve 11), and yellow light (>480 nm, for 10 min: curve 12). (B) Curve 1 is an absolute absorption spectrum of purified rhodopsin (shaded portion of the second peak in Fig. 5). This fraction was mixed with hydroxylamine to a final concentration of 10 mM and then incubated at 23°C for 7 hr, resulting in a negligible spectral change (not shown). Irradiation of the sample after the incubation with deep red light (>660 nm, for 80 min) induced no spectral change (not shown). Curve 2 is the spectrum after complete bleaching by irradiation with red light (>590 nm, for 40 min). Further irradiation with orange (>520 nm, for 20 min) or yellow light (>480 nm, for 10 min) also caused no spectral change. (*Inset*) Difference spectrum between curve 1 and curve 2. [Reprinted with permission from T. Okano, Y. Fukada, I. D. Artamonov, and T. Yoshizawa, *Biochemistry* **28,** 8848 (1989). Copyright 1989 American Chemical Society.]

equilibrated with 5 bed volumes of buffer D-20 at a flow rate of 60 ml/hr prior to the following chromatographies.

Chicken Red

The chicken red-enriched fraction obtained from the ConA–Sepharose column (e.g., fraction 5 in Fig. 3, supplemented with glycerol) is loaded onto the preequilibrated CM-Sepharose column at a flow rate of 50 ml/hr. After washing the column with 5 bed volumes of buffer D-20, the same buffer supplemented with 100 mM NaCl is used to elute chicken red, which is easily detected as a sharp peak in a continuous recording of the absorbance at 280 nm of the eluate.

Chicken Green

As described in the previous section, chicken green is enriched in the flow-through fraction from the DEAE-Sepharose column. This fraction is directly applied to the preequilibrated CM-Sepharose column, which is subsequently washed with 2 bed volumes of buffer D-20 at a flow rate of 50 ml/hr. Rhodopsin passes through the column. Then chicken green adsorbed to the column is eluted with buffer D-20 supplemented with 100 mM NaCl.

Chicken Blue

The purity and amount of chicken blue is extremely low in fractions obtained from the ConA column (e.g., fraction 2 or 3 in Fig. 3). Chicken blue-enriched fractions can be applied to the CM-Sepharose column to concentrate the pigment (10). The chromatographic procedures are the same as that described for chicken red or green (see above).

Discussion

The difference absorption maximum of chicken red was determined to be 571 nm (Fig. 4), which is slightly red-shifted from the value (562 nm) reported in digitonin solution (11, 12). On the other hand, the maximum of rhodopsin in CHAPS–PC (503 nm) was close to that in digitonin (500 nm). Because the chromophore binding site of chicken red, unlike rhodopsin, is inferred to be located near the molecular surface (13, 14), the spectral properties would be affected by the detergent more severely in chicken red than in rhodopsin. It should be noted that the absorption maximum of chicken red in CHAPS–PC (571 nm) is very close to the value in the retina (569 nm, Ref. 15) or in membranes (16), suggesting that the native conformation of chicken red is preserved in CHAPS–PC better than in digitonin. This is consistent with the previous observation that the conformation of rhodopsin (estimated from circular dischroism spectra) in CHAPS is closer to that in the native state than in digitonin (17).

The absorption maximum of chicken violet (425 nm) was estimated from the difference spectrum (Fig. 4A inset, curve 4′) between chicken violet and its photoproduct, retinal oxime plus V-photopsin (opsin moiety of chicken violet). However, this difference spectrum is distorted owing to the absorption of retinal oxime, which has an absorption maximum at 363 nm, close to that of chicken violet. To evaluate the real absorption maximum of chicken violet, the difference spectrum was corrected (2) on the assumption that the absorption spectra of various visual pigments plotted on a scale of the fourth root of the wavelength coincide in shape (in the longer wavelength region) with one another (18, 19). In this way, the absorption maximum of chicken violet was estimated to be 415 nm (Fig. 7). This value is in good agreement with those determined by analyses of electroretinograms (415 nm, Ref. 20) and early receptor potentials (413 nm, Ref. 21). This provides additional evidence that the spectral properties of visual pigments in CHAPS–PC are close to those *in vivo*.

The ratio of pigments in a chicken retina was roughly estimated from the amount (ΔOD·ml) of each pigment in the fractions from the ConA column as follows: Rhodopsin : red : green : blue : violet = 49 : 40 : 5 : 5 : 1. The highest

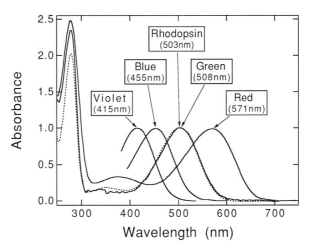

FIG. 7   Absorption spectra of chicken violet, blue, green, red, and rhodopsin. The dashed line shows the absorption spectrum of rhodopsin. The spectra of chicken blue and violet were calculated from the difference absorption spectra before and after irradiation at 4°C during the partial bleaching. Maximum absorbances in the visible region were normalized to 1.0.

content of chicken red among the cone pigments may be ascribed to double cones. In fact, microspectrophotometric (15) and immunohistochemical analyses (22, 23) showed that the red single cone and both members of the double cone contained chicken red.

Application

Chicken cone pigments purified in the CHAPS–PC system can be reconstituted in liposomes, simply by dialysis to remove CHAPS from the preparation. For instance, chicken red thus reconstituted was shown to interact efficiently *in vitro* with rod transducin (5) and rhodopsin kinase (6). Not only these biochemical properties but also the photochemical reactions of chicken red in the CHAPS–PC buffer have been investigated in detail. Laser flash photolysis and low-temperature spectrophotometry revealed that a batho-intermediate of chicken red was produced at room temperature (24), and suggested that a chloride ion bound to chicken red might dissociate from the protein moiety during the thermal conversion of batho- to lumi-intermediates (25). Thus, the purified cone pigments in CHAPS–PC are applicable to the functional analyses of cone photoreceptor cells.

Acknowledgments

We wish to express our thanks to a local poulterer, Toripin Co. Ltd., Osaka, Japan, for the kind supply of fresh chicken heads. This research was supported in part by a research grant from the Human Frontier Science Program, by a Special Coordination Fund of the Science and Technology Agency of the Japanese Government, and by Grants-in-Aid from the Japanese Ministry of Education, Science, and Culture.

References

1. G. Wald, *Nature (London)* **140**, 545 (1937).
2. T. Okano, Y. Fukada, I. D. Artamonov, and T. Yoshizawa, *Biochemistry* **28**, 8848 (1989).
3. L. M. Hjelmeland and A. Chrambach, *in* ''Methods in Enzymology'' (W. B. Jakoby, ed.), Vol. 104, p. 305. Academic Press, New York, 1984.
4. H. Matsumoto, K. Horiuchi, and T. Yoshizawa, *Biochim. Biophys. Acta* **501**, 257 (1978).
5. Y. Fukada, T. Okano, I. D. Artamonov, and T. Yoshizawa, *FEBS Lett.* **246**, 69 (1989).

6. Y. Fukada, K. Kokame, T. Okano, Y. Shichida, T. Yoshizawa, J. H. McDowell, P. A. Hargrave, and K. Palczewski, *Biochemistry* **29**, 10101 (1990).
7. T. Yoshizawa, Y. Shichida, and Y. Fukada, *Pure Appl. Chem.* **63**, 171 (1991).
8. R. S. Fager, *Vision Res.* **15**, 741 (1975).
9. L. Y. Fager, and R. S. Fager, *in* "Methods in Enzymology" (L. Packer, ed.), Vol. 81, p. 160. Academic Press, New York, 1982.
10. T. Okano, D. Kojima, Y. Fukada, Y. Shichida, and T. Yoshizawa, *Proc. Natl. Acad. Sci. U.S.A.* **89**, 5932 (1992).
11. G. Wald, P. K. Brown, and P. H. Smith, *J. Gen. Physiol.* **38**, 623 (1955).
12. H. Matsumoto and T. Yoshizawa, *in* "Methods in Enzymology" (L. Packer, ed.), Vol. 81, p. 154. Academic Press, New York, 1982.
13. H. Matsumoto, F. Tokunaga, and T. Yoshizawa, *Biochim. Biophys. Acta* **404**, 300 (1975).
14. Y. Fukada, T. Okano, Y. Shichida, T. Yoshizawa, A. Trehan, D. Mead, M. Denny, A. E. Asato, and R. S. H. Liu, *Biochemistry* **29**, 3133 (1990).
15. J. K. Bowmaker and A. Knowles, *Vision Res.* **17**, 755 (1977).
16. Y. Fukada and T. Yoshizawa, *FEBS Lett.* **149**, 117 (1982).
17. A. Kropf, *Vision Res.* **22**, 495 (1982).
18. H. B. Barlow, *Vision Res.* **22**, 635 (1982).
19. H. J. A. Dartnall, J. K. Bowmaker, and J. D. Mollon, *Proc. R. Soc. London B* **220**, 115 (1983).
20. D. V. Norren, *Vision Res.* **15**, 1164 (1975).
21. V. I. Govardovskii and L. V. Zueva, *Vision Res.* **17**, 537 (1977).
22. A. Szel, L. Takacs, E. Monostori, T. Diamantstein, I. Vigh-Teichmann, and P. Rohlich, *Exp. Eye Res.* **43**, 871 (1986).
23. Y. Shichida, Y. Taniguchi, O. Kuwata, Y. Fukada, T. Yoshizawa, S. Horiuchi, and M. Takeichi, *Exp. Eye Res.* **48**, 281 (1989).
24. H. Kandori, T. Mizukami, T. Okada, Y. Imamoto, Y. Fukada, Y. Shichida, and T. Yoshizawa, *Proc. Natl. Acad. Sci. U.S.A.* **87**, 8908 (1990).
25. Y. Imamoto, H. Kandori, T. Okano, Y. Fukada, Y. Shichida, and T. Yoshizawa, *Biochemistry* **28**, 9412 (1989).

[11]   Purification and Characterization of Bovine Transducin and Its Subunits

Tuow D. Ting, Steven B. Goldin, and Yee-Kin Ho

Introduction

Visual excitation in vertebrate rod photoreceptor cells involves a light-activated cGMP enzyme cascade in the rod outer segment (ROS). Absorption of a photon by the receptor molecule, rhodopsin, leads to the activation of a latent cGMP phosphodiesterase (PDE) that rapidly hydrolyzes cytosolic cGMP. The transient decrease in cGMP concentration causes the closure of cGMP-sensitive cation channels in the plasma membrane and results in hyperpolarization of the cell (1, 2). Signal coupling between photolyzed rhodopsin (R*) and PDE is mediated by a signal-transducing G protein called transducin (T) via a GTP-binding and hydrolysis cycle. Transducin is a trimeric protein composed of three polypeptides: T_α (39 kDa), T_β (37 kDa), and T_γ (8.5 kDa). In the dark-adapted state, T_α contains a bound GDP (T_α–GDP) and interacts with $T_{\beta\gamma}$. The T_α–GDP $\cdot$ $T_{\beta\gamma}$ complex tightly associates with rhodopsin. On photoexcitation, R* catalyzes a GTP/GDP exchange reaction converting T_α–GDP to the active form of T_α–GTP. T_α–GTP dissociates from R*/$T_{\beta\gamma}$ and activates PDE by relieving the restraint exerted by the P_γ inhibitory subunit of PDE. After the hydrolysis of the tightly bound GTP, T_α–GDP recombines with $T_{\beta\gamma}$ and is ready for another cycle of activation (3).

This chapter delineates methods for the purification of transducin and its subunits from bovine retinas. Biochemical assays for studying the various coupling functions of transducin using a reconstituted system are also described. The relative ease of obtaining large quantities of purified transducin and other components of the retinal cGMP cascade provides an ideal opportunity to elucidate the molecular mechanisms of this receptor/G-protein-coupled second-messenger system.

Purification of Transducin and Its Subunits

The purification procedure was originally developed by Fung and co-workers (4–6). Transducin and PDE are purified from crude ROS membranes prepared from frozen bovine retinas. Taking advantage of the tight binding of trans-

Methods in Neurosciences, Volume 15

ducin to R* in the absence of GTP, other peripheral membrane proteins such as PDE can be removed from photolyzed ROS membranes by repeatedly washing with low ionic strength buffer. Transducin is extracted from the washed ROS membranes with GTP. Transducin and its subunits are further purified from this extract by column chromatography. An isolation using 400 retinas typically yields more than 20 mg of transducin. Further separation of subunits generates 5 mg each of T_α and $T_{\beta\gamma}$. Based on the convenience of the purification scheme, it is recommended that a minimum of 200 retinas be used to obtain optimal yield.

Preparation of Crude Rod Outer Segment Membranes for Transducin Extraction

Fresh bovine eyes are collected from local packing companies and kept in the dark for several hours prior to dissection of the retinas under dim red light (Kodak, Rochester, NY, red No. 2 safety light filter). Bovine retinas can be stored in the dark at $-70°C$ for over 1 year without loss of enzymatic activities of the cGMP cascade. Alternatively, frozen dark-adapted bovine retinas can be purchased from supply houses (G. A. Hormel Co., Austin, MN, or J. A. Lawson Co., Lincoln, NE). Equipment required for the isolation of transducin from 400 retinas include two Du Pont (Wilmington, DE) Sorval RC5 centrifuges with SS34 rotors or Beckman Instrument (Fullerton, CA) J2-21 centrifuges with J21 rotors, 50-ml centrifuge tubes with caps, rubber policemen, and 30- to 50-ml syringes. Two liters of isolation buffer is required, which consists of 10 mM MOPS [3-(N-morpholino)propanesulfonic acid], 60 mM KCl, 30 mM NaCl, 2 mM MgCl$_2$, 0.1 mM PMSF (phenylmethylsulfonyl fluoride), and 1 mM DTT (dithiothreitol) at pH 7.5. Two sucrose solutions (500 ml each) are prepared using the isolation buffer, a 50% (w/v) solution and a 38% solution.

The isolation is carried out under dim red light to keep rhodopsin in the dark-adapted state. Four hundred frozen retinas are thawed in 200–350 ml of the 50% sucrose buffer at room temperature. The suspension is transferred to a beaker and stirred with a magnetic stirrer for about 20 min. The retinal suspension is forced twice through a 50-ml syringe (without needle) to break up the tissue, then divided equally among 16 50-ml centrifuge tubes. The volume of each tube is adjusted to 40 ml with 50% sucrose buffer. After mixing the contents by shaking, the suspension is centrifuged at 15,000 rpm (27,000 g) for 15 min at 4°C. Under these conditions, the ROS membranes float to the top of the tubes, while the remainder of the retinal membranes pellet to the bottom.

Using a rubber policeman, the floating ROS membranes are scraped off the walls of the tubes and resuspended in the supernatant. The supernatant is gently poured off without disturbing the bottom pellet and distributed equally among 28 clean 50-ml centrifuge tubes. The volume in each tube is increased to 40 ml with isolation buffer to dilute the sucrose concentration to approximately 28%. The tubes are shaken and centrifuged at 18,000 rpm (38,000 g) for 15 min. The ROS membranes sediment to the bottom of the tubes, and a small amount of lipid material floats to the top. The lipid material is discarded along with the supernatant. The ROS membrane pellets are resuspended in 150 ml of 38% sucrose isolation buffer and divided equally among 16 tubes. The volume of each tube is adjusted to 30 ml with the 38% sucrose buffer, and the tubes are centrifuged at 18,000 rpm for 45 min. The ROS membranes float to the top of the tubes and are resuspended in the supernatant.

The ROS membrane suspension is then divided among 16 clean centrifuge tubes. To reduce the sucrose concentration, the volume of each tube is increased to 45 ml with isolation buffer. After mixing, the tubes are centrifuged at 19,000 rpm (43,000 g) for 20 min to pellet the ROS membranes. The supernatants are discarded and the pellets are resuspended with 40 ml of isolation buffer. The samples are centrifuged again at 19,000 rpm for 20 min. Residual sucrose is removed by washing the ROS membranes twice more with isolation buffer. The final ROS membranes are resuspended with 40 ml of isolation buffer and divided equally among four tubes. The crude ROS membranes can be kept in the dark overnight on ice.

Extraction of transducin and PDE from crude ROS membranes is carried out under room light. Two liters of low ionic strength extraction buffer containing 5 mM Tris, 0.5 mM MgCl$_2$, 0.1 mM PMSF, and 1.0 mM DTT at pH 7.5, a 120-ml Teflon–glass homogenizer, and two 30-ml syringes fitted with 3-inch Tygon tubing are required. The crude ROS membranes are resuspended in 100 ml extraction buffer and homogenized with the Teflon–glass homogenizer by five up-and-down strokes. The homogenate is divided equally among four 50-ml centrifuge tubes, and the volume of each tube is increased to 45 ml with extraction buffer. The samples are photolyzed on ice under a desk lamp for 15 min until the red color of the suspension changes to bright orange, indicating the conversion of rhodopsin to the meta-II state (R*). Under these conditions, most of the peripheral proteins, including PDE, can be extracted by the low ionic strength buffer. However, transducin remains tightly bound to the R*-containing membrane. Thus, washing the ROS membranes repeatedly with extraction buffer differentially separates transducin from other membrane-associated proteins. To stabilize the meta-II R*, it is important to wash the membranes at 0–4°C.

After photolyzing the ROS membranes, the suspensions are centrifuged at 19,000 rpm for 30 min. The supernatants are carefully removed with a

30-ml syringe fitted with Tygon tubing and transferred to four clean 50-ml centrifuge tubes. The supernatants containing the extracted proteins are centrifuged again at 19,000 rpm for 30 min to remove residual ROS membranes. Supernatant from the second centrifugation is removed with a clean 30-ml syringe and stored on ice for subsequent chromatographic separation of PDE. The ROS membrane pellets from the two centrifugations are pooled and homogenized again with 100 ml buffer for the second extraction. This extraction process with double centrifugation is repeated a total of 6 times. Supernatants from the first four extractions are pooled for PDE purification; supernatants from the last two extractions are discarded. The final ROS membranes are saved for extraction of transducin.

The activation of transducin via the exchange of GTP leads to the dissociation of transducin subunits from R*. Under low ionic strength conditions, both T_α–GTP and $T_{\beta\gamma}$ dissociate from the ROS membranes. The soluble subunits can be separated from the ROS membranes by centrifugation. On hydrolysis of bound GTP by the intrinsic GTPase activity of T_α, T_α–GDP and $T_{\beta\gamma}$ recombine to form the heterotrimer complex, which can be purified from minor contaminants by hexylagarose chromatography. To extract transducin, the washed ROS membranes containing tightly bound transducin are homogenized in 100 ml extraction buffer containing 100 μM GTP. The homogenate is divided among four centrifuge tubes, and the volume of each tube is increased to 45 ml with GTP–extraction buffer. After centrifugation at 19,000 rpm for 30 min, the supernatants are transferred with a clean 30-ml syringe to another set of clean tubes for the second centrifugation. Prior to the second centrifugation, 50 μl of 10 mM GTP is added to all the tubes. This is a precaution since transducin hydrolyzes GTP continuously in the presence of R*, which may deplete GTP in the extraction buffer. Supernatants from the second centrifugation are removed with a clean 30-ml syringe and stored on ice for subsequent chromatographic purification of transducin. The ROS membrane pellets from both centrifugations are pooled and homogenized again with GTP–extraction buffer for another cycle of extraction. Transducin extraction is repeated 3 times, and the supernatants from these extractions are pooled for purification of transducin.

Purification of Transducin

Transducin extract containing approximately 95% pure transducin is applied to a hexylagarose column (6 × 1.5 cm, ICN ImmunoBiologicals, Lisle, IL) equilibrated with MOPS buffer (10 mM MOPS, 2 mM MgCl$_2$, 1 mM DTT, pH 7.5) at 4°C. The binding of transducin to hexylagarose forms a white band at the top of the column. After loading, the column is washed with 50

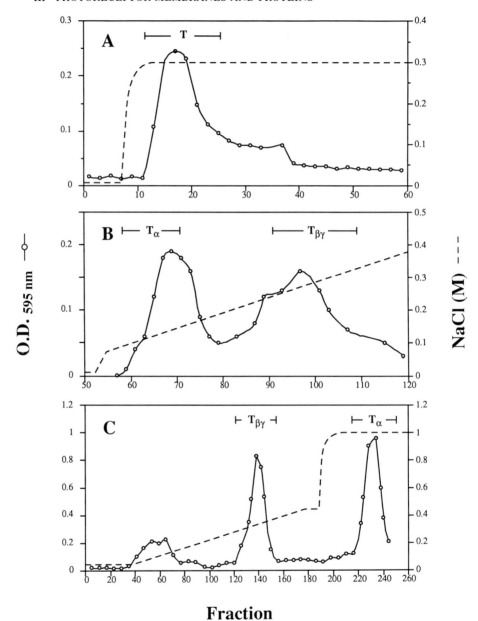

Fig. 1 Separation of transducin and its subunits. The conditions for the chromatographic separation are described in the text. The protein content was determined by the Bradford dye-binding assay monitored by the absorbance at 595 nm. (A) Purification of transducin by hexylagarose. Transducin extracted from 400 retinas in 300 ml

ml of MOPS buffer to remove unbound contaminants and free GTP. Transducin is eluted from the column with MOPS buffer containing 0.3 M NaCl. Fractions of 3 ml are collected, and the protein concentration is determined by the Bradford method (7).

The chromatogram of the hexylagarose column separation is shown in Fig. 1A. Transducin is eluted as a single peak, and the appropriate fractions are pooled and concentrated with an Amicon (Danvers, MA) concentrator (YM10 membrane) to approximately 2 ml. The final protein concentrate is clarified by centrifugation at 16,000 rpm for 15 min. Transducin can be stored in 40% glycerol at $-20°C$ for several months without loss of enzymatic activity. Purified transducin contains bound GDP and exists as T_α–GDP · $T_{\beta\gamma}$ complexes. The hexylagarose column can be regenerated by washing with 1 M NaCl and can be stored in 0.5% toluene.

Separation of T_α–GDP and $T_{\beta\gamma}$ Subunits

The T_α–GDP and $T_{\beta\gamma}$ subunits can be separated according to two established procedures using either ω-aminooctylagarose or Affi-Gel Blue chromatography as described below.

ω-Aminooctylagarose Chromatography

Transducin extract in low ionic strength buffer is applied to a ω-aminooctylagarose column (15 × 1 cm, ICN ImmunoBiologicals) equilibrated with MOPS buffer (10 mM MOPS, 2 mM MgCl$_2$, 1 mM DTT, pH 7.5). If purified transducin stored in 40% glycerol is used for this procedure, it is necessary to dilute the sample 30-fold with MOPS buffer to reduce the salt and glycerol concentration prior to loading onto the column. The column is washed with 50 ml MOPS buffer, and the proteins are eluted with a 450-ml linear NaCl

---

of extraction buffer was applied to the column. Transducin was eluted as a single peak with MOPS buffer containing 0.3 M NaCl. (B) Separation of transducin subunits by ω-aminooctylagarose. Twenty milligrams of purified transducin was applied to the column. T_α–GDP was eluted first with a peak at 0.15 M NaCl; $T_{\beta\gamma}$ was eluted later with a peak at 0.28 M NaCl. The two peaks were not completely resolved. Early fractions of the first peak containing T_α and late fractions of the second peak containing $T_{\beta\gamma}$ were collected. (C) Separation of transducin subunits by Affi-Gel Blue. Thirty milligrams of purified transducin was applied to the column, and the column was eluted with a 250-ml linear KCl gradient from 0 to 0.45 M followed with 1 M KCl. $T_{\beta\gamma}$ was eluted first during the KCl gradient, and T_α was eluted later with 1 M KCl.

gradient from 0.075 to 0.4 M in MOPS buffer. Fractions of 4 ml are collected and the protein concentration determined.

The chromatogram is shown in Fig. 1B. T_α–GDP is eluted first with a peak at 0.15 M NaCl; $T_{\beta\gamma}$ is eluted later with a peak at 0.28 M NaCl. The two peaks are not completely resolved. As shown in Fig. 1B, the early fractions of the T_α peak and the late fractions of the $T_{\beta\gamma}$ peak are collected and concentrated with Amicon concentrators. Purified T_α–GDP generally contains a small amount of $T_{\beta\gamma}$ (<1%), and $T_{\beta\gamma}$ is pure without contamination from T_α. The purified subunits are stored in 40% glycerol at $-20°C$. The overlapping fractions of T_α and $T_{\beta\gamma}$ are pooled, concentrated, and reloaded onto the ω-aminooctylagarose column for another round of separation. Similar to hexylagarose, ω-aminooctylagarose can be regenerated by washing the column with 1 M NaCl and stored in 0.5% toluene.

Affi-Gel Blue Chromatography

Transducin subunits can be separated with chromatographic media containing Cibracon blue dye such as Blue Sepharose CL-6B (Pharmacia, Piscataway, NJ), or Affi-Gel Blue (Bio-Rad Laboratories, Richmond, CA). Yamazaki and co-workers have reported the separation of frog transducin subunits using a Blue Sepharose CL-6B column eluted with a linear salt gradient (8). The following protocol describes the use of Affi-Gel Blue to separate bovine transducin subunits.

Affi-Gel Blue resin is packed in a 30 × 0.9 cm column and equilibrated with buffer containing 100 mM Tris-HCl, 6 mM MgSO$_4$, 1 mM EDTA, 1 mM DTT, and 25% glycerol at pH 7.5 (buffer A). Purified transducin stored in 40% glycerol is diluted 20-fold with buffer A and concentrated to 2 ml using an Amicon concentrator. After this buffer exchange step, transducin is applied to the Affi-Gel Blue column. The column is washed with 250 ml (10 bed volumes) of buffer A and then with 100 ml of a lower ionic strength buffer containing 10 mM Tris-HCl, 6 mM MgSO$_4$, 1 mM EDTA, 1 mM DTT, and 25% glycerol at pH 7.5 (buffer B). A flow rate of approximately 6 ml/hr is maintained by gravity flow. $T_{\beta\gamma}$ is eluted with a 250-ml linear KCl gradient from 0 to 0.45 M in buffer B; T_α is eluted with 1 M KCl in buffer B. Fractions of 2 ml are collected. Figure 1C shows the chromatogram of the Affi-Gel Blue separation. The purified subunits are concentrated with Amicon concentrators and stored in 40% glycerol at $-20°C$.

Which of the two chromatographic methods should be utilized to separate T_α–GDP from $T_{\beta\gamma}$ depends on the application. The ω-aminooctylagarose method has the advantage of a fast separation time, namely, 1 day, compared to 4 days for the Affi-Gel Blue method due to its slow flow rate. The Affi-Gel Blue method can produce pure subunits in one chromatographic run. To obtain protein yields comparable to the Affi-Gel Blue method, the ω-

aminooctylagarose method requires a second chromatographic run to separate the overlapping fractions containing both T_α–GDP and $T_{\beta\gamma}$. Only the ω-aminooctylagarose method can effectively separate T_α–Gpp(NH)p from $T_{\beta\gamma}$ as described below.

Preparation of T_α–Gpp(NH)p

T_α purified from GTP extraction is present in its latent form with tightly bound GDP, which lacks the ability to activate PDE. The active form of transducin can be obtained by substituting GTP with nonhydrolyzable analogs such as Gpp(NH)p or GTPγS. The nucleotide analogs are incorporated into purified transducin in the presence of R*. A 5-ml reaction mixture in MOPS buffer containing 15–20 mg transducin, 100 μM Gpp(NH)p (or 20 μM GTPγS), and 10 μM R* in reconstituted membranes or EDTA–urea-stripped ROS membranes is incubated on ice overnight. The R*-containing membranes are removed by centrifugation at 19,000 rpm for 20 min. The supernatant containing T_α–Gpp(NH)p is diluted 20-fold to reduce the salt concentration and applied to an ω-aminooctylagarose column for separation of T_α and $T_{\beta\gamma}$. Transducin subunits are eluted with the linear NaCl gradient described above.

Purified T_α–Gpp(NH)p shows a 1 : 1 stoichiometry of Gpp(NH)p bound per T_α and can activate the latent PDE in the absence of R* and $T_{\beta\gamma}$. T_α–Gpp(NH)p is a stable complex that can be stored in 40% glycerol at $-20°$C for over 1 year without losing the bound Gpp(NH)p. T_α–Gpp(NH)p also differs from T_α–GDP in its conformation as revealed by tryptic cleavage patterns and reactivity toward N-ethylmaleimide modification of sulfhydryl groups (6, 9).

Functional Assays for Transducin

The activation of the retinal cGMP cascade consists of two amplification stages as depicted in Fig. 2. In the first stage, R* interacts with transducin, catalyzes the exchange of GTP for bound GDP, and induces the dissociation of T_α–GTP and $T_{\beta\gamma}$ from R*. The second stage involves the activation of PDE by T_α–GTP. Because the purified T_α–Gpp(NH)p complex is capable of activating PDE in the absence of R* or $T_{\beta\gamma}$, the two amplification stages can be studied independently.

Specific assays have been developed to evaluate the individual coupling steps of the cascade cycle. The R*-catalyzed GTP exchange reaction of transducin can be monitored by a [^{3}H]Gpp(NH)p binding assay (4). The

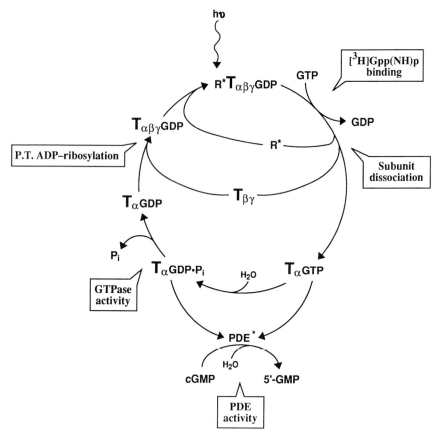

FIG. 2 Schematic of the transducin coupling cycle. The signal coupling cycle of transducin in the retinal cGMP cascade is illustrated. Biochemical assays for the various coupling steps of transducin are shown.

dissociation of T_α and $T_{\beta\gamma}$ from ROS membranes after incorporation of GTP or Gpp(NH)p can be monitored by a centrifugation method which separates soluble from membrane-bound transducin (6). The R*-mediated multiple turnover of transducin can be monitored by the continuous hydrolysis of $[\gamma\text{-}^{32}P]GTP$ (10). PDE can be activated by reconstitution with purified T_α–Gpp(NH)p. The cGMP hydrolytic activity of PDE can be measured with a pH electrode that monitors the proton release due to the hydrolysis of cGMP (11). Finally, the reassociation of T_α–GDP with $T_{\beta\gamma}$ can be assayed indirectly by the pertussis toxin-catalyzed ADP-ribosylation of T_α, which is greatly enhanced by $T_{\beta\gamma}$ (12).

As shown in Fig. 2, each coupling activity of transducin can be studied individually by a specific assay in a reconstituted system. Because purified transducin alone has no specific enzyme activity, R* and PDE are required to elicit its coupling functions. Procedures to obtain EDTA–urea-stripped ROS membranes as a source of R* and crude PDE are briefly described.

Materials for Transducin Assays

Preparation of EDTA–Urea Stripped Rod Outer Segment Membranes

The preparation is carried out at 4°C under dim red light to avoid photobleaching of rhodopsin. Crude ROS membranes prepared from 100 dark-adapted bovine retinas by sucrose flotation methods are resuspended in low ionic strength MOPS buffer (2 mM MOPS, 1 mM DTT, pH 7.5) containing 1 mM EDTA and 4 M urea. After homogenization with a Teflon–glass homogenizer, the suspension is divided equally among eight 50-ml centrifuge tubes. The volume of each tube is increased to 40 ml with MOPS–EDTA–urea buffer. The tubes are centrifuged at 19,000 rpm for 30 min at 4°C. Supernatants are removed with a 50-ml syringe and discarded. The remaining ROS membrane pellets are resuspended in MOPS–EDTA–urea buffer, homogenized, and centrifuged again. Most of the peripheral membrane proteins, such as transducin and PDE, are removed from the ROS membranes under these conditions. A total of six washes in EDTA–urea buffer is required to obtain stripped ROS membranes that are devoid of transducin and PDE activity. Finally, EDTA and urea are removed by washing the membranes 4 times with MOPS buffer. The stripped ROS membranes are stored in the dark at −70°C and used as the source of R* in the reconstitution assays.

It is important to note that the stripped ROS membranes still possess a residual nucleotide (ATP or GTP) hydrolytic activity which may not be related to transducin. It is essential that proper controls be conducted in the reconstitution assays for GTPase activity.

Preparation of Crude Phosphodiesterase

Latent PDE can be purified from the low ionic strength extract of crude ROS membranes described above. The PDE extract is applied to an 18 × 2.5 cm DEAE-Sephadex column equilibrated with MOPS buffer (10 mM MOPS, 2 mM MgCl$_2$, 1 mM DTT, pH 7.5). After washing the column with 50 ml MOPS buffer, the bound proteins are eluted with a 500-ml linear gradient of NaCl from 0.1 to 0.6 M in MOPS buffer. Fractions of 4.5 ml are collected, and protein compositions are determined by the Bradford assay and sodium dodecyl sulfate (SDS)–polyacrylamide gel electrophoresis. The chromatogram shows two broad peaks, with PDE eluting in the second peak at a NaCl concentration between 0.3 and 0.37 M. PDE fractions from the second peak are pooled, concentrated with an Amicon concentrator, and stored in 40% glycerol at $-20°C$.

The crude PDE is a latent enzyme with little cGMP hydrolytic activity, but it can be activated by trypsin treatment. SDS–polyacrylamide gel electrophoresis reveals the existence of the three polypeptides of PDE, P_α(88 kDa), P_β(84 kDa), and P_γ(14 kDa) with approximately 80% purity. Despite about 20% contamination, the crude PDE is suitable for the reconstitution assays. Further purification can be accomplished by Sephacryl S-300 or ω-aminooctylagarose chromatographies, which are not described in this chapter (13).

R^*-Catalyzed [^3H]Gpp(NH)p Binding

The [^3H]Gpp(NH)p-binding activity of transducin can be assayed by filtration on nitrocellulose filters (Millipore, Bedford, MA, HA 0.45 μm pore). The buffer used for this assay contains 10 mM MOPS, 200 mM NaCl, 2 mM MgCl$_2$, and 2 mM DTT at pH 7.5. Typically, a 30-μl reaction mixture containing 6 μM R* in stripped ROS and 30 μg transducin is incubated for 10 min at 0°C. The reaction is initiated by the addition of 30 μl of 30 μM [^3H]Gpp (NH)p. At the appropriate time, the reaction is diluted with 3 ml ice-cold buffer and immediately filtered through a nitrocellulose filter mounted on an Amicon filtration manifold. The filter is then washed twice with ice-cold buffer. The amount of radioactive nucleotide bound to transducin and retained by the nitrocellulose filter can be determined by scintillation counting. Under these conditions, the incorporation of [^3H]Gpp(NH)p is linear up to 10 min. The recovery of transducin in the nitrocellulose filter binding assays is approximately 85%. The maximal incorporation reached a stoichiometry of 0.95 mol of [^3H]Gpp(NH)p per mole of transducin. In the control experiment, binding of [^3H]Gpp(NH)p to transducin does not occur in the absence of R*.

Dissociation of Transducin from Rod Outer Segment Membranes

Activated transducin with GTP or its nonhydrolyzable analogs such as Gpp (NH)p bound to T_α dissociates from R*-containing membranes. The dissociation of transducin subunits from R* is essential for the signal amplification process by which R* is recycled for continuous activation of additional transducin molecules. The assay is performed in a buffer containing 10 mM MOPS, 2 mM MgCl$_2$, and 2 mM DTT at pH 7.5. Typically, a sample containing 100 μM R* in stripped ROS membranes and 20 μg transducin is incubated for 20 min to facilitate binding of transducin to the ROS membranes. Over

90% of the reconstituted transducin is bound to R*-containing membranes. GTP or its nonhydrolyzable analogs at various concentrations is then added. After a 5-min incubation period, solubilized transducin is separated from the membrane-bound form by centrifugation in a Beckman Airfuge (5 min at 20 psi at room temperature). Soluble transducin in the supernatant is removed, and the protein content is determined either by the Bradford assay or by SDS–polyacrylamide gel electrophoresis with subsequent Coomassie blue staining and densitometric analysis. More than 90% of the membrane-bound transducin can be released at saturating concentrations of GTP. The binding affinity of different GTP analogs to transducin can be estimated accurately by this method. As shown in Fig. 3, the dose response curves of transducin release from ROS membranes in the presence of various nucleotides indicate that the binding affinity follows the order GTPγS > Gpp(NH)p > GTP ≫ Gpp(CH$_2$)p.

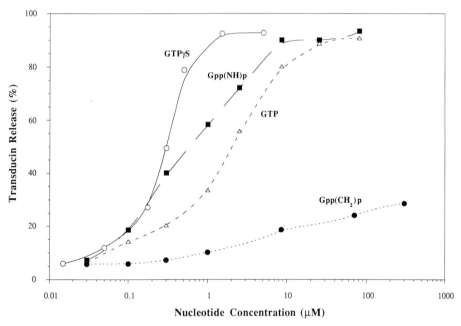

FIG. 3   Dissociation of transducin from ROS membranes. The dissociation of transducin from ROS membranes was assayed by the centrifugation method described in the text. The release of transducin from photolyzed ROS membranes was initiated by the addition of various nucleotides. Solubilized transducin was separated from the membrane-bound fractions by centrifugation in a Beckman Airfuge and then electrophoresed on a 13% polyacrylamide gel in the presence of SDS. The amount of transducin released was determined by Coomassie blue staining and densitometric analysis. The nucleotides used were GTPγS, Gpp(NH)p, GTP, and Gpp(CH$_2$)p.

R*-Catalyzed GTP Hydrolysis

Despite the intrinsic GTPase activity of T_α, purified transducin alone does not hydrolyze GTP, owing to the lack of nucleotide exchange activity. However, in the presence of R*, the turnover of transducin is accompanied by the continuous hydrolysis of GTP. Using $[\gamma\text{-}^{32}P]$GTP as substrate, the GTPase activity can be monitored by measuring the release of $[^{32}P]P_i$ using the molybdate precipitation method (14). Three solutions are required for the assay. A stop solution containing 2.5% (0.4 N) perchloric acid (PCA) and 0.56 mM KH_2PO_4 is needed for quenching the reaction. A P_i precipitation solution containing 0.0154 mM triethylamine hydrochloride (TEA-HCl) at pH 5.0 and 0.0123 mM ammonium molybdate is needed for precipitating $[^{32}P]P_i$. A wash solution containing 10 mM TEA-HCl (pH 5.0), 30 mM ammonium molybdate, 0.1 mM KH_2PO_4 and 0.20 M PCA is needed to wash the precipitates in the filtering assay. The GTPase assay is performed in a buffer containing 10 mM MOPS, 2 mM $MgCl_2$, and 2 mM DTT at pH 7.5.

Typically, a 30-μl reaction mixture containing 6 μM R* in stripped ROS membranes and 10 μg transducin is incubated at 0°C for 10 min. The reaction is initiated by the addition of 30 μl of 60 μM $[\gamma\text{-}^{32}P]$GTP. GTP hydrolysis is allowed to occur at 22°C for 5–10 min. The reaction is stopped by the addition of 1 ml of the stop solution. Inorganic phosphate is precipitated with the addition of 1 ml of the P_i precipitation solution. The sample is then vortexed and allowed to sit for at least 10 min at 4°C. The precipitates are filtered onto Whatman (Clifton, NJ) glass microfiber filters (GF/A, 2.4 cm) with an Amicon filtration manifold. After washing the filters twice with the ice-cold wash solution, the radioactivity associated with the filters is quantitated by scintillation counting. Under the experimental conditions, the GTP hydrolysis rate is linear up to 20 min.

Activation of cGMP Phosphodiesterase

Phosphodiesterase activity can be monitored by the decrease of pH of the solution caused by the hydrolysis of cGMP. The buffer used for the assay contains 10 mM MOPS, 200 mM NaCl, and 2 mM $MgCl_2$ at pH 7.5. The reaction mixture contains 25 μM R*, 10 μg transducin, 20 μg PDE, and 5 mM cGMP in a volume of 100 μl. The sample is allowed to equilibrate to achieve a baseline pH, and the reaction is initiated by the addition of 100 μl of 0.6 μM GTP or 10 μM Gpp(NH)p. The change in pH of the reaction medium is monitored by a pH microelectrode (Microelectrodes Inc., Londonderry, NH) connected to a Radiometer PHM 82 pH meter. The result is recorded on a strip chart recorder. The change in pH is converted to nanomoles of protons liberated by titrating the sample with 5-μl aliquots of 5 mM NaOH. The numbers of protons generated is then converted to the amount of cGMP hydrolyzed.

A typical result is shown in Fig. 4. In reconstitution studies with R* and transducin, PDE behaves as a latent enzyme with negligible activity in the absence of GTP. The addition of GTP or Gpp(NH)p activates PDE to hydrolyze cGMP. The kinetics of cGMP hydrolysis can be calculated from the

A   **B**

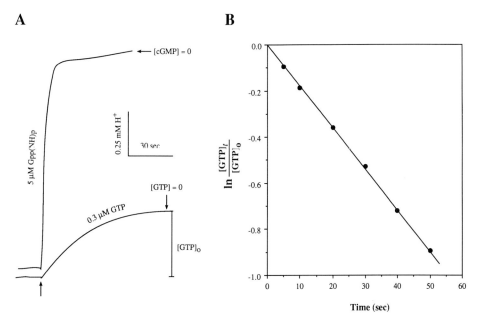

FIG. 4   Activation of cGMP phosphodiesterase by transducin. The reaction mixture contains 25 μM R*, 10 μg transducin, 20 μg PDE, and 5 mM cGMP. The reactions are initiated by the addition of GTP or Gpp(NH)p. (A) Results of the PDE activation assay as monitored by the rate of H$^+$ release due to cGMP hydrolysis using a pH microelectrode. The arrow indicates the addition of GTP or Gpp(NH)p. Total hydrolysis of the cGMP in the reaction mixture is shown by the top curve, where the cascade was activated by the addition of Gpp(NH)p. The bottom curve represents the activation of PDE by a limited amount of GTP (0.3 μM). The PDE activity was reduced slowly due to the hydrolysis of GTP by transducin. (B) First-order kinetic plot of the rate of PDE deactivation due to the hydrolysis of GTP. The values of GTP$_t$ and GTP$_0$ were determined from the experimental trace of the PDE assays described in (A). GTP$_0$ represents the total GTP content in the reaction mixture at time 0, and GTP$_t$ represents the amount of GTP remaining at time t. Hence, GTP$_t$/GTP$_0$ represents the fraction of GTP remaining at time t. The value of the slope of the linear plot of ln(GTP$_t$/GTP$_0$) versus time was used to calculate the first-order rate constant of 0.018 sec^{-1} for PDE deactivation.

initial rate of the pH change. This assay can also be used to study the relationship between GTP hydrolysis by transducin and PDE deactivation. When a limited amount of GTP (0.3 μM) is added to initiate the reaction, PDE activity increases but slowly diminishes back to the basal level. This is due to the turnover of transducin GTPase activity consuming all the added GTP. From the decay curve of PDE activity, the value for the ratio (GTP_t/GTP_0) can be determined at various time points for kinetic analysis. GTP_0 represents the total amount of GTP in the reaction mixture at time 0; GTP_t represents the amount of GTP remaining at time t. The decay process follows pseudo-first-order kinetics. A linear plot of $\ln(GTP_t/GTP_0)$ versus time is obtained as shown in Fig. 4B. The negative slope of the linear plot corresponds to the first-order rate constant of PDE deactivation due to GTP hydrolysis by transducin (15).

Subunit Interaction between T_α and $T_{\beta\gamma}$: Pertussis Toxin-Catalyzed ADP-Ribosylation

Purified T_α or $T_{\beta\gamma}$ alone does not interact with R*. The interaction requires the formation of $T_\alpha T_{\beta\gamma}$ complexes and has been studied by sedimentation and gel filtration methods. These assays generally are time consuming, and only a small number of samples can be processed at one time. However, the interaction between T_α and $T_{\beta\gamma}$ can be studied indirectly by assaying the efficiency of the ADP-ribosylation of T_α catalyzed by pertussis toxin. It has been shown that ADP-ribosylation of T_α occurs slowly in the absence of the $T_{\beta\gamma}$ subunit (12). Thus, the $T_{\beta\gamma}$ enhancement of pertussis toxin-catalyzed ADP-ribosylation of T_α can be used as an indirect measurement of the subunit interaction of transducin.

The ADP-ribosylation buffer contains 10 mM MOPS, 200 mM NaCl, 2 mM DTT, and 2 mM MgCl$_2$ at pH 7.5. The reaction is carried out by incubating a reaction mixture containing 1.0 mg/ml purified transducin, 10 μg/ml pertussis toxin (activated with 20 mM DTT at 30°C for 10 min), 1 mM [adenylate-^{32}P]NAD, and 1 mM ATP for up to 25 min at 30°C. The radioactive labeling is stopped by the addition of a 10-fold excess of nonradioactive NAD, and the sample is separated on a 13% polyacrylamide gel in the presence of SDS. The radioactivity incorporated into T_α can be revealed by autoradiography or by excising the radioactive T_α band and quantifying by scintillation counting. Under the experimental conditions, the rate of ADP-ribosylation remains linear for 50 min, and the incorporation of [^{32}P]ADP–ribose on T_α reaches a molar ratio of 1:1 in approximately 2 hr. Factors affecting the interaction between T_α and $T_{\beta\gamma}$ generally inhibit the pertussis toxin-catalyzed ADP-ribosylation reaction.

References

1. M. L. Applebury and P. A. Hargrave, *Vision Res.* **26,** 1881 (1986).
2. L. Stryer, *J. Biol. Chem.* **266,** 10711 (1991).
3. Y.-K. Ho, V. N. Hingorani, S. E. Navon, and B. K.-K. Fung, *Curr. Top. Cell. Regul.* **30,** 171 (1989).
4. B. K.-K. Fung, *J. Biol. Chem.* **258,** 10495 (1983).
5. B. K.-K.Fung, J. B. Hurley, and L. Stryer, *Proc. Natl. Acad. Sci. U.S.A.* **78,** 152 (1981).
6. Y.-K. Ho and B. K.-K. Fung, *J. Biol. Chem.* **259,** 6694 (1984).
7. M. M. Bradford, *Anal. Biochem.* **72,** 248 (1986).
8. A. Yamazaki, M. Tatsumi, D. C. Torney, and M. W. Bitensky, *J. Biol. Chem.* **262,** 9316 (1987).
9. B. K.-K. Fung and C. Nash, *J. Biol. Chem.* **258,** 10503 (1983).
10. B. K.-K. Fung and L. Stryer, *Proc. Natl. Acad. Sci. U.S.A.* **78,** 2500 (1980).
11. R. Yee and P. A. Liebman, *J. Biol. Chem.* **253,** 8902 (1978).
12. P. A. Watkins, D. L. Burns, Y. Kanaho, T.-Y. Liu, E. L. Hewlett, and J. Moss, *J. Biol. Chem.* **260,** 13478 (1985).
13. J. B. Hurley and L. Stryer, *J. Biol. Chem.* **257,** 11094 (1982).
14. Y. Sugino and Y. Miyoshi, *J. Biol. Chem.* **239,** 2360 (1964).
15. T. D. Ting and Y.-K. Ho, *Biochemistry* **30,** 8996 (1991).

[12] Purification and Characterization of Phosducin from Bovine Retina

Rehwa H. Lee and Richard N. Lolley

Introduction

Phosducin (previously called the 33K protein) is a 33-kDa phosphoprotein that is found in photoreceptors of the vertebrate retina and in pinealocytes of the pineal gland (1–3). In its native conformation, phosducin exists as a 77-kDa heterotrimeric complex with the $\beta\gamma$ subunit of transducin ($T_{\beta\gamma}$) (4). The phosducin/$T_{\beta\gamma}$ complex is present in the photoreceptor at a level similar to that of transducin (5). However, unlike transducin, which is mostly concentrated in the outer segments, the phosducin/$T_{\beta\gamma}$ complex is dispersed throughout the cytosol of photoreceptor cells (1). Although phosducin shares with the α subunit of transducin (T_{α}) the ability to bind $T\beta\gamma$, it does not show homology to T_{α} or to any other polypeptide, except that encoded by the MEKA cDNA, currently listed in protein databanks (5–7).

Phosducin is phosphorylated *in vitro* and *in situ* by protein kinase A (8, 9) and dephosphorylated by phosphoprotein phosphatase 2A (10). In photoreceptor cells, the level of phosphorylated phosducin is highest in the dark and lowest in the light (11). Acting as a $T_{\beta\gamma}$-binding protein, phosducin inhibits the light-activated GTPase and phosphodiesterase activities of a reconstituted rod outer segment (ROS) system, and its inhibition can be reversed by the addition of exogenous $T_{\beta\gamma}$ (12). These biochemical features suggest that phosducin could play a strategic role in the regulation of photoreceptor function or metabolism. The availability of purified phosducin should facilitate the investigation of its functional role in photoreceptor activities.

Assay Method

Principle

During all steps of purification, phosducin is identified by its electrophoretic mobility (33 kDa) during sodium dodecyl sulfate–polyacrylamide gel electrophoresis (SDS-PAGE) and by its ability to be phosphorylated by [γ-^{32}P]ATP in a reaction catalyzed by the catalytic subunit (C) of protein kinase A, which is purified from rabbit skeletal muscle according to Beavo *et al.* (13).

Methods in Neurosciences, Volume 15

Procedure

The phosphorylation of phosducin is carried out in a 50-μl reaction mixture containing 62.5 mM 2-(N-morpholino)ethanesulfonate (MES), pH 6.9, 2 mM magnesium acetate, 2 mM 2-mercaptoethanol, 60 μM [γ-^{32}P]ATP (specific activity 200–500 cpm/pmol), 0.1–1 μg of C, and 10–20 μl of bovine retinal fraction. The reaction is started by the addition of ATP and stopped after 10 min of incubation at 30°C by the addition of 10 μl of stopping solution, containing 25% SDS, 25% 2-mercaptoethanol, 30% glycerol, and 0.1% bromphenol blue. After standing at room temperature for at least 30 min, the samples are applied to 12.5% polyacrylamide slab gels in the presence of SDS and electrophoresed according to the conditions of Laemmli (14). The gels are stained with Coomassie blue, destained, dried, and exposed at −70°C to Cronex X-ray film (Du Pont) in X-ray cassettes lined with Lightning-plus intensifying screens (Du Pont) for visualization of ^{32}P-labeled phosphoproteins. The apparent molecular size of retinal proteins is determined, using standards purchased from Pharmacia (Piscataway, NJ). The elution profiles of phosducin from various columns are determined by densitometric scanning of the ^{32}P-labeled 33-kDa phosducin band on the film.

Purification Procedure

Materials and Reagents

Dark-adapted frozen bovine retinas are purchased from J. A. & W. L. Lawson Co. (Lincoln, NE) and stored at −70°C until used. The DEAE-cellulose (DE-52) is purchased from Whatman Co. (Hillsboro, OR), hydroxylapatite from Bio-Rad Laboratories (Richmond, CA), Q-Sepharose from LKB-Pharmacia (Piscataway, NJ), and Ultrogel AcA 44 from Sepracor Inc. (Marlborough, MA).

Ringer's buffer: 10 mM 3-(N-morpholino)propanesulfonate (MOPS), pH 7.5 (25°C), with 60 mM KCl, 30 mM NaCl, 2 mM MgCl$_2$, 1 mM dithiothreitol (DTT), and 0.1 mM phenylmethyl sulfonyl fluoride (PMSF)

Buffer A: 10 mM potassium phosphate, pH 6.8, with 5 mM DTT, 0.1 mM PMSF, and 1 mM sodium benzamidine (BZMD)

Buffer B: 150 mM potassium phosphate, pH 7.0, with 1 mM EDTA, 5 mM DTT, 0.1 mM PMSF, and 1 mM BZMD

Buffer C: 110 mM Tris, pH 7.5 (25°C), with 1 mM EDTA, 5 mM DTT, 0.1 mM PMSF, and 1 mM BZMD

Buffer D: 10 mM MOPS, pH 7.5 (25°C), with 0.2 M NaCl, 0.2 mM
    EDTA, and 2 mM DTT
Buffer E: 300 mM Tris, pH 8.0 (25°C), with 1 mM EDTA, 5 mM DTT,
    0.1 mM PMSF, and 1 mM BZMD
Buffer F: same as buffer E, except with 800 mM Tris

Purification Steps

Preparation of Crude Retinal Extract

All procedures are performed in the cold room or in an ice bath unless
otherwise noted. Four hundred dark-adapted frozen retinas are thawed at
room temperature in the dark room under dim red light to about the consistency of ice cream. (Note: All supernatants and pellets must not be exposed
to light until noted.) The retinas are ground thoroughly with a cooled mortar
and pestle on ice while adding 50–75 ml of ice-cold Ringer's buffer prepared
with 55% (w/v) sucrose. The mixture is passed through a 60-ml syringe
equipped with an 18-gauge needle; the homogenate is collected in a 1-liter
graduated cylinder, and the volume is brought to 640 ml with the same 55%
sucrose–Ringer's solution, mixed thoroughly, distributed equally to 16 50-
ml Sorvall tubes, and centrifuged in a Sorvall SS-34 rotor at 15,000 rpm
(27,000 g) for 20 min.

The material clinging to the side of the centrifuge tube is scraped with a
rubber policeman, being careful not to disturb the pellet. The supernatants
containing the suspended ROS are carefully poured off into a 1-liter graduated
cylinder. An equivalent volume of ice-cold Ringer's buffer is added, and the
material is mixed thoroughly and then distributed equally to 28 50-ml tubes
for centrifugation at 18,000 rpm for 20 min. The resultant supernatant is used
as the starting material for phosducin purification and at this point may be
exposed to light. The pellets of crude ROS are wrapped in aluminum foil
and stored at -70°C for later use in the purification of transducin or phosphodiesterase.

DEAE-cellulose Chromatography

The crude retinal extract (~1 liter) is applied to a Whatman DE-52 column
(5 × 5 cm) preequilibrated in Ringer's buffer followed by a 200-ml wash
with the same buffer. The flow-through and wash containing the sucrose and
at least one-third of the contaminating retinal proteins are discarded. The
bound proteins are then eluted with 400 ml of Ringer's buffer with 0.2 M
NaCl. The flow rate is 5 ml/min, and the eluate (400 ml) is collected in a
1-liter beaker.

Extraction at pH 5.7

The pH of the eluate is brought to 5.7 with 1 M acetic acid. The resultant protein precipitate is removed and discarded by centrifugation at 12,500 rpm for 15 min in a GSA rotor. The pH of the supernatant is immediately adjusted to 7.0 with 1 M NaOH.

Precipitation by 70% Saturated Ammonium Sulfate

Proteins in the sample are precipitated with 70% saturated ammonium sulfate by gradual addition of the salt crystals (474 g/liter) with stirring. After 30 min of additional stirring, the protein precipitate is collected by centrifugation at 12,500 rpm for 20 min, resuspended in about 50 ml of buffer A, and dialyzed overnight in 4 liters of the same buffer to remove the excess salts.

Hydroxylapatite Chromatography

The dialyzate is clarified by centrifugation. The conductivity is measured and, if necessary, adjusted with deionized water to that of buffer A before the sample is applied to a hydroxylapatite column (2.6 × 24 cm) preequilibrated in the same buffer. After a 200-ml wash with the equilibriating buffer, the bound proteins are eluted with an 800-ml linear gradient between buffer A and B. The flow rate is 0.8 ml/min, and 8-ml fractions are collected. Phosducin elutes as a broad peak centering around 75 mM potassium phosphate. Fractions containing phosducin are pooled. During this step many of the contaminating retinal proteins are removed in the flow-through and wash; the Coomassie blue-stained phosducin and β-transducin bands become discernible in the pooled fraction.

Q-Sepharose Chromatography

The pooled phosducin is applied to a Q-Sepharose column (1.6 × 15 cm) preequilibrated in buffer C at 3 ml/min. After washing with 80 ml of buffer C, elution is carried out with a 400-ml linear gradient between 0 and 0.4 M NaCl; 3-ml fractions are collected. The phosducin peak centers around 190 mM NaCl, with its elution profile coinciding with the most predominant protein peak detected by absorbance at 280 nm (Fig. 1). At this stage, the phosducin band can be readily visualized and identified by Coomassie blue staining of the SDS–polyacrylamide gel (Fig. 1, inset), along with the β subunit of transducin which appears as a 37-kDa stained band coeluting with phosducin. (The γ subunit of transducin migrates with the dye front under the SDS-PAGE conditions and thus cannot be unambiguously identified and quantified by staining.)

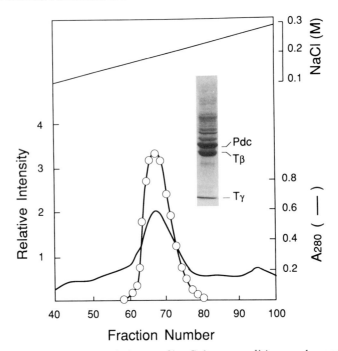

Fɪɢ. 1   Q-Sepharose column elution profile. Column conditions and procedures are as described in the text. The protein profile was monitored by absorbance at 280 nm with a ISCO UA-5 absorbance detector equipped with a type 6 optical unit. The elution profile of phosducin (○) was determined by densitometric scanning of the Coomassie blue-stained phosducin band. The identity of the phosducin band has been confirmed by a phosphorylation assay, which showed an essentially identical profile. The inset shows the Coomassie blue staining pattern of proteins in fraction 68 (Pdc, phosducin; T_β, β-transducin).

Concentration of Phosducin by Ammonium Sulfate Precipitation

The phosducin fractions are pooled (~35–40 ml), and proteins are precipitated by 70% saturated ammonium sulfate as described above and resuspended in 3 to 4 ml of buffer D.

Gel Filtration Chromatography

The concentrated phosducin sample is applied to an Ultrogel AcA 44 column (2.6 × 90 cm) preequilbrated in buffer D and eluted in the same buffer at 0.4 ml/min; 5-ml fractions are collected. The phosducin peak coincides with the single protein peak detected at 280 nm, and its elution position indicates that phosducin has a Stokes radius of about 40 Å and an apparent molecular weight of about 80,000. SDS-PAGE and Coomassie blue staining of the column fractions shows that phosducin coelutes with the $T_{\beta\gamma}$ subunit as part of a trimeric complex. Furthermore, the staining of the phosducin band and its associated β and γ bands constitutes about 95% of the total staining, indicating that the phosducin/$T_{\beta\gamma}$ complex is near homogeneity.

Dissociation of Phosducin and $T_{\beta\gamma}$ by Room Temperature Q-Sepharose Chromatography

Fractions from the Ultrogel gel column containing the phosducin/$T\beta\gamma$ complex are pooled and applied directly to a Q-Sepharose column (2.6 × 15 cm) which is preequilibrated at room temperature with buffer E. After sample application, elution is carried out with a 1.1-liter linear gradient between buffer E and F. The flow rate is 3 ml/min, and 8-ml fractions are collected. Phosducin and $T_{\beta\gamma}$ become dissociated during the elution, with the $T_{\beta\gamma}$ peak centering around 350 mM Tris, the phosducin peak around 650 mM, and the contaminating proteins eluting in between (Fig. 2). Fractions containing phosducin and $T_{\beta\gamma}$, respectively, are pooled, concentrated by ultrafiltration

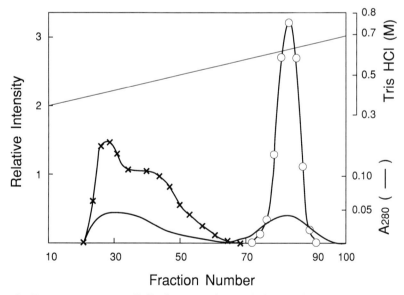

FIG. 2   Room temperature Q-Sepharose column elution profile. Column conditions and procedures are as described in the text. The elution profiles of phosducin (○) and β-transducin (×) were monitored by densitometric scanning of the Coomassie blue-stained phosducin and β-transducin bands.

over YM10 membranes (Amicon, Danvers, MA), dialyzed in buffer D with 40% glycerol, and stored at $-20°C$.

Comments

Because of the tight binding of the proteins, the procedures described result in the purification not only of phosducin but also its associated $T_{\beta\gamma}$. By careful selection of fractions from the last Q-Sepharose column, homogeneous phosducin and $T_{\beta\gamma}$ can be obtained. Using Coomassie blue-stained bovine serum albumin as the standard, it is estimated that about 3–4 mg of each protein can be routinely recovered from 400 frozen bovine retinas. It should be pointed out that, whereas the phosducin/$T_{\beta\gamma}$ complex is stable, phosducin alone is highly labile to proteolysis. Thus, it is advisable to concentrate and store the phosducin/$T_{\beta\gamma}$ complex recovered from the gel filtration column in buffer with 40% glycerol and dissociate the complex into phosducin and $T_{\beta\gamma}$ only when needed.

Properties of Bovine Transducin

The hydrodynamic properties of purified bovine retinal phosducin and phosducin/$T_{\beta\gamma}$ complex have been determined. Sedimentation velocity and gel filtration studies show that phosducin has a sedimentation coefficient of 2.7 S and a Stokes radius of 37 Å, whereas the phosducin/$T_{\beta\gamma}$ complex has a sedimentation coefficient of 4.9 S (Fig. 3) and a Stokes radius of 39.5 Å. The associated $T_{\beta\gamma}$ complex has a sedimentation coefficient of 3.3 S, but it behaves anomalously during gel filtration, apparently as a result of hydrophobic interaction with the gel matrix.

The complete amino acid sequence of bovine retinal phosducin has been determined by Edman degradation and by cDNA cloning (6, 7, 15). It is composed of 245 amino acids and has an isoelectric point of pH 4.5 (6, 11). Excluding the unidentified group which blocks its NH_2 terminus, phosducin has a calculated molecular mass of 28,185 daltons, which is considerably lower than the 33 kDa apparent molecular weight that is determined by its electrophoretic mobility during SDS-PAGE.

Phosducin is enriched with serine and threonine residues, of which serine residue 73 is the site of phosphorylation by protein kinase A, *in vitro* and *in situ* (8, 9). This phosphorylation site is conserved among phosducins of human and rat retinas and rat pineal, indicating that phosphorylation is important to the function of phosducin (3, 6, 15). It is found that the rate of phosducin phosphorylation by protein kinase A, but not dephosphorylation

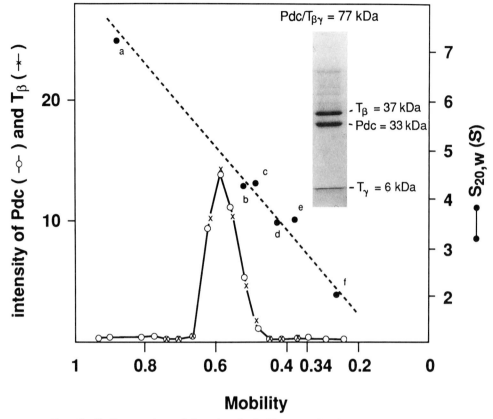

FIG. 3   Sedimentation of the phosducin/$T_{\beta\gamma}$ complex by sucrose density gradient centrifugation. Two hundred microliters of phosducin/$T_{\beta\gamma}$ complex recovered from the Ultrogel column was centrifuged on a 5–20% linear sucrose density gradient prepared in 5 mM MES, pH 6.9, 100 mM NaCl, 0.2 mM EDTA, and 15 mM 2-mercaptoethanol. The centrifugation was carried out in a Beckman SW40Ti rotor at 39,000 rpm at 4°C for 40 hr. After centrifugation, the gradient was recovered in 500-μl fractions, and the relative contents of phosducin and the β subunit of transducin in each fraction were determined by SDS-PAGE, Coomassie blue staining, and densitometric scanning of the stained phosducin (Pdc) ($\circ$) and transducin β subunit (T_β) ($\times$) bands. The sedimentation coefficient of the phosducin/$T_{\beta\gamma}$ complex ($s_{20,w} = 4.9$ S) was determined using alcohol dehydrogenase (a, 7.2 S), bovine serum albumin (b, 4.27 S), malate dehydrogenase (c, 4.3 S), horseradish peroxidase (d, 3.47 S), ovalbumin (e, 3.53 S), and myoglobin (f, 2.0 S) as standards.

by phosphatase 2A, is reduced by its being bound to $T_{\beta\gamma}$. Indeed, phosphorylation of phosducin is linked to its interaction with $T_{\beta\gamma}$, with phosphorylation of phosducin reducing its affinity for $T_{\beta\gamma}$.

Acknowledgments

This work was supported by Grants EY00395 and EY7860 from the U.S. Public Health Service, by the Retinitis Pigmentosa Foundation, and by the Veterans Administration Medical Service.

References

1. R. H. Lee, J. Whelan, R. N. Lolley, and J. McGinnis, *Exp. Eye Res.* **46,** 829 (1988).
2. A. H. Milam and S. G. Jacobson, *Opthalmology* (*Philadelphia*) **97,** 1620 (1990).
3. C. M. Craft, R. N. Lolley, M. F. Seldin, and R. H. Lee, *Genomics* **10,** 400 (1991).
4. R. H. Lee, B. Lieberman, and R. N. Lolley, *Biochemistry* **26,** 3983 (1987).
5. R. H. Lee, B. S. Lieberman, and R. N. Lolley, *Exp. Eye Res.* **51,** 325 (1990).
6. R. H. Lee, A. Fowler, J. F. McGinnis, R. N. Lolley, and C. M. Craft, *J. Biol. Chem.* **265,** 15867 (1990).
7. C.-H. Kuo, M. Akiyama, and N. Miki, *Mol. Brain Res.* **6,** 1 (1989).
8. R. H. Lee, B. M. Brown, and R. N. Lolley, *Biochemistry* **20,** 7532 (1981).
9. R. H. Lee, B. M. Brown, and R. N. Lolley, *J. Biol. Chem.* **265,** 15860 (1990).
10. R. H. Lee and B. M. Brown, *Invest. Ophthalmol. Visual Sci.* **32** (Suppl.), 1054 (1991).
11. R. H. Lee, B. M. Brown, and R. N. Lolley, *Biochemistry* **23,** 1972 (1984).
12. R. H. Lee, T. D. Ting, B. S. Lieberman, D. E. Tobias, R. N. Lolley, and Y.-K. Ho, *J. Biol. Chem.* **267,** 25104 (1992).
13. J. A. Beavo, P. J. Bechtel, and E. G. Krebs, *in* "Methods in Enzymology" (J. G. Hardman and B. W. O'Malley, eds.), Vol. 38, p. 299. Academic Press, New York, 1974.
14. U. K. Laemmli, *Nature* (*London*) **227,** 680 (1970).
15. T. Abe, H. Nakabayashi, H. Tamanoda, T. Takaqi, S. Sakuraqu, K. Yamaki, and T. Shinohara, *Gene* **91,** 209 (1990).

[13] pH Assay of Rod Outer Segment Cyclic GMP Phosphodiesterase Activity

Michael W. Kaplan and Krzysztof Palczewski

Background

The light-sensitive conductance of the plasma membrane of vertebrate photoreceptor outer segments is controlled by the cytoplasmic concentration of guanosine 3′,5′-cyclic monophosphate (cGMP). The net cytoplasmic concentration of cGMP is determined by the rate of synthesis from GTP and the rate of hydrolysis to 5′-GMP. Synthesis is catalyzed by a calcium-sensitive guanylate cyclase, whereas hydrolysis is mediated by cGMP phosphodiesterase (PDE). Hydrolysis of cGMP is initiated when inhibitory γ subunits of PDE are removed by the GTP-bound form of the α subunit of transducin, the photoreceptor-specific G protein that is activated by its interaction with photolyzed visual pigment molecules in photoreceptor disk membranes.

Liebman (1) first recognized that light-induced increases in the activity of PDE associated with rod outer segment (ROS) disk membranes can be readily monitored by measuring the generation of H^+ ions that result from the PDE-mediated hydrolysis of cGMP to 5′-GMP. Liebman and Evanczuk (2) later described how time-dependent measurements of the light-induced activity of photoreceptor PDE can be made by monitoring pH(t) of the reaction solution using a pH electrode coupled to a recording meter. Subsequently, measurements of pH have been used by a number of laboratories to monitor PDE activity and the light-activated reactions of visual transduction. In this chapter we describe the apparatus and mathematical analysis that we have used to digitally record pH(t) and to calculate $d[H^+]/dt$, the velocity of the PDE-mediated hydrolysis. We also demonstrate the effects of a number of initial conditions on the measurement of the light-induced activity of PDE, and propose a set of standard measurement conditions.

Methods

Preparation of Reaction Proteins and Membranes

The pH assay of PDE activity has been applied to homogenates of rod outer segments from frog or bovine retinas, as well as to reconstituted systems created from purified components of the visual transduction reaction sequence. Bovine ROS should be prepared from fresh retinas according to either Papermaster (3) or Schnetkamp and Daemen (4). The advantage of the second over the first method is negligible, since Ficoll must be removed before assaying PDE activity. The concentration of rhodopsin is measured spectrophotometrically in the presence of hydroxylamine, assuming a molar extinction coefficient ($\varepsilon_{498 \text{ nm}}$) of 40,600, using methods analogous to those of Wald and Brown (5). Once ROS are isolated from fresh retinas, they can be aliquoted and stored at $-80°C$ for 3–5 weeks. Frozen retinas are not suitable as starting material for isolating ROS for assays of PDE activity. Isolated ROS from frozen retinas contain significantly more contamination of retinal debris, particularly membranous material, than fresh retinas. ROS isolated from frozen retinas also contain much higher proteolytic activities, leading to proteolytic activation of PDE and to significantly more active light-independent activity.

Reconstituted systems can be prepared and assembled from purified components. Descriptions of the procedures for purifying reaction components can be found elsewhere in this volume. It is worth mentioning that rhodopsin should be in the native disk membranes rather than in reconstituted phospholipid vesicles, since the reconstituted vesicle system has, as yet, not been fully characterized. PDE can be purified as recommended by Kühn (6). Rhodopsin must be preincubated with transducin, PDE, and alternatively, rhodopsin kinase for a minimum of 40 min before assaying activity. In general, reconstituted systems are much more difficult to work with, since many more variables in such systems must be assessed and normalized.

Standard Buffer Conditions

Our standard buffer for use in assaying activity of PDE has the following composition: 100 mM KCl, 5 mM magnesium acetate, 3 mM cGMP, 100 μM GTP, 10 mM N-(2-hydroxyethyl)piperazine-N'-(2-ethanesulfonic acid) (HEPES), pH 8.0. Unless otherwise noted, all experiments described here were conducted using this buffer. The temperature of the reaction solution is maintained constant by a water-filled double-walled chamber containing circulating water from a water bath. The standard temperature for our experiments is 30°C.

Apparatus for Measuring Phosphodiesterase Activity

The general requirements and rationale for the measurement of pH changes induced by the photoactivation of rod outer segment PDE have been outlined previously in a comprehensive review by Liebman and Evanczuk (2). A pH electrode should be chosen that has fast enough response characteristics to allow the recording of time-dependent changes with high fidelity ($\tau < 0.5$ sec). We use a Ross semimicro combination electrode (Orion, Boston, MA, Model 8103) that has the required accuracy, stability, low noise, and fast response characteristics. We monitor the output of the pH electrode with a standard digital pH meter that has a low impedance analog output (Beckman, Fullerton, CA, Model Φ34). The analog signal from a dark-adapted reaction solution is sent to a low-drift differential amplifier, where an offset voltage is applied to produce an initial dark-adapted output voltage of 0 V. This output voltage is then amplified (100 or 200 times) using a dc 100-Hz bandpass amplifier to give a resolution of approximately 0.001 pH units. The amplified signal is converted to a digital format by an 11-bit analog-to-digital converter and recorded by a waveform analyzer having an appropriate time base.

Depending on the experimental conditions, a sampling rate of 10/sec to 1/sec is usually adequate to monitor light-induced pH changes. The recording apparatus should have enough memory to record data for a minimum of 100 sec in order to resolve the activation and inactivation of PDE under most conditions. These instrumentation requirements for recording data are met by a wide variety of computer-based data acquisition systems or by a digital oscilloscope with appropriate memory and digital output capabilities.

Actinic Light Source

As a source of activating light, we use a highly reproducible xenon flash lamp (Vivitar, Santa Monica, CA, Model 238) that has a half-peak duration of 1.2 msec. The intensity of the lamp is attenuated by a slit aperture and can be adjusted by changing the distance between the lamp and the sample or by inserting neutral density filters.

Data Analysis

The time-dependent output of the pH meter can be plotted as pH(t). We calibrate our measurements of pH by sequentially adding several 30- to 60-μl aliquots of calibrated 50 mM HCl (150–300 nanomoles of H$^+$) to 600 μl of sample buffer before starting each series of experiments, although the system can easily be adapted to use volumes as small as 200 μl. Others have calibrated measurements of PDE activation by back-titrating with either KOH or NaOH (2, 7). The calibrated responses of the recording apparatus and of the pH meter are used to convert measured light-induced voltage changes to plots of pH(t) for given conditions of buffering capacity of the reaction mixture. The voltage recordings can also be converted to a plot of moles of cGMP hydrolyzed as a function of time or, equivalently, changes in [H^+]. To measure the rate at which PDE converts cGMP to 5'-GMP, the velocity of the reaction can be measured or computed from the slope of the plot of changes in [H^+].

As pointed out by Barkdoll *et al.* (8), if the concentration of cGMP available for hydrolysis greatly exceeds the K_m of the reaction ($K_m \approx 1$ mM), then the velocity of the reaction is proportional to the concentration of activated PDE. Liebman and Pugh (9) demonstrated that computing $d[H^+]/dt$, the first derivative of the plot, is useful for determining the maximum rate of the PDE-mediated hydrolysis of cGMP under different experimental conditions. The plot of the first derivative is also useful for characterizing the kinetics of both the activation and the inactivation of the reaction. Barkdoll *et al.* (8) used first derivative plots of light-induced PDE activity at varying concentrations of Ca^{2+} and nucleotide triphosphates to measure t_{peak}, the time to reach the maximum rate of hydrolysis, V_{peak}, the maximum hydrolytic velocity at t_{peak}, and τ_{off}, the time constant of the decay in the reaction velocity during inactivation. Similar parameters have been used by Schmidt and Yguerabide (7, 10) to model the kinetics of PDE activation and inactivation.

We use a relatively simple algorithm to compute $d[H^+]/dt$ that is based on the method described by Savitsky and Golay (11). For any set of discrete points $Y(n)$ describing the ordinate values of a reasonably smooth, continuous function measured at a uniform interval on an abscissa (time axis), the first derivative of the function at any point N can be computed from a 25-point least-squares convolution:

$$D(N) \equiv \frac{dY(N)}{dt} = \left(\sum_{j=-12}^{12} [j \times Y(N+j)] \right)/1300$$

If necessary, noise in the plot of $D(n) = dY(n)/dt$ can be smoothed to give the function $S(n)$ by the iterative application of a 15-point least-squares smoothing convolution. For any point N, the value of the smoothed function is given by

$$S(N) = \left(\sum_{j=-7}^{7} [b_j \times D(N+j)] \right)/1105$$

where $b_0 = 167$, $b_1 = b_{-1} = 162$, $b_2 = b_{-2} = 147$, $b_3 = b_{-3} = 122$, $b_4 = b_{-4} = 84$, $b_5 = b_{-5} = 42$, $b_6 = b_{-6} = -13$, and $b_7 = b_{-7} = -78$. We have implemented these differentiation and smoothing algorithms in a simple computer program written in Microsoft QuickBasic that is available from the authors on request.

Factors Affecting Phosphodiesterase Activation and Inactivation

Prior Studies

A large number of prior studies have used the pH assay of light-induced PDE activity to document effects of varying the reaction constituents and conditions. A partial list includes varying concentrations of cGMP, ATP, GDP, GTP, Gpp(NH)p, and Ca^{2+} (2, 7–9, 12–16). Some of the effects of varying bleaching levels have also been documented (9, 12).

Effects of Initial pH of Buffer Solution

As noted by Yee and Liebman (12), PDE hydrolysis of cGMP to 5′-GMP exposes a phosphoryl acidic group (pK 6.3) that is 98% ionized at an optimum buffer pH of 8.0. At other pH values, the ionization is not as complete, and fewer H^+ ions are evolved per mole of cGMP hydrolyzed. The measured effects of initial pH of the sample buffer on apparent PDE activity are shown in Fig. 1. The maximum light-induced change in $[H^+]$ occurs at pH 8.0. The reaction also attains its highest apparent velocity at pH 8.0.

Effects of Buffer Capacity

Predictably, light-induced pH changes depend on the ionic strength and buffering capacity of the buffer used in the reaction solution. However, we have found that light-induced changes in $[H^+]$ can also depend on the concentration of the buffering molecule. A common assay buffer used in many laboratories investigating visual transduction reactions, including ours, contains 10 mM HEPES. As anticipated, when higher concentrations of HEPES are used, we observe smaller light-induced changes in pH (Fig. 2A,B). Unexpectedly, however, when appropriate calibration factors are applied to the recordings, the resulting plots show that light-induced changes in $[H^+]$ and the rate of evolution of H^+ ions actually increase when using either 50 mM or 100 mM HEPES (Fig. 2C,D). We tentatively attribute this enhanced rate of H^+ evolution at higher HEPES concentrations to a stimulation of PDE, possibly caused by the interaction of HEPES molecules with the noncatalytic cGMP binding site of PDE. An analogous stimulatory effect has been reported for dipyridamole, a drug that either stimulates or inhibits PDE depending on its concentration (17).

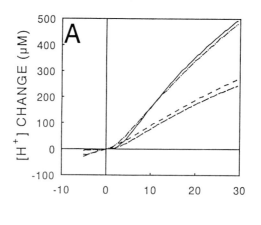

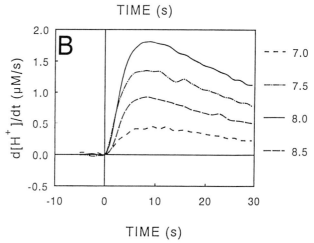

FIG. 1   (A) Light-induced changes in H^+ concentration caused by PDE-mediated hydrolysis of cGMP to 5′-GMP and (B) rate of H^+ production reflecting PDE reaction velocity for initial pH values of 7.0, 7.5, 8.0, and 8.5. The maximum rate of H^+ production occurs near pH 8.0. Note that the light-independent rate of H^+ production has been subtracted from plots of $d[H^+]/dt$ in all of the figures.

Effects of Initial Concentration of 5′-GMP

We evaluated the possibility that elevated concentrations of 5′-GMP, the hydrolysis product of cGMP, can alter the light-induced activity of PDE. As seen in Fig. 3, concentrations of up to 2 mM 5′-GMP have no significant effects on PDE-mediated hydrolysis.

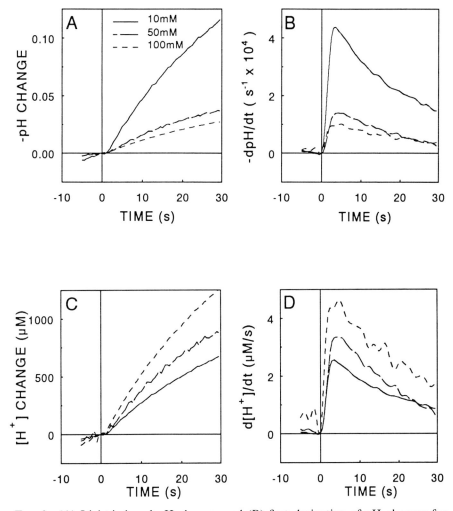

FIG. 2   (A) Light-induced pH changes and (B) first derivative of pH changes for HEPES buffer concentrations of 10, 50, and 100 mM. Increasing buffer capacity reduces the observed changes and rates of change in pH. In contrast, plots of (C) changes in [H$^+$] or (D) changes in the rate of H$^+$ production show that higher concentrations of HEPES buffer actually stimulate the light-induced, PDE-mediated hydrolysis of cGMP to 5'-GMP.

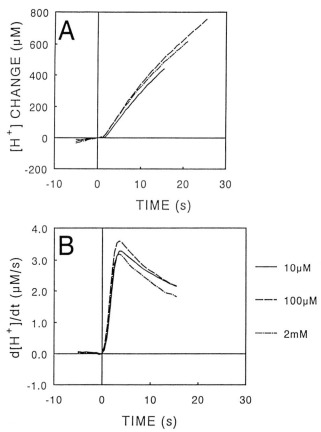

FIG. 3   (A) Light-induced changes in [H$^+$] and (B) changes in the rate of H$^+$ production in the presence of 10 μM, 100 μM, or 2 mM 5′-GMP. The product of PDE-
mediated hydrolysis of cGMP has no apparent effects on the kinetics of the reaction
at concentrations of up to 2 mM.

Effects of Fractional Bleaching Levels of Rhodopsin

We tested the effects of changing the fraction of rhodopsin bleached. Our
standard actinic flash bleaches 0.0020 of the rhodopsin in our test solution.
As seen in Fig. 4, when we decrease the fractional bleach level to 0.0012,
the rate of activation and the peak velocity of the reaction decrease proportionally; the rate of inactivation is not affected. When we increase the fractional bleach to 0.0027, the rate of activation and the peak velocity of the
reaction increases proportionally. However, we consistently find that the

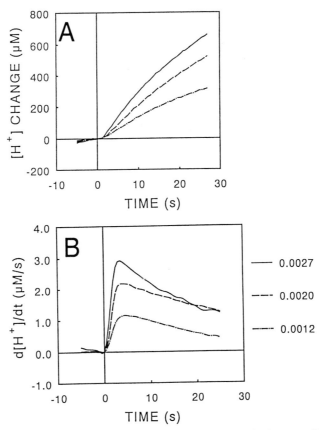

FIG. 4   (A) Light-induced changes in $[H^+]$ and (B) changes in the rate of H^+ production for fractional bleaches of 0.0027, 0.0020, and 0.0012. The maximum velocity of
PDE-mediated hydrolysis of cGMP varies nearly linearly over this range of fractional
bleaches. The activation time constant is not significantly different for the three
bleaching levels tested, but the time constant of inactivation is consistently shorter
at a fractional bleach of 0.0027 than for the lower fractional bleaches.

time constant for inactivation of the reaction is faster than at lower bleaching levels.

Effects of Temperature

The sequence of activation and inactivation of the various reactions of the
visual transduction cascade is complex and interdependent. Therefore, it is
difficult to predict *a priori* how temperature-dependent rate changes in the

multiple reactions of visual transduction will affect the overall rate of activation and inactivation of PDE. As shown in Fig. 5B, changing the temperature
of the reaction can affect activation and inactivation differently. Increasing
the temperature from 10 to 20°C substantially increases the peak velocity of
light-induced PDE hydrolysis of cGMP because the rate of increase for the
reaction is higher. However, the time constants for activation and inactivation are unchanged. Raising the temperature from 20 to 30°C does not change
the activation rate, suggesting that there is a rate-limiting step with a tempera-

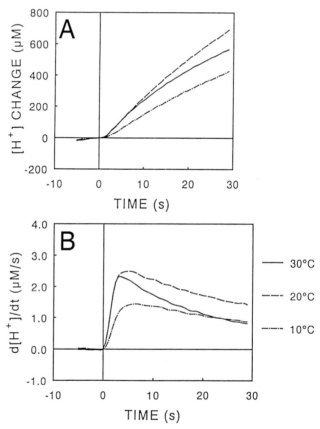

FIG. 5   (A) Light-induced changes in [H$^+$] and (B) changes in the rate of H$^+$ production for temperatures of 30, 20, and 10°C. The time constants for activation and
inactivation appear similar at 10 and 20°C, although the peak reaction velocity at
10°C is significantly lower. The rates of activation at 20 and 30°C are nearly identical,
but inactivation at 30°C is much faster than at 10 or 20°C, suggesting that rate-limiting
steps for activation and for inactivation are different.

ture dependence that saturates between the two temperatures. The time constant for inactivation, however, is substantially faster at 30 than at 20°C. Thus, the temperature dependence of the rate-limiting step for activation and the temperature dependence of the rate-limiting step for inactivation are controlled differently.

Standardizing Reaction Conditions

The examples given here demonstrate that experimental conditions must be carefully chosen and documented when using the pH assay of light-induced PDE activity. The choice of initial pH, buffer species, buffer capacity, bleaching fraction, and temperature can all affect the time-dependent characteristics of the evolution of H^+ ions when cGMP is hydrolyzed to 5'-GMP. These factors can make comparisons of results between different laboratories problematic if different experimental conditions are used. In our hands, the following standard conditions give the most reliable and reproducible results for determining the light-induced activation of PDE in bovine disk membranes: 10 mM HEPES buffer, pH 8.0, 5 mM magnesium acetate, 3 mM cGMP, 100 μM GTP, 0.0020 fractional bleach, and 30°C.

Acknowledgments

This work was supported by U.S. Public Health Service Grant EY 09339 to K.P. and grants from the Oregon Lions Sight and Hearing Foundation.

References

1. P. A. Liebman, *Ann. N.Y. Acad. Sci.* **307,** 642 (1978).
2. P. A. Liebman and T. Evanczuk, *in* "Methods in Enzymology," (L. Packer, ed.), Vol. 81, p. 532. Academic Press, New York, 1982.
3. D. S. Papermaster, *in* "Methods in Enzymology" (L. Packer, ed.), Vol. 81, p. 48. Academic Press, New York, 1982.
4. P. P. M. Schnetkamp and F. J. M. Daemen, *in* "Methods in Enzymology," (L. Packer, ed.), Vol. 81, p. 110. Academic Press, New York, 1982.
5. G. Wald and P. K. Brown, *J. Gen. Physiol.* **37,** 189 (1953).
6. H. Kühn, *in* "Current Topics in Membranes and Transport" (W. H. Miller, ed.), Vol. 15, p. 171. Academic Press, New York, 1981.
7. J. A. Schmidt and J. Yguerabide, *J. Biol. Chem.* **264,** 19790 (1989).
8. A. E. Barkdoll, III, E. N. Pugh, Jr., and A. Sitaramayya, *J. Gen. Physiol.* **93,** 1091 (1989).

9. P. A. Liebman and E. N. Pugh, Jr., *Vision Res.* **19,** 375 (1979).

10. J. Yguerabide and J. A. Schmidt, *J. Biol. Chem.* **264,** 19804 (1989).

11. A. Savitsky and M. J. E. Golay, *Anal. Chem.* **36,** 1627 (1964).

12. R. Yee and P. A. Liebman, *J. Biol. Chem.* **253,** 8902 (1978).

13. S. Kawamura and M. D. Bownds, *J. Gen. Physiol.* **77,** 571 (1981).

14. A. Sitaramayya and P. A. Liebman, *J. Biol. Chem.* **258,** 1205 (1983).

15. N. J. Cook, G. Nullans, and N. Virmaux, *Biochim. Biophys. Acta* **883,** 63 (1986).

16. A. E. Barkdoll, III, E. N. Pugh, Jr., and A. Sitaramayya, *J. Neurochem.* **50,** 839 (1988).

17. P. G. Gillespie and J. A. Beavo, *Mol. Pharmacol.* **36,** 773 (1989).

[14] Purification of Rhodopsin Kinase from Bovine Rod Outer Segments

Krzysztof Palczewski

Introduction

In vertebrate retinal rod cells, the absorption of a photon of light by rhodopsin triggers the activation of a G protein (transducin). Several hundred G proteins are activated by one molecule of photoexcited receptor (1). To terminate the signal, rhodopsin must be inactivated. The enzymatic phosphorylation of rhodopsin leads to the binding of arrestin to phosphorylated rhodopsin, which results in the turnoff of the amplification of the light signal.

In 1972–1973, three laboratories reported that rhodopsin underwent light-dependent phosphorylation by ATP in an *in vitro* reaction (2–4). The reaction was soon demonstrated to occur *in vivo* (5). Rhodopsin kinase proved to be difficult to purify and stabilize, and as a result, hindered the study of its role in the rod cell. However, since the late 1980s the enzyme has been purified, its sequence has been determined, antibodies have been raised, and the kinetics of the phosphorylation reaction has been studied (for review, see Ref. 6).

Sequence information revealed that rhodopsin kinase is a member of a novel family of protein kinases, namely, the G-protein-coupled receptor protein kinases (6, 7). It was also apparent that rhodopsin kinase could be posttranslationally modified. The C-terminal sequence of rhodopsin kinase reveals a consensus sequence for isoprenylation, CysAaaAaaXaa, which is followed by limited proteolysis of AaaAaaXaa and subsequent methylation of isoprenylated Cys. The N-terminal region contains the sequence MetAsp-PheGlySerLeuGluThr—, which could be a potential site of myristoylation at GlySerLeuGluThr, after proteolytic processing of the rhodopsin kinase native polypeptide chain. Rhodopsin kinase is known to be modified by autophosphorylation (8–10), at the N and C-terminal ends of the enzyme (11).

Several methods of purification have been developed for rhodopsin kinase (9, 12–17). Most methods are laborious and yield dilute solutions of kinase with low specific activity, often contaminated by other rod outer segment (ROS) proteins. The method described here takes advantage of a posttranslational modification of rhodopsin kinase and represents a simple, rapid, highly reproducible, and economical method for purification of the enzyme. This novel method is based on the finding that autophosphorylated forms of rho dopsin kinase bind with different affinities to heparin–Sepharose and can be separated by a salt gradient (10) (Fig. 1). The dephosphorylated form of rhodopsin kinase requires high ionic strength in order to elute it from the column, whereas the autophosphorylated form is eluted by moderate salt concentration. Rhodopsin kinase is prepared in its dephosphorylated form and bound to heparin–Sepharose; then ATP is loaded, and the kinase is allowed to undergo autophosphorylation. Autophosphorylated kinase at moderate ionic strength is specifically eluted in a one-step chromatographic procedure yielding a homogeneous protein. Use of the detergent Tween 80 (saturated with phospholipids) significantly improves both the extractability of rhodopsin kinase and its chromatographic properties.

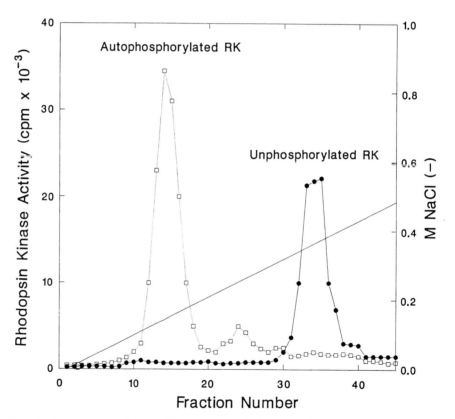

FIG. 1   Chromatographic profile of rhodopsin kinase using a heparin–Sepharose column. Chromatography of the dephosphorylated form of rhodopsin and fully phosphorylated rhodopsin kinase has been described (10). [Chromatographic profiles are adapted from J. Buczyłko, C. Gutmann, and K. Palczewski, *Proc. Natl. Acad. Sci. U.S.A.* **88,** 8715 (1991).]

Methods

All procedures should be performed on ice, or at 5°C.

Purification of Rhodopsin Kinase from Bovine Rod Outer Segments

Isolation of Rod Outer Segments

Rod outer segments are prepared from 75 fresh bovine retinas. For our preparations, eyes are obtained locally and transported to the laboratory in a light-tight container on ice. The retinas are dissected under dim red illumination. Isolation of the ROS is done under room illumination essentially as described by Papermaster (18). Extensive bleaching of rhodopsin is avoided.

Mg^{2+} Extraction

The ROS are resuspended in 50 ml (50 ml/75 retinas) of 10 mM 1,3-bis[tris (hydroxymethyl)methylamino]propane (bis-tris propane, BTP) buffer, pH 7.5, containing 5 mM $MgCl_2$, 0.5 mM benzamidine, and 20 μg/ml leupeptin. The ROS are homogenized by 5 strokes of a glass–glass homogenizer (tissue grinder, Fisher, Pittsburgh, PA, 08414B). The homogenized sample is illuminated on ice using a 150-W lamp for 2 min. The bleached suspension of ROS is centrifuged for 10 min at 47,000 g. The membrane pellet is used for the kinase extraction, while the supernatant is removed and frozen at -70°C for further p^{26} (recoverin) purification [see Polans et al. (19)].

Extraction of Rhodopsin Kinase

The extraction solution should be prepared in advance. The composition of the solution is 20 mM BTP buffer, pH 8.3, containing 0.25% Tween 80 (Sigma, St. Louis, MO, P1754), 240 mM KCl, 1 mM EDTA, 8 mg/ml phosphatidylcholine (Sigma, P3644), and 1 mM benzamidine. Before use this milky solution must be centrifuged at 30,000–47,000 g for 20 min to eliminate particles. Just prior to use in the extraction procedure, 200 mM hydroxylamine is added to the solution to obtain a final concentration of 10 mM. Rhodopsin kinase is obtained by extracting the ROS pellet 3 times with 12 ml of the extracting solution (12 ml/75 retinas). Membranes are homogenized (glass–glass homogenizer, 5 strokes) with 12 ml of extraction solution. The first homogenate is bleached using a 150-W lamp at a distance of 10 cm for 10 min at 0°C, to quench photolyzed rhodopsin. The homogenate is centrifuged at 30,000 g for 10 min. The supernatant is removed and set aside for subsequent dialysis. The pellet is resuspended in 12 ml of extraction solution and again homogenized. The second homogenate is then bleached on ice for

5 min. The homogenate is centrifuged, the supernatant removed, and the pellet resuspended and homogenized. The third homogenate is then centrifuged without any further illumination. The supernatant is removed and saved, and the pellet is discarded. Aliquots from each of the three extracts are removed to assay for kinase activity.

The three extracts are each dialyzed overnight at 4°C against 10 mM BTP, pH 7.5, containing 0.4% Tween 80. The dialysis tubing should be tied with room for volume expansion since a high salt solution is being dialyzed against a hypotonic solution. Dialysis tubing with a molecular weight cutoff of 1000 is used (Spectrum).

Purification of Rhodopsin Kinase by Heparin–Sepharose Column Chromatography

A heparin–Sepharose (Pharmacia, Piscataway, NJ) column (1 × 10 cm) is equilibrated with 10 mM BTP buffer, pH 7.5, containing 0.4% Tween 80. The column material must be degassed before pouring. The extracts containing the majority of the kinase activity are loaded onto the column (flow rate 20 ml/hr). (*Note:* If the third extract contains less than 10% of the total kinase activity, it can be discarded.) The column is washed with 10 mM BTP buffer, pH 7.5, containing 0.4% Tween 80, until the absorbance at 280 nm drops below 0.01. The column is then washed with a 10 mM BTP buffer, pH 7.5, containing 125 mM KCl, 1 mM $MgCl_2$, and 0.4% Tween 80 until the absorbance at 280 nm drops below 0.01. The column is subsequently washed with 6 ml of 10 mM BTP buffer, pH 7.5, containing 100 mM KCl, 1 mM $MgCl_2$, and 0.4% Tween 80, to avoid isocratic elution of contaminating proteins. The flow rate is then slowed to 12 ml/hr, and rhodopsin kinase is eluted with 10 mM BTP buffer, pH 7.5, containing 100 mM KCl, 1 mM $MgCl_2$, 0.4% Tween 80, and 0.2 mM ATP. Fractions (1.4 ml) are collected and assayed for kinase activity. Proteins from the fractions containing activity are visualized using sodium dodecyl sulfate–polyacrylamide gel electrophoresis (SDS-PAGE) (20) (Fig. 2). One hundred micrograms of homogeneous rhodopsin kinase can be obtained from 75 bovine retinas (Table I).

The column is regenerated by washing with 5 M urea in water followed by 1 M NaCl or 1 M KCl in buffer. Store with 0.02% azide in water if the column will sit for more than 1 or 2 weeks.

Assay of Rhodopsin Kinase Activity

Preparation of Rod Outer Segments Washed by Urea

To prepare a substrate for rhodopsin kinase, ROS are washed under dim red illumination with 5 M urea to eliminate endogenous rhodopsin kinase

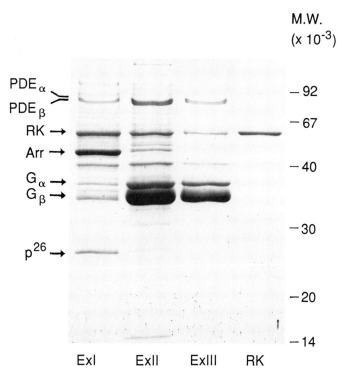

FIG. 2   Electrophoresis of rhodopsin kinase extracts and purified rhodopsin kinase. Extracts I, II, and III (12 μl) and 2 μg of purified rhodopsin kinase (purified by heparin–Sepharose chromatography and ATP elution) were loaded on the gel. PDE, Phosphodiesterase; G_α and G_β, transducin subunits; RK, rhodopsin kinase; Arr, arrestin; p^{26}, recoverin.

TABLE I   Purification of Rhodopsin Kinase

Purification step	Volume (ml)	Protein (mg)	Activity (nmol P_i/min)	Specific activity (nmol P_i/min/mg)
Rod outer segments	50.0	28.7	647.0	22.5
Mg^{2+} extract	45.0	1.6	4.7	2.9
Extract I	10.0	1.9	219.0	76.0
Extract II	11.0	1.8	189.0	105.0
Extract III	11.0	1.3	83.0	64.0
Heparin–Sepharose chromatography	20.0	0.1	55.0	555.0

activity as described by Shichi *et al.* (12). ROS from 100 bovine retinas are resuspended with 50 ml of 5 *M* urea in 10 m*M* HEPES buffer, pH 7.5. The suspension is kept for 15 min at room temperature, and membranes are collected by centrifugation (47,000 *g* for 35 min). Membranes are washed 5 times with 10 m*M* HEPES buffer, pH 7.5, containing 100 m*M* NaCl, and resuspended in the HEPES buffer at a concentration of 3.6 mg/ml. Urea-washed rhodopsin maintains its structural integrity, as determined by absorption at 500 nm, and has little or no rhodopsin kinase activity. It is important that ROS not be exposed for longer than 15 min to 5 *M* urea at room temperature, since prolonged exposure leads to a decrease in the phosphorylation of rhodopsin by the kinase.

Assay Procedure

Rhodopsin kinase activity is measured using urea-washed ROS membranes as the substrate. The reaction mixture (140–300 μl) contains 20 μ*M* urea-washed ROS, 2 m*M* MgCl$_2$, and 100 μ*M* [γ-^{32}P]ATP (100–1000 cpm/pmol) in 20 m*M* BTP buffer, pH 7.5, in a 1.6-ml Eppendorf microtube. Phosphorylation is initiated by illumination and addition of radioactive ATP, and triplicate samples are illuminated for 5, 7.5, and 10 min, to ensure that the reaction is linear with respect to the amount of rhodopsin kinase versus time. The reaction is terminated by adding 10% trichloroacetic acid (~1 ml). Protein is collected by centrifugation (14,000 g for 3 min, using an Eppendorf centrifuge, Model 5415C, Westbury, NY), and the pellet is washed repeatedly with 10% trichloroacetic acid until the counts in the wash are less than 500 cpm. The pellet is then dissolved in 400 μl of 100% formic acid and mixed with 5 ml of scintillation fluid (Ultra Gold, Packard, Meridean, CT). The activity is expressed as nanomoles of P$_i$ transferred from ATP to rhodopsin during 1 min per milligram of rhodopsin kinase.

Assessment of Purity

The purity of rhodopsin kinase should be assessed using SDS-PAGE. Additionally, the specific activity of the enzyme ranges between 500 and 800 nmol phosphate/transferred from ATP to rhodopsin during 1 min per 1 mg of rhodopsin kinase (16). The concentration of rhodopsin kinase can be determined using the micro-Bradford method (21). Because high concentrations of Tween 80 (>0.05%) interact with the dye, amino acid analysis should be applied for determination of the rhodopsin kinase concentration in a dilute solution.

Properties of Purified Rhodopsin Kinase

Stability

Rhodopsin kinase prepared by this method is stable for 1 week at 0°C. When rhodopsin kinase was stored at -20°C, improvement in stability was observed in 20% adonitol (16).

Molecular Weight and Posttranslational Modification

The molecular weight for the native polypeptide chain of rhodopsin kinase calculated from its amino acid sequence is 62,934 (7). It is important to note, however, that rhodopsin kinase may be posttranslationally modified by farnesylation at the C-terminal end and by myristoylation at the N-terminal end (7). Rhodopsin kinase also undergoes extensive autophosphorylation (3 to 4 phosphates per molecule) (10). Although these residues do not significantly influence the overall molecular weight, they may have a measurable effect on the mobility of rhodopsin kinase on hydrophobic gels or during SDS-PAGE (e.g., see Ref. 10).

Specificity

Rhodopsin kinase is a highly specific protein kinase (Table I) (22–24). It phosphorylates photolyzed rhodopsin (25), but not opsin (25) or rhodopsin (26). It is still unknown whether rhodopsin kinase phosphorylates exclusively metarhodopsin II (27) or other conformations of rhodopsin as well (28). Moreover, rhodopsin kinase phosphorylates photolyzed iodopsin (29), chicken red pigment, and agonist-occupied β-adrenergic receptor (30). Rhodopsin kinase also shows remarkable specificity toward ATP rather than GTP (Table II).

Inhibitors and Activators of Rhodopsin Kinase

Inhibitors of rhodopsin kinase include polyanions (31), some peptides derived from the surface of rhodopsin (9, 26, 31), and several nucleotides and nucleosides (32). Sangivamycin is one of the most useful inhibitors of rhodopsin kinase (33). Conversely, rhodopsin kinase is stimulated by polycations and also requires extra Mg^{2+} for maximum activity (26).

TABLE II   Specificity of Bovine Rhodopsin Kinase

Substrate	K_m (μM)	K_m/V_{max} (sec^{-1} M^{-1} × 10^{-6})	Ref.
Nucleotide			
ATP at 1 mM Mg^{2+}	1.6	0.46	16
ATP at 10 mM Mg^{2+}	5.2	0.14	16
GTP at 2 mM Mg^{2+}	1000.0	0.00001	16
Protein/peptide substrate			
Rho*[a] in native disk membranes	4.0	0.2	16
Rho* reconstituted	0.63	—	9
C-Terminal peptide (324–348)[b]	7800.0	0.000007	31

[a] Light-activated rhodopsin.
[b] Sequence derived from the C terminus of bovine rhodopsin.

Acknowledgments

I thank Drs. Janina Buczyłko and Arthur Polans for advice in the preparation of the manuscript. This research was supported by U.S. Public Health Service Grant EY 08061 and by a grant from the Human Frontiers in Science Program. The author is the recipient of a Jules and Doris Stein Research to Prevent Blindness Professorship.

References

1. M. Kahlert and K. P. Hofmann, *Biophys. J.* **59**, 375 (1991).
2. D. Bownds, J. Dawes, J. Miller, and M. Stahlman, *Nature (London) New Biol.* **237**, 125 (1972).
3. R. N. Frank, H. D. Cavanagh, and K. R. Kenyon, *J. Biol. Chem.* **248**, 596 (1973).
4. H. Kühn and W. J. Dreyer, *FEBS Lett.* **20**, 1 (1972).
5. H. Kühn, *Nature (London)* **250**, 588 (1974).
6. K. Palczewski and J. L. Benovic, *Trends Biol. Sci.* **16**, 387 (1991).
7. W. Lorenz, J. Inglese, K. Palczewski, J. J. Onorato, M. G. Caron, and R. J. Lefkowitz, *Proc. Natl. Acad. Sci. U.S.A.* **88**, 8715 (1991).
8. R. H. Lee, B. M. Brown, and R. N. Lolley, *Biochemistry* **21**, 3303 (1982).
9. D. J. Kelleher and G. L. Johnson, *J. Biol. Chem.* **261**, 4749 (1986).
10. J. Buczyłko, C. Gutmann, and K. Palczewski, *Proc. Natl. Acad. Sci. U.S.A.* **88**, 8715 (1991).
11. K. Palczewski, J. Buczyłko, P. Van Hooser, S. A. Carr, M. J. Huddleston, and J. W. Crabb, *J. Biol. Chem.* **267**, 18991 (1992).
12. H. Shichi and R. L. Somers, *J. Biol. Chem.* **253**, 7040 (1978).
13. H. Shichi, R. L. Somers, and K. Yamamoto, *in* "Methods in Enzymology"

(J. D. Corbin and J. G. Hardman, eds.), Vol. 99, p. 362. Academic Press, New York, 1983.

14. M. Feraudi, *Experientia* **39,** 586 (1983).

15. A. Sitaramayya, *Biochemistry* **25,** 5460 (1986).

16. K. Palczewski, J. H. McDowell, and P. A. Hargrave, *J. Biol. Chem.* **263,** 14067 (1988).

17. G. Okada and A. Ikai, *Anal. Biochem.* **169,** 428 (1988).

18. D. S. Papermaster, *in* "Methods in Enzymology" (L. Packer, ed.), Vol. 81, p. 81. Academic Press, New York, 1982.

19. A. S. Polans, J. Crabb, and K. Palczewski, this volume [17].

20. U. K. Laemmli, *Nature (London)* **227,** 680 (1970).

21. M. M. Bradford, *Anal. Biochem.* **72,** 248 (1976).

22. C. Fowles, R. Sharma, and M. Akhtar, *FEBS Lett.* **238,** 56 (1988).

23. B. M. Binder, M. S. Biernbaum, and M. D. Bownds, *J. Biol. Chem.* **265,** 15333 (1990).

24. K. Palczewski, J. Buczyłko, M. W. Kaplan, A. S. Polans, and J. W. Crabb, *J. Biol. Chem.* **266,** 12949 (1991).

25. H. Kühn, *Biochemistry* **17,** 4389 (1978).

26. K. Palczewski, J. H. McDowell, and P. A. Hargrave, *Biochemistry* **27,** 2306 (1988).

27. B. Seckler and R. R. Rando, *Biochem. J.* **264,** 489 (1989).

28. R. Paulsen and J. Bentrop, *Nature (London)* **302,** 417 (1983).

29. J. L. Benovic, F. Mayer, Jr., R. L. Somers, M. G. Caron, and R. J. Lefkowitz, *Nature (London)* **321,** 869 (1986).

30. Y. Fukada, K. Kokame, T. Okano, Y. Shichida, T. Yoshizawa, J. H. McDowell, P. A. Hargrave, and K. Palczewski, *Biochemistry* **29,** 10102 (1990).

31. K. Palczewski, A. Arendt, J. H. McDowell, and P. A. Hargrave, *Biochemistry* **28,** 8764 (1989).

32. K. Palczewski, N. Kahn, and P. A. Hargrave, *Biochemistry* **29,** 6276 (1990).

33. K. Palczewski, G. Rispoli, and P. B. Detweiler, *Neuron* **8,** 1 (1992).

[15] Purification of Arrestin from Bovine Retinas

Janina Buczyłko and Krzysztof Palczewski

Introduction

The binding of arrestin (also referred to as the 48K protein or S-antigen) to freshly bleached phosphorylated rhodopsin occurs rapidly (<200 msec) and quenches the activation of G protein (transducin) (1–4). We have shown that arrestin also acts in the phototransduction process by blocking rapid dephosphorylation of phosphorylated and photolyzed rhodopsin until activated rhodopsin decays (5). The dissociation of arrestin from the photoreceptor protein occurs when photolyzed rhodopsin is completely deactivated by the removal of the photoisomerized chromophore, all-*trans*-retinal (6).

The amino acid sequence of arrestin was determined first for bovine arrestin (7), and the sequence has now been determined for an additional five species. Arrestin contains a relatively high proportion of nonpolar amino acids (55%) that are assembled in a β-sheet conformation (7, 8). However, very little is known about the biochemical/biophysical and structural properties of the protein.

Arrestin is also of interest because of its ability to cause an autoimmune disease, uveoretinitis, that resembles uveitis in humans (9). Immunization of experimental animals with arrestin results in inflammation of the uvea and retina followed by destruction of retinal photoreceptor cells (reviewed in Ref. 10).

Arrestin-like proteins have been found recently in nonphotosensitive cells such as myocardium, liver, kidney, lung, and cerebellum. These proteins may be involved in the transduction of chemical signals (11), analogous to the function of arrestin in the transduction of light signals in the visual system. For example, β-arrestin has been shown to interact with the β-adrenergic receptor (12, 13) in a manner that is analogous to the interaction of arrestin with rhodopsin.

A variety of methods have been developed for the purification of arrestin. Several are based on conventional chromatographic procedures (9, 14–16) that are time consuming and often produce a mixture of intact arrestin and its proteolytic fragments. The method of Wilden *et al.* (3) utilizes the binding of arrestin to illuminated phosphorylated rhodopsin. This procedure requires the use of dark-adapted retina, gives low yield, and produces arrestin contaminated by vesicles of rod outer segment (ROS) membranes. We have developed an economical, highly reproducible, and simple method that overcomes

Methods in Neurosciences, Volume 15

the difficulties mentioned above (17). The method is based on the fact that arrestin binds the ligands heparin and phytic acid (inositol hexakisphosphate, InP_6). Thus, after arrestin is first bound to heparin–Sepharose, it is selectively eluted from the resin by phytic acid.

Methods

Purification of Bovine Arrestin by Affinity Chromatography on Heparin–Sepharose

All procedures are performed at 5°C. This procedure can be applied to bleached retinas.

Extract Preparation

Fifty frozen dark-adapted bovine retinas (obtained from Lawson, Inc., Lincoln, NE, and stored at -70°C) are thawed in a water bath at 20–25°C. The retinas are homogenized in a glass–glass homogenizer under a red safelight with 50 ml of ice cold 10 mM HEPES buffer, pH 7.5, containing 1 mM benzamidine and 20 μg/ml leupeptin (reagents can be purchased from Fisher, Pittsburgh, PA, or Sigma, St. Louis, MO). Soluble proteins are separated from retinal debris by centrifugation for 25 min at 43,700 g. The supernatant is collected and the pellet discarded.

DEAE-cellulose Chromatography

The opalescent and reddish extract (51 ml) is applied at a rate of 25 ml/hr to a 1.6 × 17 cm column of DEAE-cellulose (Whatman, Clifton, NJ, DE-52) that has been equilibrated with 10 mM HEPES buffer, pH 7.5. The column is washed with 10 mM HEPES buffer, pH 7.5, containing 15 mM NaCl, at a flow rate of 25 ml/hr until the absorbance at 280 nm drops below 0.1 and a major hemoglobin band is eluted from the column (or moves toward the end of the column; ~150 ml). The washing can be performed overnight, if convenient. Arrestin is eluted with a gradient of NaCl (240 ml total, from 0 to 150 mM NaCl containing 10 mM HEPES buffer, pH 7.5, and 0.5 mM benzamidine). The flow rate is 15 ml/hr, and 3-ml fractions are collected. Arrestin is eluted as a broad peak at about 75 mM NaCl as determined by sodium dodecyl sulfate–polyacrylamide gel electrophoresis (SDS-PAGE) and immunoblotting (Fig. 1).

Heparin–Sepharose Affinity Chromatography

Combined fractions containing arrestin from the DEAE-cellulose column (fractions 26–42, total 48 ml) are applied at a flow rate of 20 ml/hr to a 1 ×

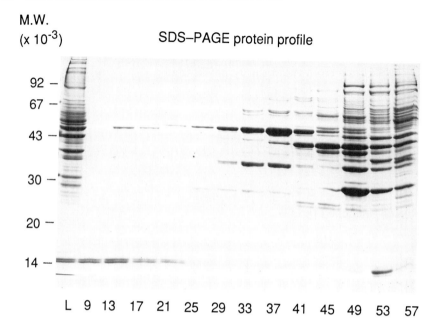

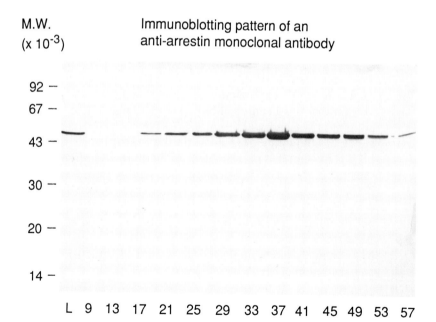

FIG. 1   DEAE-cellulose chromatography of arrestin (see text for methods). (Top) Coomassie blue-stained gel of 4 μl of the indicated fractions. (Bottom) Immunoblot

7.5 cm column of heparin–Sepharose that has been equilibrated with 10 mM HEPES buffer, pH 7.5, and 100 mM NaCl. The column is washed with 10 mM HEPES buffer, pH 7.5, containing 150 mM NaCl at a flow rate of 20 ml/hr until absorbance at 280 nm drops below 0.01 (~60 ml). Arrestin is eluted at a flow rate of 12 ml/hr by a linear gradient of InP$_6$ (phytic acid, Sigma, P-1916) in 10 mM HEPES buffer, pH 7.5, and 150 mM NaCl (70 ml total, from 0 to 8 mM InP$_6$ in the washing buffer), and 1.5-ml fractions are collected. Arrestin is eluted as a sharp peak at about 2.5 mM InP$_6$ as determined by the absorbance at 280 nm (InP$_6$ does not absorb at this wavelength), SDS-PAGE, and immunoblotting (Fig. 2). Arrestin at this stage is more than 95% pure, but the preparation contains InP$_6$, which is a competitive inhibitor of the interaction between arrestin and phosphorylated rhodopsin. Thus, careful removal of InP$_6$ is necessary. Dialysis will remove the bulk of InP$_6$, but complete removal can only be achieved by rechromatography on heparin–Sepharose with NaCl as the eluant.

Heparin–Sepharose Ion-Exchange Chromatography

To purify arrestin completely and to eliminate InP$_6$, the protein is rechromatographed on heparin–Sepharose. Fractions containing arrestin that were eluted from heparin–Sepharose by InP$_6$ (fractions 7–12, 9 ml), are dialyzed against 10 mM HEPES buffer, pH 7.5, containing 100 mM NaCl (dialyze against 1 liter buffer for 24 hr). Next, the dialyzate containing arrestin is applied at a flow rate of 13 ml/hr to a 1 × 4 cm column of heparin–Sepharose that has been equilibrated with 10 mM HEPES buffer, pH 7.5, containing 100 mM NaCl. The column is washed with HEPES buffer containing 100 mM NaCl (10 ml) at a flow rate of 13 ml/hr. Arrestin is eluted with 400 mM NaCl in the HEPES buffer as determined by absorption at 280 nm and SDS-PAGE (Fig. 3). From 50 bovine retinas, the yield is about 4 mg of homogeneous arrestin.

Assessment of Purity

The purity of arrestin should be assessed using SDS-PAGE (18). Additionally, an immunoblot analysis should be performed to evaluate the structural integrity of arrestin, since the N terminus of arrestin is susceptible to degradation (19). The extent of degradation of the N terminus of the protein can be tested

---

of the fractions from DEAE-cellulose chromatography. The staining was performed employing monoclonal antipeptide antibody C10C10 (generous gift from Dr. L. Donoso). Molecular weight standards were from Pharmacia (Piscataway, NJ). Lane L was loaded with 4 μl of extract.

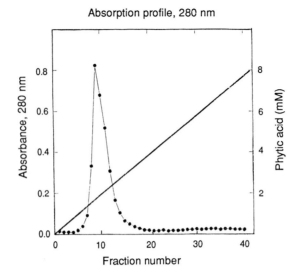

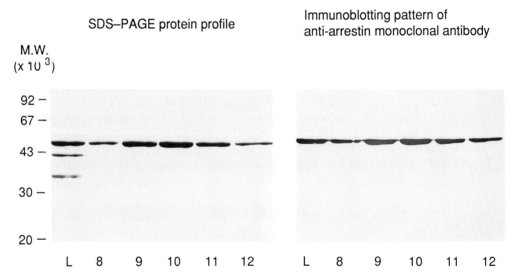

FIG. 2   Heparin–Sepharose/phytic acid chromatography of arrestin. (Top) The absorption profile was obtained from a heparin–Sepharose column (see text for details). (Bottom left) Coomassie blue-stained gel of 4 μl of the indicated fractions. (Bottom right) Immunoblot of the fractions from heparin–Sepharose. Staining was performed employing monoclonal antipeptide antibody C10C10. Lane L was loaded with 4 μl of the pooled fractions obtained from the DEAE-cellulose chromatography step.

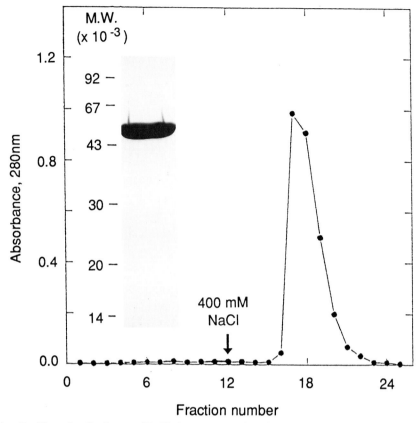

FIG. 3   Heparin–Sepharose/NaCl chromatography of arrestin. The absorption profile was obtained from a heparin–Sepharose column (see text for details). (Inset) Coomassie blue-stained gel of 4 μg of arrestin from the combined fractions (fractions 17–22).

by Edman degradation directly on the sample or on the protein blotted onto Immobilon membranes (19).

Properties of Purified Arrestin

Stability

Arrestin prepared by this method is stable for several weeks at 0°C. It is important that the buffer used for arrestin storage includes 0.02% NaN_3. We have noticed that arrestin aggregates and precipitates when exposed to very low ionic strength buffer; therefore, storing in a buffer containing 100 mM NaCl is highly recommended.

Inhibitors of Arrestin Interaction with Photolyzed and Phosphorylated Rhodopsin

We have found that heparin and dextran sulfate compete with photoactivated and phosphorylated rhodopsin to bind arrestin (20). Phytic acid and other highly phosphorylated inositols inhibit this interaction (17). The dissociation constants for arrestin and inositol phosphates are in the low micromolar range. Several other polyanions are poor inhibitors. Neither ATP, GTP, nor Ca^{2+} are ligands for arrestin, despite recent reports (discussed in Ref. 21).

Composition and Posttranslational Modification

It has been reported that bovine arrestin may contain lipids and carbohydrate moieties, covalently attached to the protein (for review, see Ref. 22). It was also reported that arrestin can be modified substoichiometrically by phosphorylation, presumably by protein kinase C (23). Mass spectroscopic analysis reveals that arrestin purified by this method does not have posttranslational modifications, other than acetylation (Fig. 4). It has been shown that all three of the cysteines in arrestin are available as free sulfhydryl groups (8, 24) rather than in disulfide linkage as previously suggested (7).

Molecular Weight

Based on the amino acid composition of arrestin obtained from the sequence of the protein, the molecular weight of arrestin is 45,275 (404 amino acids). The mass spectroscopic analysis of the native protein revealed that arrestin is acetylated on its N-terminal methionine, and that the molecular weight is $45,317.57 \pm 4.41$ (Fig.4).

Extinction Coefficient and Ultraviolet and Fluorescence Spectroscopy

The UV absorption maximum for arrestin is at 278 nm. An accurate extinction coefficient was determined by amino acid analysis. These results gave an absorbance for a 0.1% solution at 278 nm of 0.638. On a per amide basis, the molar extinction coefficients are $\varepsilon(278) = 71.5$, and $\varepsilon(190) = 10,560$ (8). The integrity of arrestin can be conveniently monitored by employing

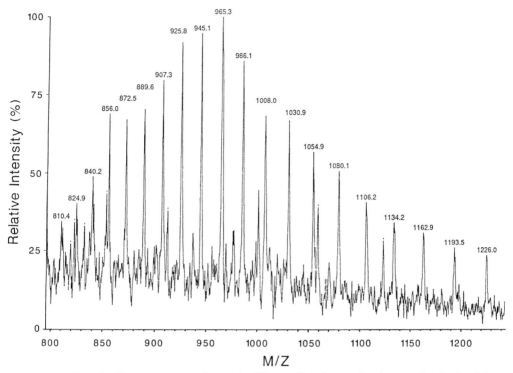

FIG. 4   Mass spectrum of arrestin. The predicted mass for the protein obtained from its sequence (7) is 45,275 daltons. If 42 daltons is added for an acetyl group, the molecular mass is then 45,317 daltons. Twenty different peaks (*m/z*) corresponding to the same mass (m = 45,317 daltons) with charges varying from +56 to +37 were identified. This verifies the molecular size of arrestin and suggests that the protein, the N terminal of which is blocked, is acetylated on its N terminus. The analysis was done by Drs. K. Walsh and L. Ericsson at the University of Washington.

fluorescence spectroscopy as described by Kotake *et al.* (25) (Fig. 5), since the emission maximum of denatured arrestin is shifted from 306 nm for the intact protein to 340 nm.

Binding Assay for Arrestin to Photolyzed and Phosphorylated Rhodopsin

A convenient assay has been developed to monitor arrestin binding to photolyzed and phosphorylated rhodopsin (17). Under red light, phosphorylated rhodopsin, which has been regenerated with 11-*cis*-retinal (30 μM; 2 to 5

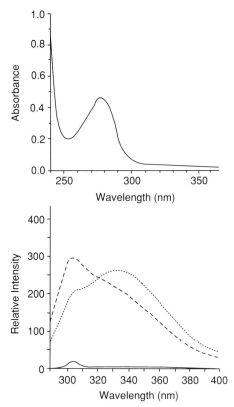

FIG. 5   UV and fluorescence spectra of arrestin. (Top) UV spectrum of arrestin (0.76 mg/ml) in 10 mM HEPES buffer, pH 7.5, containing 100 mM NaCl. (Bottom) Fluorescence spectrum (excitation at 280 nm) of arrestin (1 μM) in 10 mM HEPES buffer, pH 7.5, containing 100 mM NaCl at 25°C (dahsed line), along with those of the same sample partially denatured by incubating for 10 min at 70°C (dotted line) and buffer alone (solid line).

phosphates per molecule of rhodopsin) in 10 mM HEPES buffer, pH 7.5, containing 100 mM NaCl and 1 mM MgCl$_2$, is mixed with purified arrestin (5 μM) in a total volume of 60 μl. The sample is illuminated under a 180-W lamp for 5 min from a distance of 10 cm at 30°C. Under these conditions 45–50% of rhodopsin is bleached. The sample is centrifuged in an Airfuge (Beckman, Fullerton, CA) at 180,000 g for 2 min. The supernatant is stored for SDS-PAGE and/or protein content analysis. The pellet is washed with 180 μl of the HEPES buffer, centrifuged under the same conditions, and dissolved in 55 μl of 1% SDS containing 0.1% 2-mercaptoethanol for SDS-PAGE analysis.

Acknowledgments

We thank Drs. K. Walsh and L. Ericsson (University of Washington) for mass spectroscopy analysis of arrestin, Dr. L. Donoso (Jefferson University) for a monoclonal antibody against arrestin (C10C10), and Preston Van Hooser for excellent technical assistance. This research was supported by U.S. Public Health Service Gant EY 09339 and by a grant from the Human Frontiers in Science Program. KP is the recipient of a Jules and Doris Stein Research to Prevent Blindness Professorship.

References

1. H. Kühn, *Prog. Retinal Res.* **3,** 123 (1984).
2. U. Wilden, S. W. Hall, and H. Kühn, *Proc. Natl. Acad. Sci. U.S.A.* **83,** 1174 (1986).
3. U. Wilden, E. Wüst, I. Weyand, and H. Kühn, *FEBS Lett.* **207,** 292 (1986).
4. A. Schleicher, H. Kühn, and K. P. Hofmann, *Biochemistry* **28,** 1770 (1989).
5. K. Palczewski, J. H. McDowell, S. Jakes, T. S. Ingebritsen, and P. A. Hargrave, *J. Biol. Chem.* **264,** 15770 (1989).
6. K. P. Hofmann, A. Pulvermüller, J. Buczyłko, P. Van Hooser, and K. Palczewski, *J. Biol. Chem.* **267,** 15701 (1992).
7. T. Shinohara, B. Dietzschold, C. M. Craft, G. Wistow, J. J. Early, L. A. Donoso, J. Horwitz, and R. Tao, *Proc. Natl. Acad. Sci. U.S.A.* **84,** 6975 (1987).
8. K. Palczewski, J. H. Riazance-Lawrence, and W. C. Johnson, Jr., *Biochemistry* **31,** 3902 (1992).
9. W. B. Wacker, L. A. Donoso, C. M. Kalsow, J. A. Yankeelov, Jr., and D. T. Organisciak, *J. Immunol.* **119,** 1949 (1977).
10. I. Gery, M. Mochizuki, and R. B. Nussenblatt, *Prog. Retinal Res.* **5,** 75 (1986).
11. M. Mirashahi, F. Borgese, A. Razaghi, U. Scheuring, F. Garcia-Romeu, J. P. Faure, and R. Motais, *FEBS Lett.* **258,** 240 (1989).
12. J. L. Benovic, H. Kühn, I. Weyand, J. Codina, M. G. Caron, and R. J. Lefkowitz, *Proc. Natl. Acad. Sci. U.S.A.* **84,** 8870 (1987).
13. M. J. Lohse, J. L. Benovic, J. Codina, M. G. Caron, and R. J. Lefkowitz, *Science* **248,** 1547 (1990).
14. J. S. Zigler, M. Mochizuki, T. Kuwabara, and I. Gery, *Invest. Ophthalmol. Visual Sci.* **25,** 977 (1984).
15. C. Dorey, J. Cozette, and J. P. Faure, *Ophthalmic Res.* **14,** 249 (1982).
16. J. P. Banga, E. Kasp, S. Suleyman, E. Brown, B. A. Ellis, M. D. Sanders, and D. C. Dumonde, *Exp. Eye Res.* **44,** 199 (1987).
17. K. Palczewski, A. Pulvermüller, J. Buczyłko, C. Gutmann, and K. P. Hofmann, *FEBS Lett.* **295,** 195 (1991).
18. U. K. Laemmli, *Nature (London)* **227,** 680 (1970).
19. K. Palczewski, J. Buczyłko, N. R. Imami, J. H. McDowell, and P. A. Hargrave, *J. Biol. Chem.* **226,** 15334 (1991).
20. K. Palczewski, A. Pulvermüller, J. Buczyłko, and K. P. Hofmann, *J. Biol. Chem.* **226,** 18649 (1991).

21. K. Palczewski and P. A. Hargrave, *J. Biol. Chem.* **266,** 4201 (1991).
22. T. Shinohara, L. Donoso, M. Tsuda, K. Yamaki, and V. K. Singh, *Prog. Retinal Res.* **8,** 51 (1988).
23. I. Weyand and H. Kühn, *Eur. J. Biochem.* **193,** 459 (1990).
24. I. D. Pogozheva, T. F. Shevchenko, V. A. Livshits, and G. R. Kalamkarov, *Biol. Membr.* **6,** 1248 (1989).
25. S. Kotake, P. Hey, R. G. Mirmira, and R. A. Copeland, *Arch. Biochem. Biophys.* **285,** 126 (1991).

[16] Preparation and Characterization of Guanylate Cyclase from Vertebrate Rod Photoreceptors

Fumio Hayashi, Lara D. Hutson, Akio Kishigami, Seiji Nagao, and Akio Yamazaki

Introduction

In vertebrate rod outer segments (ROS) cGMP appears to be directly involved in the process of visual transduction. Illumination of rhodopsin leads to activation of cGMP phosphodiesterase (PDE) through transducin. The resulting fall in cytoplasmic cGMP concentration contributes to closure of cGMP-sensitive cation channels, causing the hyperpolarization of plasma membranes. Recovery of the dark state requires the resynthesis of cGMP by guanylate cyclase.

To elucidate the mechanisms for the recovery of the dark state, isolation and reconstitution of guanylate cyclase in detergent-free systems are essential. Since cGMP was first proposed to be involved in visual responses in the early 1970s, isolation of guanylate cyclase from vertebrate ROS has been attempted by many groups. Recently, we detailed the purification and basic characterization of guanylate cyclase from amphibian and bovine ROS (1). Independently, Koch (2) also reported purification of guanylate cyclase from bovine ROS. Our data about characterization of guanylate cyclase from amphibian ROS agreed closely with those obtained by Koch. However, several biochemical characteristics of amphibian guanylate cyclase differ from those of the bovine enzyme. Although these data do not prove the fundamental differences in the regulatory mechanism of guanylate cyclase between the species, we anticipate that these differences are important for elucidation of the regulatory mechanism of guanylate cyclase. Thus, in this chapter, we describe our procedures for the solubilization, stabilization, purification, and reconstitution of amphibian and bovine rod guanylate cyclase. We also describe the basic characterization of guanylate cyclase from amphibian and bovine ROS.

Solubilization and Purification of Guanylate Cyclase
Measurement of Guanylate Cyclase Activity

Guanylate cyclase is assayed by measuring the amount of $[^{32}P]cGMP$ that is derived from $[\alpha\text{-}^{32}P]GTP$ in the presence of $[^{3}H]cGMP$ (as an internal standard), 3-isobutyl-1-methylxanthine, and a GTP-generating system (1, 3). The following points should be considered for the assay of guanylate cyclase. First, the 2 mM 3-isobutyl-1-methylxanthine present in the reaction mixture does not completely inhibit endogenous PDE activity. Thus, the incubation time and protein concentration used in guanylate cyclase assays of ROS preparations should be determined carefully. Especially for frog ROS, highly activated PDE activity was detected in the ROS preparations, since an inhibitory subunit (P_γ) was released from PDE catalytic subunits by extensive washing as described below (4). In the case of toad and bovine ROS preparations, large portions of PDE (60–90%) were released by washing ROS membranes; however, the incubation time and protein concentration for the assay should be determined with caution. Second, we used alumina (ICN, Cost Mesa, CA) columns and AG1 × 2 (Bio-Rad, Richmond, CA) columns to separate $[^{32}P]cGMP$ from $[\alpha\text{-}^{32}P]GTP$ for measurement of cGMP concentration. Several high-performance liquid chromatography (HPLC) systems are also available to separate cGMP from GTP (5, 6). Our preliminary data suggest that binding of cGMP to cGMP-binding protein in a commercially available kit is affected by some proteins in the ROS preparations. Thus, we do not use a cGMP binding kit for the measurement of cGMP concentration.

Preparation of Rod Outer Segment Membranes

All procedures for ROS preparation are carried out under dim red light. Amphibian ROS membranes are prepared from dark-adapted animals as described (1). Bovine ROS membranes are prepared from dark-adapted frozen retinas (7). ROS membranes from 50 retinas are illuminated and washed 7 times each by passage through a 21-gauge needle with 7 ml of the following buffers: (a) buffer A, which is 10 mM Tris-HCl, pH 7.5, 5 mM dithiothreitol (DTT), 5 mM MgSO$_4$, 1 mM [ethylenebis(oxyethylenenitrilo)]tetraacetic acid (EGTA), 0.1 mM phenylmethylsulfonyl fluoride (PMSF), 0.0025% (v/v) butylated hydroxytoluene (BHT); (b) buffer B, which is 100 mM Tris-HCl, pH 7.5, 5 mM DTT, 5 mM MgSO$_4$, 1 mM EGTA, 0.1 mM PMSF, and 0.0025% BHT; (c) buffer C, which is 10 mM Tris-HCl, pH 7.5, 5 mM DTT, 1 mM EGTA, 0.1 mM PMSF, and 0.0025% BHT; (d) buffer B containing 500 μM GTP; and (e) buffer D, which is 5 mM Tris-HCl, pH 7.5, 5 mM DTT, 1 mM EGTA, 0.1 mM PMSF, and 0.0025% BHT. In the toad and bovine preparations, PDE is extracted specifically in step c. Toad and bovine PDEs are purified from these PDE preparations by a single step column chromatography as described (7). The α subunit and β,γ subunits of transducin are extracted in steps d and e, respectively. These subunits are also purified from these preparations by a single step column chromatography as described (7).

Solubilization of Guanylate Cyclase

Amphibian Guanylate Cyclase

Washed ROS membranes from 100 retinas are suspended in 20 ml of buffer E [20 mM Tris-HCl, pH 7.5, 1 mM DTT, 0.1 mM PMSF, 0.005% BHT, and 5% (v/v) Triton X-100] and incubated for 3 hr at 0°C. Crude guanylate cyclase preparations are obtained by centrifugation at 4°C for 30 min (100,000 g). Only negligible guanylate cyclase activity is found in the pellet fractions. Glycerol (25%, v/v, final concentration) and MnCl$_2$ (2 mM final concentration) are added to the supernatants for stablization of the enzyme. MnCl$_2$ is also required for the subsequent column chromatography. When we developed this method (1), Lubrol PX was used for the extraction of guanylate cyclase; however, Lubrol PX is no longer commercially available.

Bovine Guanylate Cyclase

Following extraction of lipids and membrane-bound proteins with detergents, guanylate cyclase is extracted from cytoskeletal elements with detergents containing 1 M KCl (2). We modified this method as follows. After washing ROS membranes from 100 retinas as described above, ROS membranes are suspended in 20 ml of buffer F (20 mM Tris-HCl, pH 7.5, 1 mM DTT, 1 mM EGTA, 0.1 mM PMSF, 5 μM pepstatin, and 5 μM leupeptin) containing 5% Triton X-100, incubated for 3 hr at 0°C, and centrifuged at 4°C for 30 min (100,000 g) The pellet containing guanylate cyclase is incubated overnight at 0°C in 20 ml of buffer F containing 1 M KCl and 5% (v/v) n-dodecyl-β-D-maltoside. Guanylate cyclase is obtained by centrifugation at 4°C for 30 min (100,000 g).

It should be emphasized that n-dodecyl-β-D-maltoside should be used for this solubilization method. As shown in Fig. 1, Triton X-100 and Nonidet P-40 are less effective for the solubilization of guanylate cyclase from cytoskeletal elements, although these detergents show an equivalent or higher ability to extract the enzyme from ROS membranes washed with detergent-free buffers (8, 9). Following solubilization of the enzyme, glycerol and MnCl$_2$ are added to the supernatant for stabilization and subsequent column chromatography.

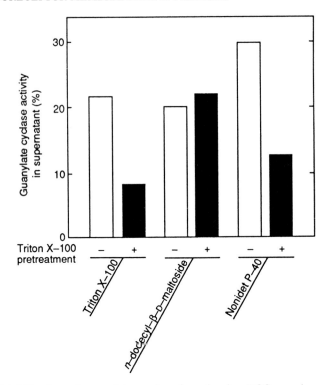

FIG. 1   Solubilization of guanylate cyclase from bovine ROS membranes. Washed ROS membranes (12.3 mg of protein) from 20 retinas were divided into two portions. Each portion was suspended in 4 ml of buffer F or buffer F containing 5% (v/v) Triton X-100. Following incubation for 3 hr at 0°C, the samples were subjected to centrifugation (100,000 g) at 4°C for 30 min. Each pellet was washed twice with 2 ml of buffer F or buffer F containing 5% Triton X-100. Then each pellet was divided into three portions, and each portion was suspended in 700 μl of buffer F containing 5% detergent and 1 M KCl. Detergents used were Triton X-100, n-dodecyl-β-D-maltoside, and Nonidet P-40. Following incubation overnight at 0°C, supernatants and pellets were prepared by centrifugation (100,000 × g) at 4°C for 30 min. Pellets were suspended in 700 μl of buffer F containing 1 M KCl and each detergent. Equal amounts (80 μl) of the supernatant and pellet mixtures were used for assay of enzyme activity.

Purification of Guanylate Cyclase

Prior to the application of bovine guanylate cyclase to a GTP–agarose affinity column, the guanylate cyclase preparation is dialyzed overnight at 4°C against

1 liter (three changes) of buffer G (20 mM Tris-HCl, pH 7.5, 1 mM DTT, 2 mM MnCl$_2$, 0.1 mM PMSF, 0.005% BHT, 0.2% Triton X-100, and 25% glycerol). The guanylate cyclase preparations from amphibian ROS do not require dialysis. The guanylate cyclase preparations are then applied to a GTP–agarose column (7 × 30 mm, Sigma) that has been equilibrated with buffer G. The column is washed with 30 ml of buffer G, and guanylate cyclase is eluted with a GTP gradient in buffer G, as shown in Fig. 2. Approximately 30% of the applied activity is recovered from the column. Sometimes a TSK DEAE-5-PW (7.5 × 75 mm) column (Bio-Rad) chromatography step is conducted prior to GTP affinity column chromatography (12). If so, peak fractions are dialyzed as described above prior to GTP–agarose column chromatography.

In the GTP–agarose column chromatographies, only one prominent protein band [resolved by sodium dodecyl sulfate–polyacrylamide gel electrophoresis (SDS-PAGE)] around 110 kDa is eluted with GTP gradients (Fig. 2). The activity of guanylate cyclase coincides exactly with the protein concentration profile. Based on the analysis of silver-stained protein bands on the gels, the purity of the enzyme appears to be 95% or better. In addition to the 110-kDa protein, we occasionally observe minor proteins of 250, 155, 65, and/or 35 kDa by SDS–PAGE. The identification of guanylate cyclase is confirmed using other chromatographic analysis of the purified enzymes, such as TSK DEAE-5-PW and concanavalin A (ConA)–Sepharose column chromatography (1). The enzyme activity correlates only with the 110-kDa proteins in these chromatographies.

Reconstitution of Bovine Guanylate Cyclase

Incorporation of purified proteins into liposomes provides a method by which to investigate the regulatory mechanisms of membrane-bound enzymes in a detergent-free system. Such methodology may be particularly useful in studying rod guanylate cyclase, since it would allow the enzyme to interact with protein regulators and component proteins of the PDE cascade.

Following purification of guanylate cyclase from bovine ROS by GTP–agarose column chromatography, 350 μl of guanylate cyclase fractions in buffer G is mixed in the described order with 7 μl of buffer H (1.43 M NaCl, 286 mM Tris-HCl, pH 7.5, 28.6 mM MnCl$_2$, and 14.3 mM DTT), 50 μl of phosphatidylcholine solution, and 93 μl of 10% Triton X-100. The phosphatidylcholine solution is prepared by suspending soybean phosphatidylcholine (Sigma, St. Louis, MO) buffer G (125 mg/ml) and dissolving with sonication (~10 min) under a stream of N$_2$ at 20°C in a Benson sonic bath

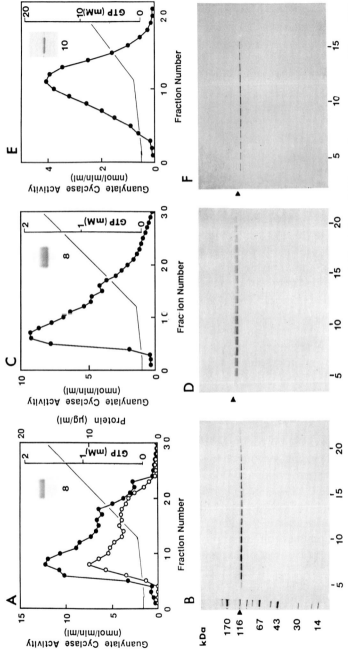

FIG. 2   Purification of guanylate cyclase. Guanylate cyclase was solubilized from ROS membranes prepared from 220 toad retinas (A, B), 70 frog retinas (C, D), and 100 bovine retinas (E, F). Chromatography was performed on GTP–agarose, and guanylate cyclase was eluted with GTP as described in the text. After GTP–agarose column chromatography, 10 μl of each fraction was used for the measurement of enzyme activity (●) (A, C, E). The protein profile of each fraction (40 μl) was analyzed by SDS-PAGE (B, D, F). The protein concentration (○) in each fraction of toad enzyme is shown in A. Insets in A, C, and E show enlarged photographs of the protein band from fractions 8 (toad and frog) or 10 (bovine). In these experiments, buffers containing Lubrol PX were used; however, equivalent chromatograms were obtained by using buffers containing Triton X-100.

(Danbury, CT). The final concentration of each component in the mixture is 20 mM Tris-HCl, pH 7.5, 1 mM DTT, 2 mM MnCl$_2$, 20 mM NaCl, 2% Triton X-100, and 12.5 mg/ml phosphatidylcholine.

After incubation for 30 min at 0°C, 450 μl of the mixture is applied to an Extractigel column (7 × 30 mm, Pierce Chemical Co., Rockford, IL) which has been equilibrated with buffer I (20 mM Tris-HCl, pH 7.5, 1 mM DTT, 2 mM MnCl$_2$, 20 mM NaCl, and 0.1 mM PMSF). The liposomes containing guanylate cyclase are eluted with Buffer I. The turbid liposome fraction is eluted with the first 1 ml of buffer I. Then, 333 μl of glycerol is added to the fraction (1 ml), and the mixture is incubated for 30 min at 0°C. Buffer I (12 ml) is then added to the mixture, which is subjected to centrifugation for 2 hr at 4°C (300,000 g) using a Beckman (Fullerton, CA) TL100 centrifuge. The pellet is suspended in 500 μl of buffer I using a 21-gauge needle. Incorporation of the enzyme in the liposomes is 10–35% of the applied protein judging from the activity measured. Part of the loss in enzyme activity after liposome incorporation might be due to the inaccessibility of the catalytic site inside the liposomes.

Characterization of Guanylate Cyclase

Basic Characterization

As shown in Table I, amphibian and bovine guanylate cyclase have almost the same characteristics. In addition, our study (1) indicates that amphibian and bovine guanylate cyclase show specific binding to ConA–Sepharose, indicating that the enzymes are glycoproteins. However, several biochemical characteristics of amphibian guanylate cyclase differ from those of the bovine enzyme: (1) the bovine enzyme shows tighter binding to GTP–agarose columns than the amphibian enzyme (Fig. 2); (2) the purified amphibian enzyme shows a doublet band in silver-stained gels, whereas the bovine enzyme shows a singlet; (3) the amphibian enzymes are released from ROS membranes by detergents in the absence of KCl, whereas detergents with 1 M KCl are required for the solubilization of the bovine enzyme; and (4) the bovine enzyme exhibits positive cooperativity with respect to MnGTP, but the amphibian enzyme does not.

It is interesting to note that several isoforms were found for guanylate cyclase purified from both amphibian and bovine ROS (1). Toad isoforms may be separated by both GTP–agarose and ion-exchange column chromatography. The isoforms exhibit different kinetic properties. Although we cannot exclude the possibility that the isoforms are products of different genes, the simplest explanation is that the polymorphism may be due to

TABLE I   Molecular Properties of Rod Guanylate Cyclase

Property	Amphibian[a]	Bovine
Molecular weight	110,000 and 115,000	110,000[a,b]
Specific activity[c]	0.8–1.4	0.1–0.7[b]
$K_m (\mu M)$	85–160	274[b]
K_i for Gpp(NH)p[d]	95–105	—
K_i for pyrophosphate (μM)	30–45	—
Ca^{2+} effect	No	No[a,b]
ANF effect[e]	No	—
Isoforms	2–3	5[a]
Positive cooperativity with MnGTP	No	Yes[b] (Hill coefficient $n = 1.6 \pm 0.1$)

[a] Data from Ref. 1.
[b] Data from Ref. 2.
[c] Units are μmol cGMP formed/min/mg protein.
[d] Guanosine 5-(β,γ-imido)triphosphate.
[e] Atrial natriuretic factor.

posttranslational modifications of the enzyme, such as phosphorylation and prenylation.

Protein Regulator for Guanylate Cyclase

In addition to the polymorphism of guanylate cyclase, published data (8–12) suggest the possibility of multiple regulatory mechanisms of guanylate cyclase in vertebrate rod photoreceptors. In crude ROS preparations, Ca^{2+} regulates guanylate cyclase activity; however, no positive data have been obtained to show that Ca^{2+} directly regulates purified guanylate cyclase (1, 2). Thus, it is reasonable to suggest that a Ca^{2+}-sensitive factor(s) contributes to differences between crude preparations and the purified enzyme.

Koch and Stryer (10) reported that a factor is required for the Ca^{2+}-sensitive activation of bovine guanylate cyclase. This factor stimulates guanylate cyclase activity at low concentrations of Ca^{2+}; however, in the presence of a higher Ca^{2+} concentration, the factor becomes nonfunctional as an activator of bovine guanylate cyclase. The amino acid sequence has been published, and the factor was named recoverin (13).

In frog ROS preparations, we also found a factor with the same properties as the factor in bovine ROS, as shown in Fig. 3. Without washing with an EGTA-containing buffer, ROS membranes show higher guanylate cyclase

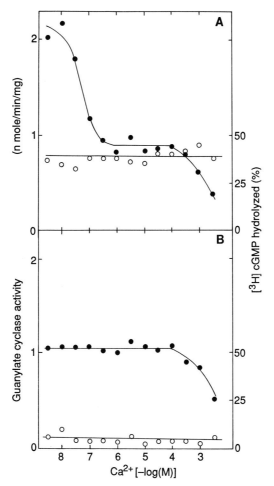

FIG. 3   Effect of Ca^{2+} on guanylate cyclase activity in frog ROS membranes. Intact ROS were prepared from five dark-adapted *Rana catesbeiana* using Percoll (Pharmacia, Piscataway, NJ) gradients in buffer J (10 mM Tris-HCl, pH 7.5, 5 mM $MgCl_2$, 1 mM $CaCl_2$, 115 mM NaCl, 2.5 mM KCl, and 10 mM glucose) as described (14). Following the removal of Percoll from the ROS membranes by washing with buffer J (5 times), the membranes were divided into two portions. One portion (A) was suspended in 2 ml of buffer J and washed with 2 ml of buffer J (3 times). The other portion (B) was washed (3 times) with buffer K (5 mM Tris-HCl, pH 7.5, 1 mM DTT, and 1 mM EGTA) and then suspended in 2 ml of buffer J. Guanylate cyclase (●) and PDE (○) activities were measured, and free Ca^{2+} concentrations were calculated as described (14). A value of $4.4 \times 10^7 \ M^{-1}$ was taken as the apparent binding constant of EGTA for Ca^{2+}.

activity in the presence of lower concentrations of Ca^{2+}, and the activity is decreased in the presence of higher concentrations of Ca^{2+} (Fig. 3A). However, once ROS membranes are washed with an EGTA-containing buffer, the Ca^{2+}-dependent changes in guanylate cyclase activity are not detected (Fig. 3B). The change in guanylate cyclase activity is not sensitive to calmodulin or to calmodulin inhibitors. These data suggest that guanylate cyclase activity in amphibian rods may be regulated in the same fashion as guanylate cyclase in bovine ROS. However, it is not clear whether a recoverin-like protein (26 kDa) found in the amphibian ROS plays a role in our observation, since addition of the recoverin-like protein did not stimulate guanylate cyclase in the presence of low concentration of Ca^{2+}.

Alternatively, the Ca^{2+}-dependent inhibition of guanylate cyclase in vertebrate ROS may result from inhibition of guanylate cyclase activity by pyrophosphate. Guanylate cyclase activity both in purified vertebrate preparations (1) and in crude ROS preparations from vertebrate (9) and invertebrate retinas (14) was shown to be inhibited by pyrophosphate. In addition, pyrophosphatase has been reported to be sensitive to Ca^{2+} (9). Our data (1) indicate that the pyrophosphate-dependent inhibition of guanylate cyclase activity may differ for the various isoforms of guanylate cyclase.

Conclusion

In summary, we describe a simple purification method for vertebrate rod guanylate cyclase and basic characterization of the purified enzyme. Recently, the amino acid sequence encoding the human retinal guanylate cyclase has been published (15). Sequence of peptides derived from bovine guanylate cyclase which we purified is homologous to the human guanylate cyclase (unpublished observation). By enabling more precise characterization of rod guanylate cyclase, the techniques described in this chapter should provide a better understanding of the molecular mechanisms of recovery of the dark state in vertebrate rod photoreceptors.

Acknowledgments

We are indebted to Dr. Hitoshi Shichi for the use of laboratory equipment. We also thank Carolyn Otto for proficient editorial assistance. This work was supported by National Institutes of Health Grants EY 07546 and EY 09631. A.Y. is the recipient of a Jules and Doris Stein Professorship from Research to Prevent Blindness.

References

1. F. Hayashi and A. Yamazaki, *Proc. Natl. Acad. Sci. U.S.A.* **88,** 4746 (1991).
2. K.-W. Koch, *J. Biol. Chem.* **266,** 8634 (1991).
3. K. Nakazawa and M. Sano, *J. Biol. Chem.* **249,** 4207 (1974).
4. A. Yamazaki, F. Hayashi, M. Tatsumi, M. W. Bitensky, and J. S. George, *J. Biol. Chem.* **265,** 11539 (1990).
5. L. J. Reysz, A. G. Carroll, and H. W. Jarrett, *Anal. Biochem.* **166,** 107 (1987).
6. A. Yamazaki, M. Tatsumi, D. C. Torney, and M. W. Bitensky, *J. Biol. Chem.* **252,** 9316 (1987).
7. A. Yamazaki, T. Tatsumi, and M. W. Bitensky, *in* "Methods in Enzymology" (J. D. Corbin and R. A. Johnson, eds.), Vol. 159, p. 702. Academic Press, San Diego, 1988.
8. Y. Horio and F. Murad, *J. Biol. Chem.* **266,** 3411 (1991).
9. S. Hakki and A. Sitaramayya, *Biochemistry* **29,** 1088 (1990).
10. K.-W. Koch and L. Stryer, *Nature (London)* **334,** 64 (1988).
11. R. Lolley and E. Racz, *Vision Res.* **22,** 1481 (1982).
12. I. M. Pepe, I. Panfoli, and C. Cugnoli, *FEBS Lett.* **203,** 73 (1986).
13. A. M. Dizhoor, S. Ray, S. Kumar, G. Niemi, M. Spencer, D. Brolley, K. A. Walsh, P. P. Philipov, J. B. Hurley, and L. Stryer, *Science* **251,** 915 (1991).
14. P. R. Robinson and R. H. Cote, *Vis. Neurosci.* **3,** 1 (1989).
15. A. W. Shyjan, F. J. de Sauvage, N. A. Gillett, D. V. Goeddel, and D. G. Lowe, *Neuron.* **9,** 727 (1992).

[17] Calcium-Binding Proteins in the Retina

Arthur S. Polans, John Crabb, and Krzysztof Palczewski

Introduction

In the 100 years since Sydney Ringer first demonstrated the requirement of calcium for the preservation of heart muscle contractibility, calcium has been implicated in a wide variety of physiological processes. Some of these processes, such as bone formation and fibrin polymerization during blood clotting, depend on adequate concentrations of extracellular calcium. Considerable information has been obtained about the actions of vitamin D and certain hormones in the regulation of extracellular calcium. However, the realization that calcium also acts intracellularly has spurred investigations of its role as a second messenger in an assortment of cellular activities. It was not until the discovery of troponin C, however, that the diverse intracellular actions of calcium might be explained by the presence of different, high-affinity calcium-binding proteins (1, 2).

Intracellular calcium-binding proteins generally are classified into two, structurally distinct groups (3). The first group currently consists of over 170 proteins, including calmodulin, troponin C, and the S-100 proteins. These proteins share a common structural motif, the EF hand, which is comprised of 12 or 14 amino acids contributing 6–8 oxygen atoms to the coordination of calcium (4). This calcium-binding loop is flanked by two α helices. Studies of secondary structure reveal conformational changes of the protein that occur on binding calcium; these changes are thought to underlie the interactions with effector molecules (4). The second group of calcium-binding proteins, the annexins, interact with phospholipids in a calcium-dependent manner, and they contain structural regions that resemble mutated EF hands (5). The nonconserved regions of the annexins are potential sites for specialized reactions, including phosphorylation by protein kinase C or tyrosine kinases (6). This group of proteins has been described in the literature by a variety of names, including calpactins, calelectrins, and chrombindins.

The function of some calcium-binding proteins is known. On binding calcium, calmodulin can activate a diverse set of enzymes, including adenylate cyclase, protein kinases, and cyclic nucleotide phosphodiesterases (7). Other binding proteins regulate the diffusion and buffering of intracellular calcium (2). The majority of calcium-binding proteins, however, are of unknown

Methods in Neurosciences, Volume 15

function. Nonetheless, these proteins most often are expressed in a cell-specific manner and, therefore, are thought to be involved in specialized functions of the cell (8). Further, the portions of their sequences not involved in calcium binding remain highly conserved, suggesting that these regions may be important for interacting with effector molecules (9).

In the retina, calcium is thought to act as a modulator of light adaptation. Alterations in calcium concentration effect the recovery phase of the photoresponse, as well as the sensitivity of the cell to a flash of light in the presence of background illumination (10). It has been suggested that guanylate cyclase is one site of calcium action in the photoreceptor (11). A calcium-binding protein, designated recoverin, has been shown to activate guanylate cyclase as the calcium concentration is lowered from approximately 400 to 40 nM (12, 13). This corresponds to the range over which the calcium concentration diminishes in a rod cell on illumination. Recoverin is a member of the EF hand group of calcium-binding proteins and was identified recently as the autoantigen in the paraneoplastic degenerative disease of the retina known as cancer-associated retinopathy (14). In this regard, abnormalities in calcium binding proteins have been noted for several neurodegenerative diseases (15).

Although the function of recoverin might be determined, other calcium-binding proteins present in the retina, such as calmodulin, parvalbumin, calbindin, and calretinin, are of unknown function (8, 9). These calcium-binding proteins may have roles related to the specialized functions not only of photoreceptors but other retinal neurons as well. In this chapter, we discuss the purification and partial characterization of some of the major retinal calcium-binding proteins. These data, it is hoped, will encourage further investigation of the functions of these proteins, as well as the identification of new calcium-binding proteins.

Methods and Results

Purification of Recoverin and Visinin

Preparation of Retinal Homogenates

Fifty freshly dissected or frozen bovine retinas are disrupted in 35 ml of buffer (50 mM HEPES, 1 mM EDTA, 100 mM NaCl, pH 7.5, containing 1–2 μg/ml each of leupeptin, pepstatin, and aprotinin) using two passes of a 1-inch Teflon homogenizer followed by six passes with a glass on glass tissue grinder. Retinal homogenates of human tissue can be prepared similarly. Eyes from 40- to 49-day-old Cornish cross chickens are dissected, and the retina with attached pigment epithelium and choroid are homogenized as described for bovine tissue. These same procedures were used previously with isolated rod outer segments (14).*

Retinal homogenates are centrifuged at 39,000 g for 20 min at 4°C using a JA-17 rotor (Beckman Instruments, Fullerton, CA). All procedures up to this step are performed under dim red illumination. The retinal extracts are adjusted to yield a final concentration of 2 mM CaCl$_2$.

Phenyl-Sepharose Chromatography

Prior to preparing the retinal extracts, a Phenyl-Sepharose (Pharmacia Fine Chemicals, Piscataway, NJ) column (1 × 4 cm) is prepared and equilibrated at 4°C with 50 mM HEPES, 2 mM CaCl$_2$, 100 mM NaCl, pH 7.5, for at least 3 hr prior to use. The extract from 150 or fewer retinas can be processed through this column. Larger columns should be avoided with that amount of sample owing to excessive retention of recoverin. The sodium dodecyl sulfate–polyacrylamide gel electrophoresis (SDS-PAGE) protein staining pattern of an aliquot of the soluble extract is shown in Fig. 1 (lane a). The remaining extract is applied to the column, which is washed with equilibrating buffer at a rate of 15 ml/hr until the A_{280} returns to baseline. This washing step usually extends overnight. The majority of extractable protein runs unretarded through the column (Fig. 1, lane b) or elutes during washing of the column (Fig. 1, lane c). Bound proteins are eluted with 50 mM HEPES, 10 mM EDTA, 100 mM NaCl, pH 7.5, at the same flow rate. Fractions (1 ml each) are collected, and aliquots are subjected to SDS-PAGE. The eluted material consists primarily of four proteins, including bovine recoverin (Fig. 1, lane d). Following the same procedures, a retinal homogenate from chicken yields two principal proteins, one of which is visinin (Fig. 1, lane e). EGTA can substitute for EDTA during the elution, and concentrations of 1 mM were found to be effective.

Mono Q Chromatography

Protein fractions from the Phenyl-Sepharose eluate are combined and dialyzed using 1000 MW cutoff tubing against 10 mM 1,3-bis[tris(hydroxymethyl)methylamino]propane (BTP) buffer, pH 8.4. Aliquots containing 0.5–1.0 mg of protein are applied to a Mono Q column (HR 5 × 50 mm; Pharmacia Fine Chemicals) equilibrated with 10 mM BTP buffer, pH 8.4. The column is developed with a linear gradient of NaCl (0–0.25 M) during 20 min at a rate of 0.5 ml/min. Fractions (0.5 ml each) are collected, and aliquots are analyzed by SDS-PAGE and Western blot staining. Bovine

---

* A portion of the methods section pertaining to our chromatographic procedures and amino acid analyses of proteins originally appeared in the *Journal of Cell Biology* (14).

kDa

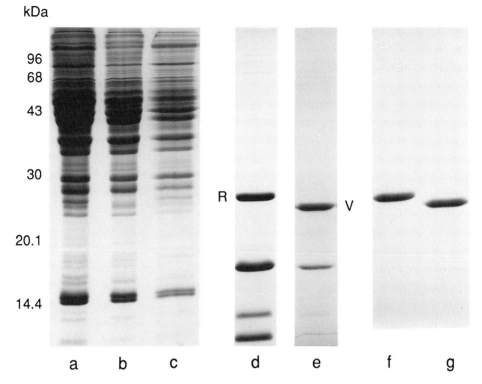

FIG. 1   Purification of recoverin and visinin by Phenyl-Sepharose and Mono Q column chromatography. Bovine retinas were extracted with EDTA, and the soluble fraction (after adjusting the calcium concentration) was applied to a Phenyl-Sepharose column. An aliquot of the soluble extract was separated by SDS-PAGE, and the protein staining pattern is shown in lane a. Protein which did not bind to the Phenyl-Sepharose column is shown in lane b, and protein which could be washed from the column is shown in lane c. Bound material could be eluted with EDTA and is shown in lane d. Chicken retinas were processed the same way, and the final eluate from the Phenyl-Sepharose column is shown in lane e. The letters R and V indicate the positions of recoverin and visinin at 26 and 24 kDa, respectively. The material eluted from the Phenyl-Sepharose column, depicted in lanes d and e, was further purified by Mono Q chromatography. Lane f shows recoverin purified from the bovine preparation, and lane g from the chicken preparation shows purified visinin. Molecular size standards (lane not shown) were phosphorylase b (96 kDa), bovine serum albumin (68 kDa), ovalbumin (43 kDa), carbonic anhydrase (30 kDa), soybean trypsin inhibitor (20.1 kDa), and α-lactalbumin (14.4 kDa).

recoverin and chicken visinin elute at approximately 100 mM NaCl and are shown in Fig. 1 (lanes f and g, respectively).

Amino Acid Sequence Analysis

Purified bovine recoverin and chicken visinin are cleaved with endoproteinase Lys-C (Boehringer-Mannheim Biochemicals, Indianapolis, IN), and lysyl peptides are isolated by narrow-bore reversed-phase high-performance liquid chromatography (RP-HPLC) (Vydac, Hesperia, CA) as described elsewhere (14). Peptides are sequenced (16) with an Applied Biosystems (Foster City, CA) gas-phase sequencer (Model 470) equipped with an on-line phenylthiohydantoin amino acid analyzer (Model 120). Phenylthiocarbamylamino acid analysis is performed with an Applied Biosystems automatic system (Models 420H/130/920). Following these procedures, the identities of bovine recoverin and chicken visinin are confirmed (see Ref. 14 and Fig. 2).

Antibody Production

Antisera are raised in New Zealand White rabbits by subcutaneous immunizations with 50–100 μg of purified bovine recoverin or chicken visinin mixed with an equal volume of Freund's complete adjuvant. Animals are boosted at 1- to 2-week intervals with 10–25 μg of purified protein mixed with Freund's incomplete adjuvant. In some experiments antibodies are affinity-purified by elution from Western blots of purified bovine recoverin or chicken visinin (17).

```
              130                              150
Visinin    I F K M I P E E E R L Q L P E D E N S P Q K R A D K L W A Y F N K
               : : : : : : : : : : : : : : : : :             : : : : : :
           M I P E E E R L Q L P E D E N S P Q K           L W A Y F N K


              170                              190
Visinin    G E N D K I A E G E F I D G V M K N D A I M R L I Q Y E P K K
                     : : : : : : : : : :     : : : : : : : : : : : :
           I A E G E F I D G V M   N D A I M R L I Q Y E P K
```

FIG. 2   Identification of visinin by partial amino acid sequence analysis. The partial amino acid sequence of visinin (top line), as deduced from its nucleotide sequence (Yamagata *et al.*, *Neuron.* **2,** 469–476, 1990), is compared with the amino acid sequences of four peptides from the purified 24-kDa protein obtained from our experiments with chicken retina. Both are given in single-letter code [see *Eur. J. Biochem.* **5,** 151–153 (1968)]. The double dots indicate identical amino acids. This confirms the identity of visinin obtained by our procedures.

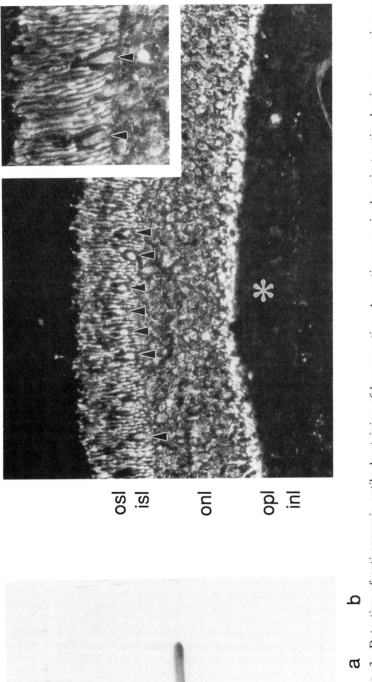

osl
isl

onl

opl
inl

a   b

FIG. 3 Detection of antirecoverin antibody staining of human retina. An antiserum raised against native bovine recoverin was used to stain Western blots of purified bovine recoverin (lane a) and chicken visinin (lane b) by procedures described in the text. The antiserum labeled only recoverin. Cryosections of formaldehyde-fixed human retina were incubated with a 1 : 1000 dilution of antiserum and subsequently incubated with a biotinyl-goat anti-rabbit IgG and streptavidin–Texas red conjugate. While the inner retina is devoid of label (asterisk), the outer retina is stained intensely. Arrows indicate labeled cone cells, which are shown at higher magnification in the inset. osl, Outer segment layer; isl, inner segment layer; onl, outer nuclear layer; opl, outer plexiform layer; inl, inner nuclear layer.

Western Blot Analysis

Proteins are resolved using a 0.75 mm, 15% polyacrylamide gel containing glycerol and transferred to Immobilon membranes essentially following the procedures described elsewhere (18). Western blots are rinsed with 20 mM Tris-HCl, 150 mM NaCl, pH 8.2, and nonspecific sites are saturated by incubation for 45 min at 37°C with 5% (w/v) bovine serum albumin (BSA) in TBST (10 mM Tris-HCl, pH 8.0, 150 mM NaCl, 0.05%, v/v, Tween 20). Blots typically are incubated with primary antisera or affinity-purified antibodies for 1 hr in TBST containing 1% (w/v) BSA and 1% (v/v) normal goat serum. After three 10-min washes with TBST, blots are incubated for 30 min with an alkaline phosphatase-conjugated goat anti-rabbit immunoglobulin G (IgG) at dilutions of 1:5000 to 1:7500 using TBST containing BSA and normal goat serum. After washing with TBST, antibody binding is detected using 5-bromo-4-chloro-3-indolyl phosphate (BCIP) and nitro blue tetrazolium (NBT) as substrates following the manufacturer's recommended procedures (Promega, Madison, WI).

Fluorescence Light Microscopy

Cryosections of acrylamide-embedded retina are prepared as described elsewhere (18). Sections are blocked for 1 hr with 1% (w/v) BSA and 1% (v/v) normal goat serum in 0.1 M sodium phosphate buffer, pH 7.4. Sections typically are incubated with antisera or affinity-purified antibodies for 1 hr in 0.1% (w/v) BSA, 0.1% (v/v) normal goat serum in phosphate buffer. After several washes, sections are incubated with a biotinyl-goat anti-rabbit IgG at a dilution of 1:500. After further washing, sections are incubated for 1 hr with a 1:100 dilution of streptavidin–Texas red conjugate (Amersham Corp., Arlington Heights, IL). After dehydrating with ethanol and clearing with xylene, sections are coverslipped and viewed with a Zeiss Universal fluorescence light microscope using ×25 and ×40 neofluar objectives.

Antibodies generated against native recoverin label bovine recoverin (Fig. 3, lane a) but not chicken visinin (Fig. 3, lane b) on Western blots. The antibodies stain the photoreceptors of the human retina from the outer segments to the synaptic processes (Fig. 3). Importantly, both rods and cones are labeled (Fig. 3, inset). Antibodies specific for visinin label the cone-dominant chicken retina (Fig. 4A) but not human retina (Fig. 4B). These data indicate that visinin is not present in the human retina, and that differences between recoverin and visinin probably reflect species differences rather than rod–cone differences. This conclusion has been supported by other lines of evidence obtained in our laboratories.

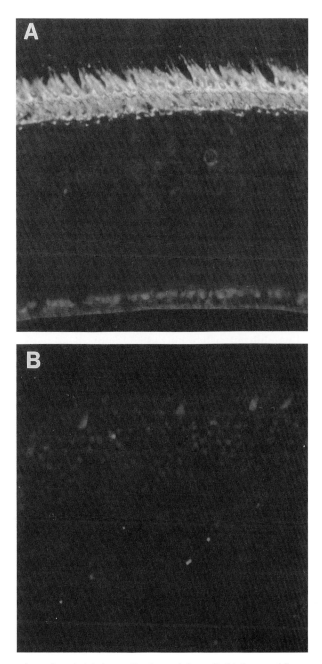

FIG. 4   Detection of antivisinin antibody staining of chicken and human retinas. An affinity-purified antibody to chicken visinin labeled cryosections of chicken retina (A) but not human retina (B), following the procedures given in the text and in the legend to Figure 3.

Purification of Calmodulin and S-100 Related Proteins

In addition to bovine recoverin and chicken visinin, Phenyl-Sepharose chromatography yields at least three other calcium-binding proteins that can be purified to apparent homogeneity in a single chromatographic step.

Phenyl-Sepharose Eluate

The retinal extract from 100 bovine eyes is applied to a Phenyl-Sepharose column, and the eluate is obtained by the addition of EDTA, as described above. The relevant fractions are combined, dialyzed against water, and lyophilized.

Reversed-Phase High-Performance Liquid Chromatography

The sample is redissolved in 2 ml of 0.1% (v/v) trifluoroacetic acid (TFA) in water (buffer A), and an aliquot of 400–500 μl is loaded onto a 4.6 × 150 mm C_4 column (Phenomonex W-Porex 5, Torrance, CA). The gradient is developed at 0.6 ml/min using buffer A and buffer B (80% CH_3CN, 0.08%, v/v, TFA) with a program extending over 95 min: 0–45% buffer B, 5 min; 45–68% buffer B, 85 min; 68–95% buffer B, 90 min; 95–100% buffer B, 95 min. Aliquots (0.5 ml each) are collected and either dialyzed against water and lyophilized or lyophilized and neutralized with 0.1 M Tris base prior to electrophoresis. Purified proteins are cleaved and subjected to partial amino acid sequence analysis as described above.

The RP-HPLC profile obtained for the separation of the bovine Phenyl-Sepharose eluate is shown in Fig. 5. Fractions obtained from each of the peaks are subjected to SDS-PAGE. Peak I contains an abundant 17-kDa protein (Fig. 5 inset, lane a) that is identified by partial amino acid sequence analysis as calmodulin. Peak II contains the 13-kDa protein (Fig. 5 inset, lane b) that was present in the bovine Phenyl-Sepharose eluate (Fig. 1, lane d). Peak III consists of the 9-kDa protein (Fig. 5 inset, lane c), also seen in the Phenyl-Sepharose eluate of Fig. 1 (lane d); a protein of the same molecular weight is isolated in peak V. The 9-kDa proteins of peaks III and V may differ in the posttranslational modification of the same polypeptide chain or in the extent of bound calcium. Alternatively, the two peaks may represent the separation of distinct proteins. Partial amino acid sequencing and other analyses indicate that the 13- and 9-kDa proteins are S-100 related proteins. The multiple peaks identified as IV in the chromatogram of Fig. 5 contain recoverin. Again, the separation of recoverin into distinct peaks may reflect differences in posttranslational modifications or bound calcium. Efforts are now underway to characterize the structure and function of the 13- and 9-kDa proteins and to localize each in the retina.

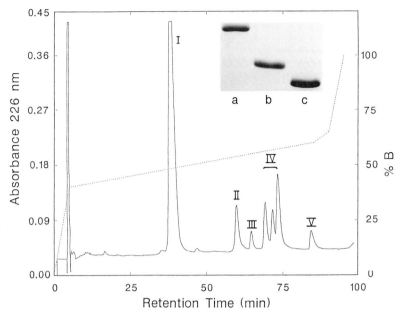

FIG. 5 Reversed-phase HPLC purification of a bovine retinal Phenyl-Sepharose eluate. Protein eluted from the Phenyl-Sepharose column by the addition of EDTA (Fig. 1) was dialyzed, lyophilized, and further separated on a C_4 column, as described in the text. Five major fractions were identified, and the constituent proteins were characterized by SDS-PAGE (inset). Peak I contained a 17-kDa protein (lane a). Peak II contained a 13-kDa protein (lane b), and peaks III and V contained a 9-kDa protein (lane c). The complex fraction IV contained recoverin.

Conclusions

Calcium-binding proteins that share significant structural features are found throughout the four kingdoms, indicating that a primordial gene has been reiterated at various stages of evolution in order to harness calcium for a diverse set of biological processes. Biochemical and immunocytochemical studies have demonstrated that several calcium-binding proteins are present in the retina (8, 9). One of these, recoverin, may have a direct role in mediating some light adaptational events in photoreceptors (12, 13). Visinin may act similarly in the cone-dominant chicken retina.

The role of calmodulin in photoreceptors is not as well documented. Although biochemical measurements indicate that calmodulin is present in photoreceptors (19, 20), immunocytochemical methods, thus far, have failed to support this conclusion. However, calmodulin is known to complex with spectrin, which is present in rod cells (21), and binding to an effector molecule may interfere with the immunocytochemical detection. Calmodulin appears to function by regulating specific enzymatic reactions in a calcium-dependent manner. Aside from regulating effector molecules, calmodulin and other calcium-binding proteins also may act as buffers of calcium. Calmodulin, for example, has four calcium binding sites with apparent affinities of 10^6–10^7 M^{-1}. These affinities, along with its apparent abundance in cells, indicate that calmodulin should bind most free calcium in a dark-adapted photoreceptor. This buffering capacity may protect the cell from the cytotoxic effects of elevated calcium. Additionally, the buffering capacity of these proteins might slow any response initiated by the reduction of intracellular calcium that occurs on illumination (10).

The S-100 proteins, like calmodulin, are highly conserved (22) and are often found as hetero- or homodimers (23). The retinal Phenyl-Sepharose eluate contains two proteins that are of the same molecular weight as S-100 subunits. Like calmodulin, the S-100 proteins supposedly exert their biological effects by regulating other molecules in a calcium-dependent manner. In other tissues, S-100 proteins regulate adenylate cyclase activity, and the homodimeric disulfide-bonded form of S-100β induces neurite extension (for review, see Ref. 24). In the presence of microtubule-associated proteins, both S-100α and S-100β can cause the calcium-dependent depolymerization of microtubules and inhibit their further assembly (25). S-100 proteins also can block the phosphorylation of protein kinase C substrates (26). Whereas the 13- and 9-kDa proteins can be isolated by Phenyl-Sepharose chromatography of total retinal extracts, they are not obtained from isolated rod outer segments. It is not yet known whether these proteins are present in other regions of the photoreceptor and/or other retinal neurons.

Calbindin has been localized by several laboratories, including our own, to cone cells, as well as inner retinal neurons in a species-specific manner (8, 27, 28). Additionally, in human retina, we have observed calretinin immunoreactivity to a small degree in cone cells but to a larger extent in the inner retina; a similar pattern was observed in monkey (9). We have purified both proteins following published procedures (29, 30). If calcium is a major modulator of light adaptation in the retina, then the presence of calbindin and calretinin exclusively in cone cells may explain some of the differences in the adaptational properties between rods and cones.

More calcium-binding proteins, undoubtedly, will be discovered in the retina. Although the function of these proteins has eluded description in the brain, the accessibility and well-characterized physiology of retinal neurons makes the retina a promising site for elucidating the role of these proteins in the central nervous system.

Acknowledgments

This work was supported by grants (to A. S. Polans) from the National Eye Institute (NIH EY 07089), the National Retinitis Pigmentosa Foundation, Inc., and from the Oregon Lions Sight and Hearing Foundation. Further support included (to J. Crabb) National Institutes of Health Grants EY 06603, CA 37589, and (to K. Palczewski) EY 08061.

References

1. S. Ebashi, *J. Biochem.* (*Tokyo*) **48**, 150 (1960).
2. R. H. Kretsinger, *in* "Neuroscience Research Progress Bulletin," Vol. 19, MIT Press, Cambridge, Massachusetts, 1981.
3. C. W. Heizmann and W. Hunziker, *Trends Biochem. Sci.* **16**, 98 (1991).
4. N. C. J. Strynadka and M. N. G. James, *Annu. Rev. Biochem.* **58**, 951 (1989).
5. M. R. Crompton, S. E. Moss, and M. J. Crumpton, *Cell* (*Cambridge, Mass.*) **55**, 1 (1988).
6. E. F. Sato, Y. Tanaka, K. Edashige, J. Sasaki, M. Inoue, and K. Utsumi, *in* "Novel Calcium-Binding Proteins" (C. W. Heizmann, ed.), p. 567. Springer-Verlag, Berlin, 1991.
7. A. R. Means, J. S. Tash, and J. G. Chafouleas, *Physiol. Rev.* **62**, 1 (1982).
8. M. R. Celio, *Neuroscience* **35**, 375 (1990).
9. J. Rogers, *in* "Novel Calcium-Binding Proteins" (C. W. Heizmann, ed.), p. 251. Springer-Verlag, Berlin, 1991.
10. E. N. Pugh, Jr., and T. D. Lamb, *Vision Res.* **30**, 1923 (1990).
11. K. W. Koch and L. Stryer, *Nature* (*London*) **334**, 64 (1988).
12. A. Dizhoor, S. Ray, S. Kumar, G. Niemi, M. Spencer, D. Brolley, K. Walsh, P. P. Philipov, J. B. Hurley, and L. Stryer, *Science* **251**, 915 (1991).
13. H. G. Lambrecht and K. W. Koch, *EMBO J.* **10**, 793 (1991).
14. A. S. Polans, J. Buczylko, J. Crabb, and K. Palczewski, *J. Cell Biol.* **112**, 981 (1991).
15. A. M. Iacopino and S. Christakos, *Proc. Natl. Acad. Sci. U.S.A.* **87**, 4078 (1990).
16. J. W. Crabb, C. M. Johnson, S. A. Carr, L. G. Armes, and J. C. Saari, *J. Biol. Chem.* **263**, 18678 (1988).
17. M. D. Burton, L. T. Onstott, and A. S. Polans, *Anal. Biochem.* **183**, 225 (1989).
18. A. S. Polans and M. D. Burton, *Invest. Ophthalmol. Visual Sci.* **29**, 1523 (1988).
19. S. Nagao, A. Yamazaki, and M. Bitensky, *Biochemistry* **26**, 1659 (1987).
20. R. E. Kohnken, J. G. Chafouleas, D. M. Eadie, A. R. Means, and D. G. McConnell, *J. Biol. Chem.* **256**, 12517 (1981).
21. S. Wong and R. S. Molday, *Biochemistry* **25**, 6294 (1986).
22. B. Moore, *in* "Neuronal and Glial Proteins" (P. J. Marangos, I. C. Campbell, and R. M. Cohen, eds.), p. 137. Academic Press, San Diego, 1984.
23. T. Isobe, T. Nakajima, and T. Okuyama, *Biochim. Biophys. Acta* **494**, 222 (1977).

24. D. C. Hilt and D. Kligman, *in* ''Novel Calcium-Binding Proteins'' (C. W. Heizmann, ed.), p. 65. Springer-Verlag, Berlin, 1991.
25. J. Baudier, C. Briving, J. Deinum, K. Haglid, L. Sorskog, and M. Wallin, *FEBS Lett.* **147,** 165 (1982).
26. J. Baudier, C. Bronner, D. Klingman, and R. D. Cole, *J. Biol. Chem.* **264,** 1824 (1989).
27. R. Pochet, M. Parmentier, D. E. M. Lawson, and J. L. Pasteels, *Brain Res.* **345,** 251 (1985).
28. M. Parmentier, M. Ghysens, F. Rypens, D. E. M. Lawson, J. L. Pasteels, and R. Pochet, *Gen. Comp. Endocrinol.* **65,** 399 (1987).
29. K. Maruyama, K. Ebisawa, and Y. Nonomura, *Anal. Biochem.* **151,** 1 (1985).
30. L. Winsky and D. M. Jacobowitz, *in* ''Novel Calcium-Binding Proteins'' (C. W. Heizmann, ed.), p. 277. Springer-Verlag, Berlin, 1991.

[18]   Preparation and Characterization of Protein Kinase C from Rod Outer Segments

Alexandra C. Newton

Introduction

Structure, Function, and Regulation of Protein Kinase C

The Ca^{2+}/lipid-dependent enzyme protein kinase C transduces extracellular signals that provoke the turnover of the inositol phospholipids (1). Receptor-mediated hydrolysis of phosphatidylinositol bisphosphate generates two second messengers: the water-soluble head group inositol trisphosphate and the lipid backbone diacylglycerol. Inositol trisphosphate mobilizes intracellular Ca^{2+}, causing cytosolic protein kinase C to translocate to the plasma membrane, where it is activated by diacylglycerol. Activity is also dependent on phosphatidylserine, an acidic, aminophospholipid located exclusively on the inner leaflet of the plasma membrane (2). The activated kinase phosphorylates a wide variety of proteins, in addition to catalyzing its autophosphorylation by an intrapeptide reaction (3). Protein kinase C is also activated by potent tumor promoters, phorbol esters, which replace the diacylglycerol requirement for activity (4).

Mounting evidence suggests that a major function of protein kinase C is the desensitization of cells to extracellular information by receptor phosphorylation. For example, phosphorylation of the epidermal growth factor (EGF) receptor by protein kinase C inhibits the intrinsic tyrosine kinase activity of the EGF receptor, a function essential for transducing the growth factor signal (5). Desensitization of the β-adrenergic receptor (6), serotonin 5-HT_{1A} receptor (7), and the nicotinic acetylcholine receptor (8) may also result, in part, from protein kinase C activation. Not all protein kinase C-catalyzed phosphorylations of receptors are negative modulators: phosphorylation of the vitamin D receptor (9) appears to couple the receptor to its effectors.

Protein kinase C is a single polypeptide with a molecular mass of approximately 80 kDa: the kinase region is located in the 45-kDa carboxy-terminal domain, whereas the membrane-binding region is confined to the 35-kDa amino terminus of the peptide. Protein kinase C is a family of functionally similar proteins; to date, nine different mammalian isozymes of the protein have been described (2). Of these isozymes, α, βI, βII, and γ are dependent on Ca^{2+} for activity, whereas the more recently discovered δ, ε, ζ, η, and θ are Ca^{2+}-independent kinases. All members of the family are activated by phosphatidylserine and diacylglycerol. A photoreceptor-specific isozyme from *Drosophila* has been cloned (10).

Protein Kinase C in Rod Outer Segments

The abundance of protein kinase C in rod outer segments (11) and the light-induced turnover of phosphatidylinositol bisphosphate (12) suggest that the enzyme is involved in rod outer segment function. Protein kinase C phosphorylates rhodopsin in intact retinas, a phosphorylation that is most pronounced at low levels of illumination (13). Enzymological studies have revealed that protein kinase C has the same affinity for unbleached and bleached rhodopsin (13) and that the phosphorylation inhibits the light-dependent coupling of rhodopsin to transducin (14). Based on the foregoing observations, two biochemically distinct desensitizing phosphorylations have been proposed for rhodopsin (13): the protein kinase C-catalyzed phosphorylation that mediates desensitization to low levels of light, and the rhodopsin kinase-catalyzed phosphorylation that dominates at high levels of light. Modification by two different kinases, one dominating at low agonist concentrations (modifying unliganded and liganded receptor) and the other at high agonist concentrations (modifying liganded receptor only), has also been proposed to provide two adaptive mechanisms for the β-adrenergic receptor (15).

Assay for Protein Kinase C

Substrate

The initial rate of incorporation of the γ-phosphate of $[\gamma\text{-}^{32}P]ATP$ into saturating amounts of the synthetic peptide FKKSFKL-NH$_2$ (16) provides an excellent measure of protein kinase C activity since this peptide is not recognized detectably by other kinases in rod outer segments. One peptide unit of protein kinase C activity is defined as 1 nmol ^{32}P incorporated per minute into saturating amounts of protein kinase C-selective peptide. Commercially available histone H1 is the standard protein kinase C substrate and can be substituted at a final concentration of 20 μM in the assay described below; reactions are allowed to proceed for 3 min at 30°C. The Ca^{2+}/lipid-independent activity is significantly higher when histone is used as a substrate, however, as it is phosphorylated by other rod outer segment kinases (see Fig. 3).

Lipid

Sonicated suspensions of bovine brain L-α-phosphatidylserine (1.4 mM) and sn-1,2-dioleoylglycerol (76 μM) are prepared by drying a chloroform mixture of the lipids under N$_2$, hydrating in 20 mM Tris, pH 7.4 (30°C), and sonicating briefly (30 sec in bath sonicator at room temperature) to disperse lipid. In the experiments presented, lipid was purchased from Avanti Polar Lipids (Birmingham, AL).

Assay

Sample containing protein kinase C (typically 10 μl in buffer containing 1 mM EDTA, 1 mM EGTA) is diluted into a solution containing 100 μM leupeptin, 2 mM dithiothreitol (DTT), 20 mM Tris, pH 7.4 (30°C), to a final volume of 48 μl. To this is added lipid (8 μl of 1.4 mM phosphatidylserine, 76 μM diacylglycerol) and 8 μl of 5–10 mM CaCl$_2$ (CaCl$_2$ is added so that the concentration of free Ca^{2+} in the assay mixture is 200–400 μM). To measure protein kinase C-independent activity, 16 μl of a solution containing 1 mM EDTA, 1 mM EGTA, pH 9, is substituted for the lipid and Ca^{2+}. The reaction is initiated by addition of 16 μl of a solution containing 0.25 mg/ml protein kinase C-selective peptide, 100 μM [γ-^{32}P]ATP (0.14 Ci/mmol ATP), 50 mM MgCl$_2$, 20 mM Tris, pH 7.4, and samples are incubated at 30°C for 10 min. Thus, in an assay of a 10-μl column fraction, the 80-μl incubation medium contains 50 μg/ml protein kinase C-selective peptide, 50 μM leupeptin, 1 mM DTT, 140 μM phosphatidylserine, 7.6 μM diacylglycerol, 0.5 mM CaCl$_2$, 0.125 mM EDTA, 0.125 mM EGTA, 20 μM ATP, 10 mM MgCl$_2$, and 20 mM Tris, pH 7.4. The reaction is quenched by the addition of 25 μl of a solution containing 0.1 M ATP, 0.1 M EDTA, pH 7, and aliquots (85 μl) are spotted on Whatman (Hillsboro, OR) P-81 ion-exchange papers (8 cm^2). Papers are washed 4 times, for 5 min per wash, in a total of 2 liters of 0.4% (v/v) phosphoric acid, followed by a quick rinse in ethanol. Radioactivity is detected by scintillation counting of samples in 2.5 ml scintillation fluid. Phosphate incorporation into the protein kinase C-selective peptide is linear with time for the first 10 min of the assay.

Autophosphorylation is detected by omitting substrate from the phosphorylation assay and quenching reactions with sodium dodecyl sulfate (SDS)–polyacrylamide gel electrophoresis sample buffer. Rhodopsin phosphorylation is assayed similarly except that receptor (80 nM) reconstituted in phosphatidylserine–diacylglycerol (95:5, mol %) membranes is in-ed in the assay (13). Samples are analyzed by SDS–polyacrylamide gel electrophoresis followed by autoradiography. Radioactive bands are excised from dried gels and ^{32}P incorporation quantified by liquid scintillation counting.

Purification of Protein Kinase C from Bovine Rod Outer Segments

Rod outer segments are obtained from bovine retinas (typically 60) and separated by sucrose density centrifugation, following a modification of Zimmerman and Godchaux (17). The time between slaughtering and lysis of rod outer segments is minimized (≤6 hr) because of the lability of protein kinase C. Sucrose density gradient-isolated rod outer segments are resuspended in 10 ml homogenization buffer containing 10 mM EGTA, 2 mM EDTA, 21 μM leupeptin, 0.2 mM phenylmethylsulfonyl fluoride (PMSF), 1 mM DTT, 20 mM Tris, pH 7.4, at 4°C and incubated on ice for 20 min, with frequent gentle stirring, to effect osmotic lysis. Freeze–thawing is not recommended as this procedure denatures some of the protein kinase C. The sample is centrifuged at 200,000 g for 60 min at 4°C. The supernatant, referred to as rod outer segment (ROS) cytosol, is chromatographed as described below.

Chromatography

All chromatographic procedures are performed at 4°C using a fast protein liquid chromatography (FPLC) system. Because of the susceptibility of protein kinase C to proteolysis by calpain, which copurifies with protein kinase C on Q Sepharose (18), leupeptin is included in all buffers. The column buffer is 1 mM DTT, 1 mM EDTA, 1 mM EGTA, 21 μM leupeptin, 10% glycerol, 20 mM Tris, pH 7.4 (4°C).

Q Sepharose
The ROS cytosol is diluted 1.5-fold in column buffer (to ensure that the conductivity of the sample is comparable to that of the column buffer) and applied to a Q Sepharose (Pharmacia, Piscataway, NJ) column (9 ml) at a flow rate of 2 ml/min. The column is washed until the absorbance reading returns to zero (4 column volumes); approximately half the ROS cytosolic protein does not bind to the column. Protein kinase C is eluted at a flow rate of 1 ml/min with a 10-column volume gradient consisting of 55 ml of a 0–0.25 M KCl gradient and 33 ml of a 0.25–1.00 M KCl gradient (Fig. 1).

Under these conditions, 60% of protein kinase C elutes as a sharp peak at approximately 100 mM KCl, with the remaining 40% of activity continuing to elute up to 175 mM KCl. Typically, 90% of the protein kinase C activity is recovered from the Q Sepharose column. Rhodopsin kinase elutes at a slightly higher salt concentration than protein kinase C (110 mM KCl under

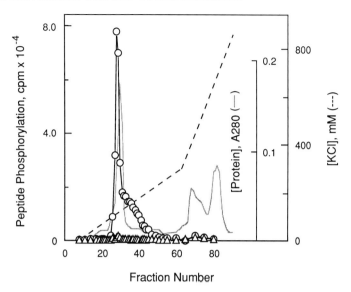

FIG. 1   Q Sepharose chromatography of bovine rod outer segment protein kinase C. Phosphorylation of the protein kinase C-selective peptide was measured in the presence of Ca^{2+} and lipid (○) or in the presence of chelator (△). The KCl concentration and absorbance at 280 nm are indicated.

these conditions), and care should be taken when pooling not to include these fractions if high purity of protein kinase C is desired. Arrestin copurifies with protein kinase C on this column, and it is responsible for the large UV absorbance that peaks two fractions after the peak of protein kinase C activity. Fractions containing protein kinase C but not rhodopsin kinase (i.e., fractions 25–29 in the profile shown in Fig. 1) are pooled and applied directly onto the next column. Other protein kinase C-containing fractions (fractions 30–45; Fig. 1) are pooled and stored at −20°C in 50% glycerol.

Phenyl-Superose

Pooled Q Sepharose fractions are diluted with an equal volume of column buffer containing 2.8 M KCl to bring the KCl concentration to 1.5 M KCl. The sample is loaded onto a 5/5 Phenyl-Superose (Pharmacia) column at a flow rate of 0.5 ml/min and washed until the UV absorbance returns to 0. Arrestin does not bind to this column and is washed off in 10 column volumes. The sample is eluted at a flow rate of 0.5 ml/min with a 10-ml gradient of 1.5–0 M KCl (Fig. 2). Protein kinase C elutes at approximately 0.24 M KCl. Any contaminating rhodopsin kinase present elutes several fractions later at 0 M KCl. Because arrestin and most other proteins from the Q Sepharose

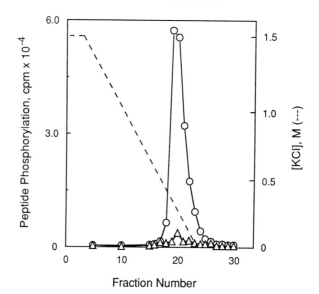

FIG. 2   Phenyl-Superose chromatography of pooled Q Sepharose fractions. Phosphorylation of the protein kinase C-selective peptide was measured in the presence of Ca^{2+} and lipid ($\bigcirc$) or in the presence of chelator ($\triangle$).

pool do not bind to the Phenyl-Superose column, over 500-fold purification is achieved in this step. Protein kinase C, migrating with an apparent molecular mass of 85 kDa, is the major protein in the peak fraction (fraction 19), with minor bands of 23 and 40 kDa detected by silver staining. Fractions are stored at $-20°C$ in column buffer diluted with glycerol to a final concentration of 50%. A summary of a protein kinase C preparation from the cytosol of bovine rod outer segments (from 62 retinas) is presented in Table I. The yield can be increased if the suspending medium in which the retinas are vortexed to break off the rod outer segments is included in the purification; many soluble rod outer segment proteins, including protein kinase C, are released into the medium during rod outer segment isolation.

Characterization of Rod Outer Segment Protein Kinase C

Figure 3 shows that phosphorylation of the protein kinase C-selective peptide and histone H1 by rod outer segment protein kinase C depends on both Ca^{2+}

TABLE I   Purification of Protein Kinase C from Bovine Rod Outer Segments

Fraction	Protein (mg)	Activity (peptide units)	Specific activity (peptide units/mg)	Yield[a] (%)	Purification[b] (-fold)
ROS cytosol:					
10 ml, from 62 retinas	6.8	5.6	0.8	100	1
Q Sepharose:					
5.3 units ROS cytosol loaded onto column					
Fractions 25–55	—	4.4	—	83 (79%)	—
Fractions 25–29	0.8	2.2	2.8	42 (39%)	3.4
Phenyl-Superose:					
1.2 units of Q Sepharose fractions 25–29 loaded onto column					
Fractions 18–24	—	1.0	—	87 (18%)	—
Fractions 19–20	0.0004	0.6	1.5×10^3	54 (11%)	1.8×10^3

[a] Yield is expressed relative to the material loaded onto the column; values in parentheses indicate yield relative to activity in ROS cytosol.
[b] Purification is expressed relative to the specific activity of ROS cytosol.

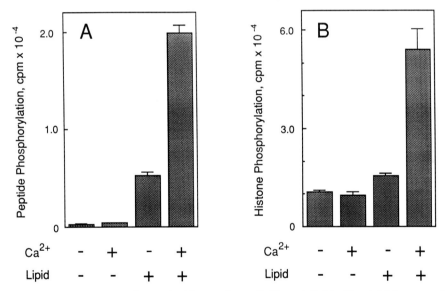

FIG. 3   Dependence of protein kinase C on Ca^{2+} and lipid. The initial rates of phosphorylation of (A) the protein kinase C-selective peptide and (B) histone H1 were measured in the absence or presence of free Ca^{2+} (250 μM) and in the absence or presence of phosphatidylserine–diacylglycerol (95 : 5, mol %). Data are shown as means ± S.E.

and lipid.* Thus, rod outer segment protein kinase C belongs to the family of Ca^{2+}-dependent protein kinase C that comprises the isozymes α, β, and γ. Biochemical data indicate that the enzyme is most similar to the α isozyme (20, 21), whereas immunological data suggest that rod outer segment protein kinase C is a novel isozyme (21).

Rhodopsin is an excellent substrate for rod outer segment protein kinase C (Fig. 4). The enzyme catalyzes the phosphorylation of unbleached and bleached rhodopsin with similar kinetics and to a final stoichiometry of 1 mol phosphate per mole rhodopsin. The K_m for the phosphorylation of unbleached and bleached rhodopsin reconstituted in phosphatidylserine–diacylglycerol membranes is 40 nM receptor (13). Enzymological data support the hypothesis that the protein kinase C-catalyzed phosphorylation of rhodopsin will dominate at low bleach levels, whereas the rhodopsin kinase-catalyzed phosphorylation will dominate at high bleach levels.

Summary

Approximately 2000-fold purification of protein kinase C is achieved by sequential anion-exchange and hydrophobic chromatography of bovine rod outer segment cytosol. Biochemical and immunological data indicate that the rod outer segment enzyme represents a novel Ca^{2+}-dependent protein kinase C, possibly a photoreceptor-specific isozyme. Although the function of the enzyme in regulating the structure and function of photoreceptors remains to be elucidated, evidence supports a role for the enzyme in desensitization to low levels of illumination (13).

Acknowledgments

The author is grateful to Sungsoon Park for isolating rod outer segments, Yelena Hobbie and Jeff Orr for assistance in chromatography, and David Williams for helpful discussions. This work was supported by a Searle Scholars Award from the Chicago Community Trust and by Grant EY 08820 from the National Institutes of Health.

---

* As with other Ca^{2+}-dependent isozymes, some Ca^{2+}-independent protein kinase C activity is observed at the high concentrations of phosphatidylserine (95 mol %) used in the assay described. The Ca^{2+}-independent activity is not detected in a detergent–lipid mixed micellar assay, where the phosphatidylserine concentration required for maximal activity is 10 mol % (19).

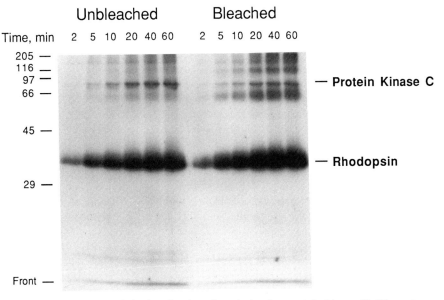

FIG. 4   Time course of rhodopsin phosphorylation by protein kinase C. The autoradiogram shows ^{32}P incorporation from $[\gamma\text{-}^{32}P]ATP$ into unbleached and bleached rhodopsin (80 nM) reconstituted in phosphatidylserine–diacylglycerol (95 : 5, mol %) after incubation with protein kinase C (3 nM) and $CaCl_2$ (1 mM) for 2 to 60 min at 30°C. Protein kinase C was purified from bovine retinas (13). Autophosphorylated protein kinase C and phosphorylated rhodopsin bands are indicated.

References

1. Y. Nishizuka, *Science* **233**, 305 (1986).
2. A. C. Newton, *Annu. Rev. Biophys. Biomol. Struct.* **22**, 1 (1993).
3. A. C. Newton and D. E. Koshland, Jr., *J. Biol. Chem.* **262**, 10185 (1987).
4. M. Castagna, Y. Takai, K. Kaibuchi, K. Sano, U. Kikkawa, and Y. Nishizuka, *J. Biol. Chem.* **257**, 7847 (1982).
5. C. Cochet, G. N. Gill, J. Meisenhelder, J. A. Cooper, and T. Hunter, *J. Biol. Chem.* **259**, 2553 (1984).
6. D. J. Kelleher, J. E. Pessin, A. E. Ruoho, and G. L. Johnson, *Proc. Natl. Acad. Sci. U.S.A.* **81**, 4316 (1984).
7. J. R. Raymond, *J. Biol. Chem.* **266**, 14747 (1991).
8. J. E. G. Downing and L. W. Role, *Proc. Natl. Acad. Sci. U.S.A.* **84**, 7739 (1987).
9. J.-C. Hsieh, P. W. Jurutka, M. A. Galligan, C. M. Terpening, C. A. Haussler, D. S. Samuels, Y. Shimizu, N. Shimizu, and M. R. Haussler, *Proc. Natl. Acad. Sci. U.S.A.* **88**, 9315 (1991).

10. E. Schaeffer, D. Smith, G. Mardon, W. Quinn, and C. Zuker, *Cell* (*Cambridge, Mass.*) **57,** 403 (1989).
11. D. J. Kelleher and G. L. Johnson, *J. Cyclic Nucleotide Protein Phosphorylation Res.* **10,** 579 (1985).
12. A. Ghalayini and R. E. Anderson, *Biochem. Biophys. Res. Commun.* **124,** 503 (1984).
13. A. C. Newton and D. S. Williams, *J. Biol. Chem.* **266,** 17725 (1991).
14. D. J. Kelleher and G. L. Johnson, *J. Biol. Chem.* **261,** 4749 (1986).
15. W. P. Hausdorff, M. G. Caron, and R. J. Lefkowitz, *FASEB J.* **4,** 2881 (1990).
16. B. R. Chakravarthy, A. Bussey, J. F. Whitfield, M. Sikorska, R. E. Williams, and J. P. Durkin, *Anal. Biochem.* **196,** 144 (1991).
17. W. F. Zimmerman and W. Godchaux III, *in* "Methods in Enzymology" (L. Packer, ed.), Vol. 81, p. 52. Academic Press, New York, 1982.
18. S. M. Azarian, C. L. Schlamp, and D. S. Williams, *J. Cell Sci.,* in press.
19. R. M. Bell, Y. Hannun, and C. Loomis, *in* "Methods in Enzymology" (P. M. Conn, ed.), Vol. 124, p. 353. Academic Press, New York, 1986.
20. G. Wolbring and N. J. Cook, *Eur. J. Biochem.* **201,** 601 (1991).
21. A. C. Newton and D. S. Williams, manuscript submitted.

[19] Simultaneous Purification and Characterization of the cGMP-Gated Cation Channel and the $Na^+/Ca^{2+},K^+$-Exchanger

Neil J. Cook

Introduction

The cGMP-gated cation channel and the $Na^+/Ca^{2+},K^+$-exchanger are two integral membrane proteins of paramont importance in the process of vertebrate phototransduction (1, 2). They are both localized in the plasma membrane of the rod photoreceptor outer segment (1, 2). Under conditions of darkness, a significant proportion of cGMP-gated channels is open and mediates a constant inward flow of cations, primarily Na^+ and Ca^{2+}. Sodium ions diffuse toward the inner segment, where they are actively extruded via a Na^+,K^+-ATPase. Calcium ions are extruded directly from the outer segment by the $Na^+/Ca^{2+},K^+$-exchanger. Under physiological conditions this protein couples an inwardly directed Na^+ electrochemical gradient and an outwardly directed K^+ electrochemical gradient to the transport of Ca^{2+} against its electrochemical gradient with a stoichiometry of $4Na_o^+ : 1Ca_i^{2+}, 1K_i^+$.

Illumination of the photoreceptor cell results in activation of a well-characterized enzymatic cascade which leads to the hydrolysis of cGMP. A decrease in the cytosolic concentration of free cGMP results in channel closure and hyperpolarization of the photoreceptor cell. Because the $Na^+/Ca^{2+},K^+$-exchanger continues to operate independently of light, illumination also leads to a decrease in the cytosolic Ca^{2+} concentration, an event important in recovery and reestablishment of the preillumination state of the photoreceptor cell. Clearly, an understanding of the structures of the cGMP-gated channel and the $Na^+/Ca^{2+},K^+$-exchanger and an understanding of how they execute their functions are essential to obtain complete elucidation of vertebrate phototransduction at the molecular level. A mandatory step toward this goal has been the purification and identification of the two transport proteins followed by their molecular cloning. In this chapter, we describe the techniques that we have developed for the solubilization and purification of both the cGMP-gated channel and the $Na^+/Ca^{2+},K^+$-exchanger, as well as methods for the investigation of their functional properties by reconstitution into liposomes (3, 4).

Methods in Neurosciences, Volume 15

Methods

Rod Outer Segment Membrane Preparation

We routinely prepare rod outer segment membranes from bovine retinas using a discontinuous sucrose gradient procedure (5). This method is rapid and yields highly pure rod outer segment membranes.

Purification

Reagents

Hypotonic wash buffer: 10 mM HEPES–KOH, pH 7.4; 1 mM dithiotheitol; 2 mM EDTA

Solubilization buffer: 10 mM HEPES–KOH, pH 7.4; 1 mM dithiothreitol; 10 mM CaCl$_2$; 0.1 M KCl; 1.1% (w/v) CHAPS; 0.22% (w/v) asolectin

DEAE wash buffer: 10 mM HEPES–KOH, pH 7.4; 1 mM dithiothreitol; 10 mM CaCl$_2$; 0.1 M KCl; 0.8% (w/v) CHAPS; 0.16% (w/v) asolectin

DEAE elution buffer: 10 mM HEPES–KOH, pH 7.4; 1 mM dithiothreitol; 10 mM CaCl$_2$; 0.75 M KCl; 0.8% (w/v) CHAPS; 0.16% (w/v) asolectin

AF Red elution buffer: 10 mM HEPES–KOH, pH 7.4; 1 mM dithiothreitol; 10 mM CaCl$_2$; 1.8 M KCl; 0.8% (w/v) CHAPS; 0.16% (w/v) asolectin

Concanavalin A (Con A) equilibration buffer: 10 mM HEPES–KOH, pH 7.4: 1 mM dithiothreitol; 10 mM CaCl$_2$; 1 mM MnCl$_2$; 0.1 M KCl; 0.8% (w/v) CHAPS; 0.16% (w/v) asolectin

Con A elution buffer: 10 mM MgCl$_2$; 1 mM HEPES–KOH, pH 7.4; 1 mM dithiothreitol; 10 mM CaCl$_2$; 0.1 M α-methylmannoside; 0.8% (w/v) CHAPS; 0.16% (w/v) asolectin

Reconstitution buffer: 10 mM HEPES–KOH, pH 7.4; 1 mM dithiothreitol; 2 mM CaCl$_2$; 0.5% (w/v) CHAPS; 1.84% (w/v) asolectin; this buffer must be sonicated until a homogeneous suspension is obtained

Dialysis buffer: 10 mM HEPES–KOH, pH 7.4; 100 mM KCl; 2 mM CaCl$_2$

All solubilization and chromatography buffers are filtered (nitrocellulose, 0.45 μm pore size) before use and adjusted to contain the following protease inhibitors: diisopropylfluorophosphate (0.1 mM), aprotonin (2 μg/ml), leupeptin (2 μg/ml), and pepstatin (2 μg/ml). Asolectin (soybean phosphatidylcholine, type IV-S; Sigma, St. Louis, MO), is treated with butyrated hydroxytoluene and α-tocopherol before use (6).

Solubilization

Rod outer segment membranes containing 50 mg rhodopsin are treated to remove peripheral proteins in complete darkness by suspension in hypotonic wash buffer followed by centrifugation at 150,000 g for 30 min. This procedure is performed 3 times, and the pellet is then suspended in 50 ml solubilization buffer. After intermittent vortexing over a period of 15 min, the suspension is centrifuged at 150,000 g for 30 min. The resulting supernatant is then used for column chromatography at 4°C under normal light conditions.

DEAE Chromatography

The solubilized membranes are directly applied at a flow rate of 0.5 ml/min to a column (0.9 × 4 cm) packed with DEAE-Fractogel TSK (Merck, Darmstadt, Germany), that has been equilibrated with DEAE wash buffer. The column is then washed with DEAE wash buffer, and, after the absorbance at 280 nm of the effluent has returned to the baseline level, the column is eluted with DEAE elution buffer.

Affinity Chromatography on AF Red–Fractogel TSK

The protein fraction eluted from the DEAE column is directly applied at a flow rate of 0.2 ml/min to a column (0.9 × 6 cm) packed with AF Red–Fractogel TSK (Merck) that has been equilibrated with DEAE elution buffer. The protein fraction that does not bind to the column is collected, and the column is then washed with DEAE elution buffer. After the absorbance at 280 nm has returned to baseline level, the column is eluted with AF Red elution buffer to yield essentially pure channel protein complex.

Lectin Affinity Chromatography

The protein fraction that does not bind to the AF Red column is directly applied at a flow rate of 0.4 ml/min to a column (0.9 × 6 cm) packed with Con A–Sepharose 4B (Pharmacia, Uppsala, Sweden) that has been equilibrated with Con A equilibration buffer. After washing with equilibration buffer until the absorbance at 280 nm has returned to baseline level, the column is eluted with Con A elution buffer to yield essentially pure $Na^+/Ca^{2+},K^+$-exchanger.

The purification procedures for the cGMP-gated channel and the $Na^+/Ca^{2+},K^+$-exchanger are schematically represented in Fig. 1. In a typical experiment starting with rod outer segment membranes containing approxi-

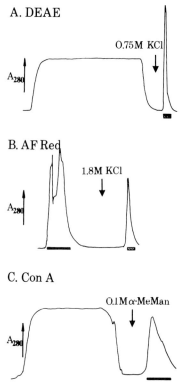

FIG. 1 Chromatographic purification of the cGMP-gated channel and the $Na^+/Ca^{2+},K^+$-exchanger from bovine rod outer segments. (A) DEAE-Fractogel TSK chromatography; (B) AF Red-Fractogel TSK chromatography; (C) Concanavalin A–Sepharose 4B chromatography. In A–C, the abscissa represents the absorbance of the column effluent at 280 nm (not to scale between chromatograms), and the ordinate represents effluent volume. Column fractions containing the cGMP-gated channel are underlined with hatched bars, and those containing the $Na^+/Ca^{2+},K^+$-exchanger are underlined with solid bars.

mately 50 mg rhodopsin, the procedure yields 10–30 μg of both proteins in purified form.

Functional Reconstitution

Reconstitution of the purified channel or exchanger protein into Ca^{2+}-containing asolectin liposomes is achieved using a CHAPS dialysis procedure (6). One milliliter of reconstitution buffer is added per milliliter of purified protein extract and incubated for 30 min on ice. The suspension is then placed in presoaked dialysis tubing (i.d. 1-8/32, Medicell, London, UK) and dialyzed for a total of 48 hr against three changes of dialysis buffer (total volume 5 liters). A transmembrane Ca^{2+} gradient can then be established by a further overnight dialysis step against Ca^{2+}-free dialysis buffer. The release of calcium, either by the addition of cGMP in the case of the channel protein or by the addition of Na^+ in the case of the exchanger protein, can then be spectroscopically determined using the metallochromic dye arsenazo III. More recently, we have succeeded in reconstituting the $Na^+/Ca^{2+},K^+$-exchanger into Na^+-containing liposomes (5). The addition of such liposomes to a cuvette containing Ca^{2+} and arsenazo III in the absence of Na^+ results in the dilution of extraliposomal Na^+ and the establishment of an electrochemical Na^+ gradient across the liposomal membrane. This results in Ca^{2+} uptake that can be readily measured spectroscopically.

Molecular Characterization

cGMP-Gated Channel

Sodium dodecyl sulfate (SDS)–polyacrylamide gel electrophoresis of the purified channel protein extract is shown in Fig. 2 (lane A). As well as the 63-kDa channel protein, the extract also typically exhibits a 240-kDa component not essential for channel activity (3). We have recently shown that this protein is a cytoskeletal component immunologically related to spectrin and that it is directly associated with the channel complex (7). The channel therefore presumably exists as a homooligomer (probably a tetramer or pentamer) of the 63-kDa polypeptide. The channel protein binds the lectin concanavalin A, and it has been shown to be N-glycosylated at one site only (8).

Complementary DNA for the channel protein has been cloned and sequenced, and transcripts of the cDNA have been shown to lead to the expression of cGMP-gated channel activity in *Xenopus* oocytes (9). The channel protein sequence was found to correspond to a protein with a molecular mass of 79.6 kDa; the difference between this value and that deduced from SDS–polyacrylamide gel electrophoresis can be explained by the observation that the channel protein is post- or cotranslationally modified by the removal of a 92-amino acid peptide at its N terminus (10). From the sequence alone it is unclear in which channel "superfamily" the cGMP-gated channel belongs, namely, ligand-gated channels which consist of pentamers of subunits exhibiting four putative transmembrane α helices or voltage-gated channels which exhibit four subunits (or domains), each of which possesses six putative

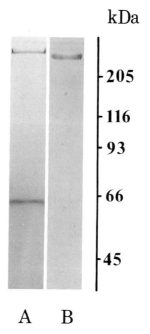

FIG. 2 SDS–9% polyacrylamide gel electrophoresis of the cGMP-gated channel purified extract (lane A) and the $Na^+/Ca^{2+},K^+$-exchanger purified extract (lane B).

transmembrane helices. Topological studies have revealed that the N terminus is localized intracellularly (10) and that the amino acid sequence 321–339 is localized extracellularly, with Asn-327 being N-glycosylated (11). Together with the observation that the C terminus must be localized intracellularly since it contains the cGMP binding site (9), these results have permitted the proposal of topological models for the cGMP-gated channel within the rod outer segment plasma membrane (11).

$Na^+/Ca^{2+},K^+$-Exchanger

The purified $Na^+/Ca^{2+},K^+$-exchanger has an apparent molecular mass of 230 kDa as determined by SDS–polyacrylamide gel electrophoresis (Fig. 2, lane B). The exchanger is probably functional as a monomer, although it does have a tendency to form aggregates in the absence of disulfide reducing agents. The $Na^+/Ca^{2+},K^+$-exchanger is extensively glycosylated and binds the lectins concanavalin A, wheat germ agglutinin, and *Ricinus communis* lectin (after neuraminidase treatment in order to remove terminal sialic acid residues) (4, 12, 13). Neuraminidase treatment alone reduces the apparent molecular mass of the exchanger by about 15 kDa (13). It is also conceivable that the exchanger protein is O-glycosylated, since during gas-phase sequencing of two peptides that we suspect to be localized extracellularly, three Thr residues and one Ser did not give detectable signals (14).

We have succeeded in obtaining partial amino acid sequences after purifying and sequencing peptides arising from cyanogen bromide cleavage of the purified $Na^+/Ca^{2+},K^+$-exchanger. Corresponding oligonucleotide probes were prepared and used to clone the cDNA of the exchanger (14). The corresponding amino acid sequence was found to code for a protein with a molecular mass of approximately 130 kDa. The difference between this value and that observed on SDS–polyacrylamide gel electrophoresis could be due to the extensive glycosylation of the exchanger protein or to abnormal migration of this membrane protein on SDS–polyacrylamide gels (or a combination of these factors). The N terminus of the purified $Na^+/Ca^{2+},K^+$-exchanger was found to begin at Asp-66; it is not yet clear whether the 65 N-terminal amino acids constitute a cleavable signal sequence or whether this proteolysis is an artifact that occurs during chromatographic purification. Based on preliminary topological data, we have proposed a model for the folding of the $Na^+/Ca^{2+},K^+$-exchanger across the rod outer segment plasma membrane (14): the exchanger has a long, heavily glycosylated N-terminal region exposed extracellularly that is followed by a cluster of five transmembrane helices. This is followed by a large hydrophilic, cytosolic loop and then a further cluster of six transmembrane helices. The model terminates with a short, hydrophilic C-terminal region exposed on the intracellular side of the membrane.

Functional Characterization

cGMP-Gated Channel

Using our reconstitution procedure, we were able to investigate several functional properties of the purified cGMP-gated channel protein using Ca^{2+} [or Mg^{2+} (15)] as the transported ion. Furthermore, by fusing channel-containing proteoliposomes with an artificial lipid bilayer formed across the orifice of a Teflon septum, it was possible to investigate several conductive properties of the purified cGMP-gated channel (16). These results are summarized in Table I (17–22), and are compared with the properties of the cGMP-gated channel within its native membrane. It can be seen that the purified channel protein exists in a physiologically relevant condition and exhibits many of the properties of the cGMP-gated channel *in situ*. There are, how-

TABLE I   Comparison of Functional Properties of Purified and
Reconstituted cGMP-Gated Channel with Those of Rod
Photoreceptor Channel *in Situ*

Property	Reconstituted[a–d]	*In situ*[e–i]
K_m cGMP (μM)	11–31	5–67
Cooperativity cGMP (n)	2.3–3.4	1.7–3.0
Unit conductance (pS)	26	25
Substates (pS)	<10	8–10
Ion selectivity	$Na^+ > K^+ > Rb^+ > Cs^+$	$Na^+ > K^+ > Rb^+ > Cs^+$
l-cis-Diltiazem	Insensitive	Sensitive

[a] Cook *et al.* (6).
[b] Cook *et al.* (3).
[c] Hanke *et al.* (16).
[d] Wohlfart *et al.* (15).
[e] Fesenko *et al.* (17).
[f] Zimmerman *et al.* (18).
[g] Stern *et al.* (19).
[h] Zimmerman and Baylor (21).
[i] Haynes *et al.* (22).

ever, two properties of the reconstituted channel that are consistently different: the K_m value of the purified channel for cGMP is generally lower than values reported for the cGMP-gated channel in the native membrane, and the purified and reconstituted channel has a markedly reduced sensitivity to the blocker *l-cis*-diltiazem. These phenomena can probably be explained by the observation (23) that, in the native membrane, the cGMP-gated channel exists in two forms with different cGMP-sensitivities and pharmacological behaviors. One form is activated by low concentrations of cGMP ($K_m \sim 10$–20 μM) and is not blocked by *l-cis*-diltiazem. The second form is activated by high concentrations of cGMP ($K_m \sim 170$ μM) and is almost completely blocked by *l-cis*-diltiazem. It is conceivable that we have succeeded in isolating only the first of the two forms, or that during isolation the second form of the channel protein has undergone some modification (e.g., dephosphorylation) leading to its conversion to the first form. Further work is required to clarify this issue.

$Na^+/Ca^{2+},K^+$-Exchanger

Using the reconstitution procedure described here, we were able to investigate several modes of operation of the $Na^+/Ca^{2+},K^+$-exchanger. The electrogenicity, reversibility, and K^+ dependence of the $Na^+/Ca^{2+},K^+$-exchanger can all be demonstrated using the reconstituted, purified protein. We have reported that the Na^+ binding site of the exchanger is specific for Na^+ (4), that the K^+ binding site can also bind other cations [with a selectivity of $K^+ \geq Rb^+ > Cs^+ > Li^+$ (5)], and that the only divalent cation transported by $Na^+/Ca^{2+},K^+$-exchanger is Ca^{2+} [Mg^{2+} is not transported (15)]. Our results therefore provide confirmation that many transport properties of the rod outer segment plasma membrane are intrinsic to the $Na^+/Ca^{2+},K^+$-exchanger, and they have led to the discovery of some transport properties of this protein that had not been demonstrated *in situ*.

Using the purified and reconstituted $Na^+/Ca^{2+},K^+$-exchanger, we were also able to characterize many of the kinetic properties of this transport protein. These are summarized in Table II (24–27) and are compared with the $Na^+/Ca^{2+},K^+$-exchanger *in situ*. The K_m values we determined for Na^+ and K^+ are comparable to the values reported for the exchanger protein in its native membrane; however, we did find a higher degree of cooperativity for the Na^+ dependence and a lower turnover number for the purified and reconstituted exchanger. Our experimentally determined n value [3.01 (range 2.50–3.42); n was determined from Hill plots and denotes the number of sodium ions exchanged for one calcium ion] does, however, correlate well with the accepted stoichiometry of the $Na^+/Ca^{2+},K^+$-exchanger (four Na^+ exchanged for one Ca^{2+}) since Hill plots are generally believed to underestimate the degree of cooperativity. Our lower turnover number (115 Ca^{2+} transported/sec) may be an artifact of the reconstitution procedure (e.g., the phospholipids employed may not be as suitable as those present in the native

TABLE II   Comparison of Functional Properties of Purified and Reconstituted $Na^+/Ca^{2+},K^+$-Exchanger with Those of Rod Photoreceptor Exchanger *in Situ*

Property	Reconstituted[a]	*In situ*
K_m Na^+ (mM)	26.1	30–93[c–e]
Cooperativity Na^+ (n)	3.01	2.0–2.3[c–e]
K_m K^+ (mM)	1.0	1.2–1.5[f]
K_m Ca^{2+} (μM)	n.d.[b]	5.0[g]
Turnover number (Ca^{2+}/sec/exchanger)	115	250–750[h]

[a] Friedel *et al.* (5).
[b] n.d., Not determined.
[c] Schnetkamp (23).
[d] Schnetkamp and Bownds (24).
[e] Lagnado *et al.* (25).
[f] Schnetkamp *et al.* (26).
[g] Barrios *et al.* (27).
[h] Calculated from Schnetkamp and Bownds (24) as described by Friedel *et al.* (5).

rod outer segment membrane). In any case, we believe our results clearly demonstrate that the purified and reconstituted $Na^+/Ca^{2+},K^+$-exchanger exists in a physiologically relevant form, and that the methods described here will constitute a valuable system for the investigation of the functional properties of this important transport protein.

Discussion

The cGMP-gated cation channel and the $Na^+/Ca^{2+},K^+$-exchanger have been solubilized and purified in a functional form using the zwitterionic detergent CHAPS (28). This detergent was selected because of its net neutrality (which thereby permits ion-exchange chromatography) and its high critical micellar concentration (which permits functional reconstitution by dialysis). We have found that the presence of protease inhibitors, together with calcium and exogenous phospholipid, in all chromatography buffers greatly improves the stability of both proteins in detergent solution.

We have modified our original procedure (3) for the purification of the cGMP-gated channel by slightly decreasing the concentration of KCl (from 0.15 to 0.1 M) when applying solubilized rod outer segment membranes to the DEAE-Fractogel TSK column. This improvement was found to increase significantly the yield of the cGMP-gated channel at this step without having any noticeable effect on the degree of purification. Over the years we have found that the purification of the cGMP-gated channel on AF Red–Fractogel TSK gives rather variable yields, presumably because of variation between batches of this affinity matrix. In many cases it can be observed that the high-salt elution step is insufficient to elute all of the channel protein from the column; we found that it was possible to elute additional channel protein from the column under denaturing conditions with detergent buffer containing 6 M urea.

Although we have successfully used Con A lectin chromatography for the final purification of the $Na^+/Ca^{2+},K^+$-exchanger, other lectin matrices (e.g., immobilized wheat germ agglutinin) were also found to give good results. Chromatography of solubilized rod outer segment membranes on immobilized *Ricinus communis* lectin, after pretreatment of the membranes with neuraminidase, was also found to lead to purification of the $Na^+/Ca^{2+},K^+$-exchanger to approximately 60% purity (13).

In conclusion, the procedures described here permit the rapid purification of tens of micrograms of the cGMP-gated channel and $Na^+/Ca^{2+},K^+$-exchanger proteins. The purification procedures are rapid and can be carried out within one working day. The availability of both proteins in their purified forms will greatly facilitate studies directed at the structure and regulation of these transport proteins. A reconstitution procedure is described that permits the investigation of the functional properties of both proteins after purification. This strategy offers two important advantages over *in situ* studies. First, the transport protein can be studied in its purified form. All functional properties observed are therefore intrinsic to the protein under investigation and cannot be attributed to other transport mechanisms. Second, it is possible to impose completely defined conditions (e.g., ion concentrations) on the system, thereby greatly simplifying data interpretation. We believe that our results testify to the immense value of the reconstitution procedure and that the methods developed here will continue to provide a unique system for functional studies of the cGMP-gated channel and the $Na^+/Ca^{2+},K^+$-exchanger.

Acknowledgments

This work was supported by the Deutsche Forschungsgemeinschaft (SFB 169, Projekt C3), the Fonds der Chemischen Industrie, and the Max-Planck Gesellschaft. The author thanks U. Benjamin Kaupp (Jülich, Germany) and Robert S. Molday (Vancouver, Canada) for fruitful collaborations during the course of this work and Nadik Abdulaev for valuable comments on the manuscript.

References

1. K.-W. Yau and D. A. Baylor, *Annu. Rev. Neurosci.* **12,** 289 (1989).
2. P. P. M. Schnetkamp, *Prog. Biophys. Mol. Biol.* **113,** 177 (1989).
3. N. J. Cook, W. Hanke, and U. B. Kaupp, *Proc. Natl. Acad. Sci. U.S.A.* **84,** 585 (1987).
4. N. J. Cook and U. B. Kaupp, *J. Biol. Chem.* **263,** 1382 (1988).
5. U. Friedel, G. Wolbring, P. Wohlfart, and N. J. Cook, *Biochim. Biophys. Acta* **1061,** 247 (1991).
6. N. J. Cook, C. Zeilinger, K.-W. Koch, and U. B. Kaupp, *J. Biol. Chem.* **261,** 17033 (1986).
7. L. L. Molday, N. J. Cook, U. B. Kaupp, and R. S. Molday, *J. Biol. Chem.* **265,** 18690 (1990).
8. P. Wohlfart, H. Müller, and N. J. Cook, *J. Biol. Chem.* **264,** 20934 (1989).
9. U. B. Kaupp, T. Niidome, T. Tanabe, S. Terada, W. Bönigk, W. Stühmer, N. J. Cook, K. Kangawa, H. Matsuo, T. Hirosi, T. Miyata, and S. Numa, *Nature* (*London*) **342,** 762 (1989).
10. R. S. Molday, L. L. Molday, A. Dosé, I. Clark-Lewis, M. Illing, N. J. Cook, E. Eismann, and U. B. Kaupp, *J. Biol. Chem.* **266,** 21917 (1991).
11. P. Wohlfart, W. Haase, R. S. Molday, and N. J. Cook, *J. Biol. Chem.* **267,** 644–648 (1992).

12. D. A. Nicoll and M. L. Applebury, *J. Biol. Chem.* **264,** 16207 (1990).
13. D. Reid, U. Friedel, R. S. Molday, and N. J. Cook, *Biochemistry* **29,** 1601 (1990).
14. H. Reiländer, A. Achilles, U. Friedel, G. Maul, F. Lottspeich, and N. J. Cook, *EMBO J.* **11,** 1689–1695 (1992).
15. P. Wohlfart, R. Vienhues, and N. J. Cook, *Biochim. Biophys. Acta* **1022,** 283 (1990).
16. W. Hanke, N. J. Cook, and U. B. Kaupp, *Proc. Natl. Acad. Sci. U.S.A.* **85,** 94 (1988).
17. E. E. Fesenko, S. S. Kolesnikov, and A. Lyubarsky, *Nature (London)* **313,** 310 (1985).
18. A. L. Zimmerman, G. Yamaka, F. Eckstein, D. A. Baylor, and L. Stryer, *Proc. Natl. Acad. Sci. U.S.A.* **82,** 8813 (1985).
19. J. H. Stern, U. B. Kaupp, and P. MacLeish, *Proc. Natl. Acad. Sci. U.S.A.* **83,** 1163 (1986).
20. A. L. Zimmerman and D. A. Baylor, *Nature (London)* **321,** 70 (1986).
21. L. W. Haynes, A. R. Kay, and K.-W. Yau, *Nature (London)* **321,** 66 (1986).
22. K.-W. Koch, N. J. Cook, and U. B. Kaupp, *J. Biol. Chem.* **262,** 14415 (1987).
23. P. P. M. Schnetkamp, *J. Physiol. (London)* **373,** 25 (1986).
24. P. P. M. Schnetkamp and M. D. Bownds, *J. Gen. Physiol.* **89,** 481 (1987).
25. L. Lagnado, L. Cervetto, and P. A. McNaughton, *Proc. Natl. Acad. Sci. U.S.A.* **85,** 4548 (1989).
26. P. P. M. Schnetkamp, D. K. Basu, and R. T. Szerencsei, *Am. J. Physiol.* **257,** C152 (1989).
27. B. Barrios, D. A. Nicoll, and K. D. Philipson, *Biophys. J.* **57,** 180a (1990).
28. L. M. Hjelmeland, *Proc. Natl. Acad. Sci. U.S.A.* **77,** 6368 (1980).

Section IV

Molecular Biology of Photoreceptor Cells

[20] Construction of Directional cDNA Libraries from Human Retinal Tissue/Cells and Their Enrichment for Specific Genes Using an Efficient Subtraction Procedure

Anand Swaroop

Introduction

The identification of genes that are specifically expressed in retinal cell types should provide molecular insights into the development of visual function. A major requirement for cloning and characterizing these novel genes is the ability to generate high-fidelity cDNA libraries from retinas at different stages of development and from individual retinal cell types. Subtraction methods can then be used to enrich for cell- or tissue-specific clones in a cDNA library. Described here are step-by-step protocols for constructing directional cDNA libraries from human retinal tissues/cells and isolating specific clones by an efficient subtraction cloning procedure.

Construction of cDNA Libraries

Choice of Vector

Lambda (λ) phage is the vector of choice for generating cDNA libraries because of high efficiency of cloning and ease in storage and screening. However, plasmid vectors are more versatile and have several unique features. Certain plasmid vectors (e.g., Bluescript) contain multiple cloning sites, T3 and T7 RNA polymerase promoters, and an f1 origin of replication. The subtraction cloning procedure, described in this chapter, uses cDNA libraries in the Bluescript plasmid vector. However, direct construction of cDNA libraries in Bluescript requires a larger amount of poly (A)$^+$ RNA because of lower cloning efficiency. The clones in the phage λzap II (Stratagene, La Jolla, CA) can be converted to Bluescript, but transfer of the complete cDNA library generates bias based on size because of the single-stranded phage step. We, therefore, prefer to generate cDNA libraries in Charon BS lambda vector (1). These libraries can be transferred to Bluescript plasmid in one simple step without significant bias.

Materials

Biochemicals, Reagents, and Enzymes

The reagents are purchased from the following suppliers: $p(dT)_{12-18}$ and deoxynucleoside triphosphate (dNTP) solutions, Pharmacia (Piscataway, NJ); RNasin, Promega Corp. (Madison, WI); $[\alpha\text{-}^{32}P]dCTP$, Amersham (Arlington Heights, IL); nuclease-free bovine serum albumin (BSA), phenol, 1-kb ladder, transformation-competent cells, Moloney murine leukemia virus (MMLV) reverse transcriptase, and *Escherichia coli* RNase H, GIBCO–BRL (Grand Island, NY); low melting point agarose, FMC Bioproducts (Rockland, ME); Gigapack Gold packaging extract, Stratagene; calf intestine alkaline phosphatase (CIP), Boehringer-Mannheim (Indianapolis, IN); oligonucleotide 5′GCTTGAATTCAAGC3′, custom synthesis; all other enzymes, New England Biolabs (Beverly, MA).

Host Bacteria

Escherichia coli K802 rec A⁻ is obtained from American Type Culture Collection (Rockville, MD, Cat. No. 47026).

Phage

Charon BS (+) and (−) are available from the author [Departments of Ophthalmology and Human Genetics, University of Michigan, Kellogg Eye Center, 1000 Wall Street, Ann Arbor, MI 48105; phone (313) 936-9547, fax (313) 936-2340]. Vector arms (under the trade name Lambda BlueMid) can also be obtained from Clontech (Palo Alto, CA).

Solutions

First-strand buffer (5×): 250 mM Tris-Cl, pH 8.3 (at room temperature); 375 mM KCl; 15 mM MgCl$_2$; 50 mM dithiothreitol (DTT); 0.5 mg/ml BSA

Second-strand buffer (5×): 125 mM Tris-Cl, pH 7.5; 500 mM KCl; 25 mM MgCl$_2$; 25 mM DTT; 0.5 mg/ml BSA

T4 DNA polymerase buffer (10×): 670 mM Tris-Cl, pH 8.7 (at room temperature); 67 mM MgCl$_2$; 100 mM 2-mercaptoethanol; 166 mM (NH$_4$)$_2$SO$_4$; 67 μM (ethylenedinitrilo)tetraacetic acid (EDTA)

*Alu*I Methylase buffer (10×): 0.5 M Tris-Cl, pH 7.5; 0.1 M EDTA; 50 mM 2-mercaptoethanol

10× Ligation buffer: 0.5 M Tris-Cl, pH 7.5; 0.1 M MgCl$_2$; 10 mM ATP; 0.5 mg/ml BSA; 100 mM DTT

SM: Per liter, 5.8 g NaCl, 2 g MgSO₄, 50 ml of 1 *M* Tris-Cl (pH 7.5), 5
ml of 2% gelatin solution, and water to make up to 1 liter; autoclave

All other common solutions are described in the molecular cloning manual (2).

Procedure

An outline of the method for cDNA library construction is shown in Fig. 1.
The step-by-step protocol is as follows.

Preparation of Phage Arms

Digest 20–50 μg of Charon BS phage DNA with *Hind*III and then *Eco*RI
for several hours. Dephosphorylate the arms to reduce the background. Add
1–2 units of alkaline phosphatase directly after the digestion. Incubate at
37°C for 30 min, add 1/10 volume of 0.5 *M* [ethylenebis(oxyethylenenitrilo)]te-
traacetic acid (EGTA) and incubate at 65°C for 45 min. Extract twice with
buffer-saturated phenol, twice with a mixture of phenol and chloroform (1 : 1,
v/v), and once with a mixture of chloroform and isoamyl alcohol (24 : 1,
v/v). Add 1/10 volume of 3 *M* sodium acetate (pH 5) and 2 volumes of 100%
ethanol. Microcentrifuge to collect the DNA, wash with 70% ethanol, dry
in a SpeedVac concentrator, and dissolve in 25 μl of TE8 (10 m*M* Tris-Cl,
pH 8.0; 1 m*M* EDTA). Test the arms for the generation of background
plaques (2).

Preparation of RNA

Prepare total RNA from tissues and cells by the protocol of Chomczynski
and Sacchi (3) and isolate poly(A)⁺ RNA by passing the total RNA through
an oligo(dT) cellulose column (2). The FastTrack kit from Invitrogen (San
Diego, CA) can also be used to obtain mRNA directly.

Preparation of cDNA

First-Strand cDNA Synthesis

Place 0.5–5.0 μg of poly(A)⁺ RNA in a 0.5-ml Eppendorf tube and add 2.5
μg of p(dT)₁₂₋₁₈ and water to make up the total volume to 20 μl. Incubate
at 90°C for 2–3 min and chill quickly on ice. To the tube, add the following
in order: 11 μl of first-strand buffer (5×), 2.75 μl of dNTP mix (each 10
m*M*), 1.5 μl of RNasin, 17.25 μl of water, and 2.5 μl of MMLV reverse
transcriptase (200 units/μl). Mix, then remove 5 μl to another tube containing

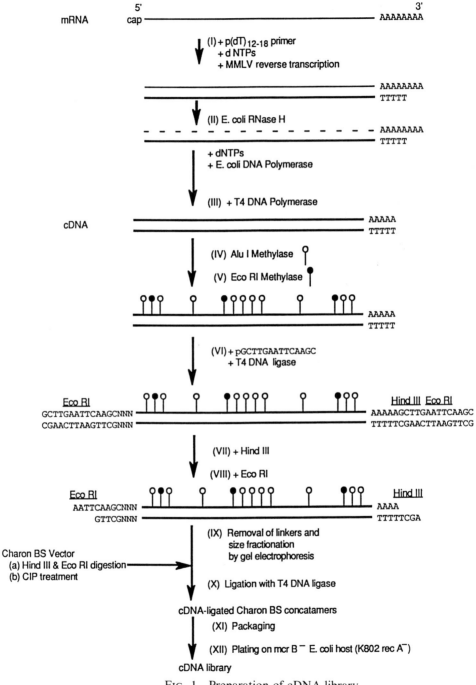

FIG. 1   Preparation of cDNA library.

1–5 μCi of [α-^{32}P]dCTP that has been dried *in vacuo*. This will serve as the test reaction. Incubate both the first-strand and test reaction tubes at 37°C for 2 hr. Add 1 μl of 0.5 M EDTA (pH 8.0) and 44 μl of TE8 to the test reaction, and store at −20°C until ready for analysis. Transfer the first-strand reaction tube to ice and directly proceed to second-strand synthesis.

Second-Strand Synthesis

To the 50 μl first-strand mixture, add the following: 250 μl water, 80 μl second-strand buffer (5×), 7.5 μl of dNTP mix (each 10 mM), 10 μl of *E. coli* DNA polymerase I (10 units/μl), and 1.75 μl of *E. coli* RNase H (2 units/μl). Mix. Place a 40-μl aliquot in another Eppendorf tube with 0.5 μl (5 μCi) of [α-^{32}P]dCTP (test reaction for second strand synthesis). Incubate both the tubes at 15°C for 5 hr and then transfer to ice. To the test reaction tube, add 2 μl of 0.5 M EDTA and 7.5 μl of TE8 and store at −20°C for further analysis. Add 10 μl of 0.5 M EDTA to the second-strand reaction tube. Extract once with phenol–chloroform (1 : 1, v/v) and once with chloroform–isoamyl alcohol (24 : 1, v/v). To the supernatant, add 125 μl of 7.5 M ammonium acetate and 2.5 volumes of 100% ethanol. Store overnight at −20°C.

Quality and Yield of cDNA

To assess the quality of the cDNA synthesis before proceeding to the next step, the first- and second-strand cDNAs are analyzed by alkaline gel electrophoresis using a 10- to 20-μl aliquot from the labeled test reactions (2). The second-strand test reaction product can also be analyzed by neutral agarose gel electrophoresis. Use labeled markers (e.g., 1-kb ladder) during electrophoresis to determine the size of the cDNAs. To obtain the yield of the first- and second-strand cDNA synthesis, take 10 μl from each test reaction tube and spot on separate glass fiber filters. Dry the filters in air or under an infrared lamp. Count the filters in scintillation solution to determine the total radioactivity (total cpm). The incorporation of radioactivity in cDNA is measured after precipitation with 10% trichloroacetic acid (TCA). For this, spot 10 μl from each test reaction on two separate glass fiber filters. Wash the filters in a petri dish with chilled TCA solution 3 to 4 times (each wash, 2–3 min). In the end, wash the filters with 95% ethanol and dry under an infrared lamp. Count the radioactivity after adding scintillation solution.

$$\text{First-strand yield } (\mu\text{g}) = \frac{\text{cpm incorporated}}{\text{total cpm}} \times 33$$

$$\text{Second-strand yield } (\mu\text{g}) = \frac{\text{cpm incorporated}}{\text{total cpm}} \times 132$$

The multiplication factors, 33 and 132, are calculated only for the first- and second-strand reactions described here. The amount of first-strand cDNA should be between 20 and 50% of the poly(A)$^+$ RNA. The yield of the second-strand cDNA is usually more than 80%. To estimate the amount of total double-stranded cDNA, multiply the second-strand yield by 2.

Trimming of cDNA Ends

Microcentrifuge the second-strand cDNA reaction to obtain the cDNA pellet. Wash the cDNA with 70% ethanol, dry in a SpeedVac, and dissolve in 42.5 μl of water. Add 5 μl of T4 DNA polymerase buffer (10×), 1 μl of dNTP mix (10 mM each), 0.5 μl of BSA (20 μg/μl) and 1 μl of T4 DNA polymerase (5–10 units). Mix and incubate at 37°C for 30 min. Add 150 μl of TE8 and extract once with phenol–chloroform (1 : 1, v/v) and once with chloroform–isoamyl alcohol (24 : 1, v/v). Add ammonium acetate to 2 M final concentration and precipitate the cDNA with 2.5 volumes of 100% ethanol. Store at −20°C overnight or freeze on dry ice for 30 min.

Methylation

Microcentrifuge to obtain the cDNA pellet, wash once with 70% ethanol, dry in a SpeedVac, and dissolve in 20 μl of water. Add 2.5 μl of 10× AluI methylase buffer, 1 μl of S-adenosylmethionine (2.5 mM, prepared fresh by diluting 2.5 μl of 32 mM stock to 32 μl with water), and 1.2 μl of AluI methylase (5 units/μl). Incubate at 37°C for 60 min. Then add 60 μl of water, 8.75 μl of 1 M Tris-Cl (pH 8.0), 2 μl of 5 M NaCl, 2.5 μl of 2.5 mM S-adenosylmethionine, and 1.5 μl of EcoRI methylase (40 units/μl). Incubate at 37°C for 1–2 hr and then add 93 μl of water, 3 μl of 1 M MgCl$_2$, 1 μl of BSA (20 μg/μl), 1.5 μl of dNTP mix (each 10 mM), and 1 μl of Klenow DNA polymerase enzyme (5 units/μl). Incubate at 37°C for 15–20 min. Then extract once with phenol–chloroform (1 : 1, v/v) and once with chloroform–isoamyl alcohol (24 : 1, v/v) before ethanol precipitation in the presence of ammonium acetate. Store overnight at −20°C.

Linker Ligation and Digestion with HindIII and EcoRI

The blunt-ended and methylated cDNA is pelleted by centrifugation and dissolved in 6 μl of water. To this, add 1–2 μg of kinased oligonucleotide (pGCTTGAATTCAAGC) and adjust the volume with water to 10 μl. Add 1.2 μl of ligation buffer (10×) and 0.8 μl of T4 DNA ligase (400 units/μl). Incubate overnight at 15°C. Inactivate the ligase by heating at 65°C for 15 min. The ligation of the oligonucleotide will generate a HindIII site at the 3′ end of cDNA because of the poly(A) tail (see Fig. 1). The cDNA should now be digested with *Hin*dIII and *Eco*RI. For this, add 5 μl of *Hin*dIII digestion buffer (10×), 31 μl of water, and 2 μl of *Hin*dIII (10 units/μl) to the linker-ligated cDNA. Incubate for 2–3 hr at 37°C, then increase the NaCl concentration to 100 mM and the volume to 100 μl before adding 2 μl of *Eco*RI (20 units/ml). Incubate again for 2–3 hr. Precipitate the cDNA with 100% ethanol. Dissolve the pellet in 20 μl of TE8.

Size Selection and Removal of Unligated Linkers

Prepare a 1% low melting agarose gel and electrophorese the cDNA at 50 V until the bromphenol blue dye is about 5 cm from the origin. Using a clean, sharp blade, cut the agarose gel containing cDNAs of desired size (e.g., more than 0.7 kb), and purify the cDNA from the gel by phenol extraction using standard procedures (2). Use only long-wavelength UV light when viewing the agarose gel.

Ligation to Phage Arms

Dissolve the linker-ligated cDNA in 20 μl of water. Generally, two concentrations of cDNAs should be used for ligation to Charon BS phage arms. Place 0.7–1 μg of phage arms in separate tubes and ligate these to 2 or 10 μl of cDNA in a total volume of 12 and 15 μl, respectively. After adding appropriate volumes of 10× ligation buffer and T4 DNA ligase, incubate the reaction mixtures overnight at 12°C.

Packaging

Take 4 μl from each ligation mixture for packaging of phage molecules. Gigapack-Gold packaging extract (Stratagene) is preferred because of its high efficiency. Store the packaged mixture at 4°C. The number of independent plaques after packaging is determined by titrating the phage on *E. coli* K802 rec A$^-$. The desired number of independent plaques is 1×10^6 for cells in culture and $3–5 \times 10^6$ for tissues. The remaining ligation mixture can also be packaged to increase the depth of the library.

Amplification of cDNA Library

The unamplified library can be used to screen for desired cDNA clones. However, one needs to amplify the library to prepare a stock for long-term storage and future screenings. Between 50,000 and 100,000 plaques per large NZ agar petri dish are plated on 20 to 40 petri dishes (2). After the lysis is complete, the phage are collected in 10–15 ml of SM per plate. Aliquots of about 1 ml from the combined SM from all the plates serve as stocks of the library, which can be stored at 4°C without significant loss of titer. Most of the remaining library stock may be used to prepare the phage DNA by standard procedures (2).

Transfer of Library to Bluescript Plasmid

Overview

The cDNA library (or individual clones) in Charon BS vector can be transferred to the Bluescript KS plasmid without generating significant bias. The digestion of Charon BS library DNA with *Not*I will release the Bluescript plasmid that harbor cDNA inserts (1). The linear plasmid molecules are recircularized by self-ligation under low DNA concentrations (~10–20 μg phage DNA per milliliter of ligation volume) and used for transforming *E. coli* competent cells.

Procedure

About 20 μg of phage library DNA is digested with the restriction enzyme *Not*I for 4–6 hr. Inactivate the enzyme by incubating at 65°C for 30–60 min, then increase the volume of digestion reaction to 898 μl with water and add 100 μl of ligation buffer (10×) and 2 μl of T4 DNA ligase. Incubate for 6 hr to overnight at 12°C. Add 1/10 volume of sodium acetate (pH 5) and precipitate the DNA with 100% ethanol. After centrifugation, wash the DNA pellet with 70% ethanol, dry, and dissolve it in 25 μl of water. Use 1 μl of this DNA for transformation of Max-efficiency DH5α cells (from BRL, Gaithersburg, MD), or XL-1 blue cells (from Stratagene). We prefer to use electro-transformation (with the electroporation apparatus from Bio-Rad, Richmond, CA, or ECM 600 from BTX Inc., San Diego, CA) since it is less expensive than Max-α cells, and gives high efficiency. One may have to perform 15–25 transformations to obtain the desired number of plasmid clones (>2 × 10^6 for cells, >4 × 10^6 for tissues). After transformation and 1 hr of incubation at 37°C, take 1 and 10 μl for plating. Add 4 ml of LB medium and ampicillin (50 μg/ml) to the remaining transformation mixture in each tube. Grow the cells overnight at 37°C. Combine cultures from all transformation tubes, and freeze 1-ml aliquots as plasmid library stocks with 20% glycerol at −70°C. Part of the culture can be used to prepare double-stranded plasmid DNA or single-stranded (ss) DNA for subtraction procedure.

Subtraction Procedure

Materials

Biochemicals and Enzymes

The reagents are purchased from the following suppliers: bio-11-UTP, Enzo Diagnostics (New York, NY); columns for separating free biotinylated nucleotides, glycogen, and RNase-free DNase I, Boehringer-Mannheim; ribonucleotide solutions, Pharmacia; Vectrex–avidin, Vector Laboratories (Burlingame, CA); Max-efficiency DH5α cells and T7 and T3 RNA polymerases, GIBCO–BRL; restriction enzyme *Not*I, New England Biolabs; RNasin, Promega Corp.; R408 helper phage, Stratagene.

Media

To make 2× YT; dissolve Bacto-tryptone (16 g), yeast extract (10 g), and NaCl (10 g) in 800 ml of water. Adjust to pH 7–7.5. Make up to 1 liter with water.

Solutions

Transcription buffer (5×): 0.2 M Tris-Cl, pH 7.5 (at 37°C); 30 mM MgCl$_2$; 10 mM spermidine; 50 mM NaCl

Vectrex–avidin (VA) binding buffer: 100 mM Tris-Cl, pH 7.5; 150 mM NaCl; 0.5% sodium dodecyl sulfate (SDS)

Procedure

Overview

The steps of the subtraction protocol (4) are schematically shown in Fig. 2. In the example, a human retinal cDNA library is enriched for specific genes by subtraction against a JY lymphoblastoid cell line library. Such a subtraction will only remove most of the constitutively expressed genes. In brief, ssDNA from the retinal library is hybridized to biotin-labeled JY RNA that is complementary in orientation to the cDNA inserts in retinal ssDNA. The eluant, obtained after incubating the hybridization mixture with the avidin matrix, is enriched for retinal ssDNAs that do not find their complement in JY RNA. The ssDNA molecules can be used directly to transform *E. coli* competent cells and to obtain a subtracted library enriched for specific genes.

Preparation of Single-Stranded DNA

The cDNA library in Bluescript plasmid (as derived from Charon BS phage library) should be in an F episome containing host (e.g., XL-1 blue or

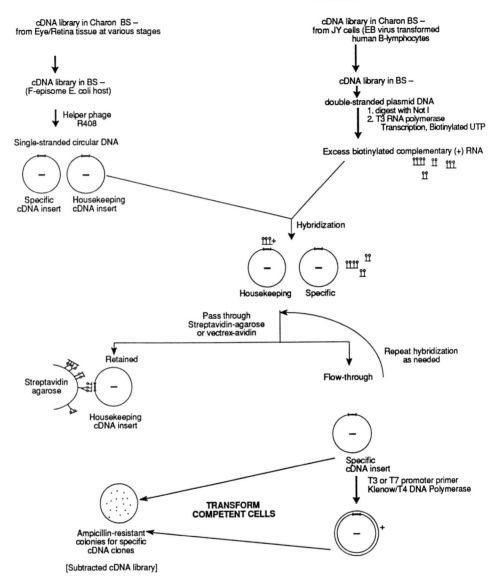

FIG. 2   Subtraction cDNA cloning. [Modified from A. Swaroop, J. Xu, N. Agarwal, and S. M. Weissman, *Nucleic Acids Res.* **19**, 1954 (1991), by permission of Oxford University Press.]

DH5αF′), so that the ssDNA can be prepared using helper phage. Bluescript plasmid can be secreted as a single-stranded phage because of the presence of origin sequences from the f1 phage needed for packaging and replication (5). Detailed procedures for preparing ssDNA from Bluescript and from filamentous phages have been described in several manuals (2, 5).

About 1 ml of an overnight culture from a plasmid retinal cDNA library is used to inoculate 10 ml of 2× YT medium. Shake at 37°C. Add about 20-fold excess of helper phage to cells when the OD_{600} of the culture is between 0.3 and 0.5. Shake at 37°C for another 8 hr. Centrifuge the culture to pellet the cells, transfer the supernatant to another tube, and spin again. Place the supernatant in a fresh tube and add 0.25 volumes of 20% polyethylene glycol (PEG) in 3.5 M ammonium acetate (pH 7.5). After mixing, incubate at room temperature for 15–20 min. Centrifuge at 12,000 g for 20 min. Remove the supernatant carefully. Centrifuge again for 3–5 min and remove the remaining supernatant completely. Dissolve the pellet in 500–1000 μl TE8. Extract 2–3 times with phenol–chloroform (1 : 1, v/v) and once with chloroform–isoamyl alcohol (24 : 1, v/v), Vortex for at least 30 sec during each extraction. To the aqueous phase, add 0.75 volumes of 7.5 M ammonium acetate and 3 volumes of chilled ethanol (100%). Incubate on ice for 15–20 min. Pellet the ssDNA, wash with 70% ethanol, dry in a SpeedVac, and dissolve the pellet in 100–200 μl of water. Analyze an aliquot of the ssDNA by agarose gel electrophoresis. Use 1 μl for each transformation or electroporation. Optimize the efficiency of transformation by using a known amount of ssDNA from Bluescript plasmid. As a reference, generally 5×10^5 to 5×10^6 ampicillin-resistant colonies are obtained with 1 μg of ssDNA.

Preparation of Biotinylated RNA

The biotinylated RNA for subtraction is prepared from the JY cDNA library in Bluescript plasmid. One has to know the orientation of the inserts in the two cDNA libraries (retina and JY) in order to generate complementary hybridizing species. Based on the direction of f1 origin of replication in Bluescript KS, one can generate ssDNA in the (+) or (−) orientation. If both libraries are constructed in Charon BS (−), the plasmid libraries will be in Bluescript KS (−). Here the rescued ssDNA will have the sense strand of cDNA. The complementary biotinylated RNA from the JY library can then be prepared with T3 RNA polymerase. (Note that the orientation of the cDNA insert is opposite to the β-galactosidase open reading frame.) For this, linearize about 20 μg of the JY plasmid library DNA with the restriction enzyme *Not*I. Extract once each with phenol, phenol–chloroform (1 : 1, v/v), and chloroform–isoamyl alcohol (24 : 1, v/v). Precipitate the DNA with ethanol after adding 1/10 volume of 3 M sodium acetate, pellet, and dissolve in 25 μl water. Check the concentration by measuring the OD_{260} and staining the gel with ethidium bromide after electrophoresis. (The library DNA can be linearized with *Sal*I or *Kpn*I restriction enzymes if T7 RNA polymerase is to be used for generating biotinylated RNA.)

To about 1 μg of linear library DNA, add 10 μl of transcription buffer (5×), 1.2 μl of 0.25 M DTT, 1 μl of RNasin, 5 μl of ribonucleotide ATP + GTP + CTP mix (20 mM each), 8 μl of bio-11-UTP (20 mM), and water to make up to 46 μl. Start the reaction by adding 4 μl of T3 RNA polymerase. Incubate for 2 hr at 37°C. Remove the DNA template by digesting with 0.7 μl of RNase-free DNase I (40 units/μl) and incubating the reaction at 37°C for 10–15 min. Then add 2 μl of 0.5 M EDTA and 100 μl of water. Pass through a Sephadex G-50 or equivalent column to remove free nucleotides. Collect the RNA and check the concentration by measuring the OD_{260} and performing gel electrophoresis. Store at -70°C until ready to use.

Preparation of Buffer-Saturated Vectrex–Avidin

About 250 mg of vectrex–avidin (VA) is needed for each subtraction reaction. Suspend the VA in 10 ml of binding buffer containing 50 μg/ml denatured sonicated salmon testes DNA that has been extracted twice with phenol–chloroform (1 : 1, v/v). Agitate at room temperature for 30 min using an Adams nutator (Cat. No. 14-062, Fisher Scientific, Springfield, NJ). Centrifuge for 1 min to pellet the VA. Decant and repeat the above steps. Wash the VA 3 times with binding buffer without salmon testes DNA and resuspend in 500 μl of binding buffer.

Hybridization

For subtraction hybridization, ssDNA from a retina library is annealed to a molar excess (5 to 200-fold) of biotinylated JY RNA that has the complementary orientation.

1. Place 0.2–1 μg of retinal ssDNA and 10–50 μg of JY biotinylated RNA in a 0.5-ml Eppendorf tube. Add water to 100 μl, then add 10 μl of 3 M sodium acetate (pH 5) and 300 μl of 100% ethanol. Store overnight at -20°C.
2. Centrifuge the sample, wash the pellet twice with 70% ethanol, dry in a SpeedVac, and dissolve the pellet in 8 μl of water. To this, add 10 μl of 1 M sodium phosphate (pH 7.2), 1 μl of 0.2 M EDTA, and 1 μl of 20% SDS. Mix and heat at 65°C for 5–10 min. Take up the solution in a 50- or 100-μl capillary. Seal the ends of the capillary carefully by using a flame. Place the sealed capillary in boiling water for 5 min, then quickly transfer to a water bath set at 60 or 65°C and incubate overnight.

Separation of Unannealed Single-Stranded DNA

1. Dilute the hybridization mixture to 200 μl with VA binding buffer. Heat at 60°C for 5–10 min and cool to room temperature.
2. Add about 100 mg of buffer-saturated VA and incubate for 30–60 min at room temperature with constant shaking on an Adams nutator. Collect the supernatant by spinning the tube for 10 sec. Wash the VA with 100–200 μl of binding buffer. Centrifuge and combine the two supernatants.
3. To the combined supernatant, add about 100 mg of fresh buffer-saturated VA. Incubate again for 30–60 min at room temperature with constant shaking. Spin and collect the supernatant.
4. Add 1 μl glycogen (20 μg/μl), 40 μl of 3 M sodium acetate (pH 5), and 1 ml of 100% ethanol. Mix and leave overnight at −20°C.

Transformation

Centrifuge to pellet the subtracted ssDNA, wash with 70% ethanol, dry, and dissolve in 50 μl of water or TE8. Use 1 or 2 μl for transformation of Max-efficiency DH5α cells or for electroporation of competent *E. coli* to obtain the subtracted library.

Notes and Comments

1. For recommended reading for cDNA library construction, see Refs. 6–8.
2. The quality of poly(A)$^+$ RNA should be checked by Northern analysis before starting the cDNA synthesis. A sharp band on probing the Northern blot with any gene (e.g., β-actin) is indicative of good quality RNA.
3. All precautions for working with RNA (2) should be observed during the first two steps of cDNA library construction and during the subtraction procedure.
4. Eppendorf tubes, tips, distilled water, and common solutions should be autoclaved for 90 min. Use disposable individually wrapped pipettes.
5. [α-^{32}P]dCTP may be added during the total second-strand reaction. This helps in estimating the yield of double-stranded cDNA in subsequent steps.
6. Oligonucleotide 5'GCTTGAATTCAAGC3' should be checked before ligation to cDNA, by self-ligation followed by EcoRI digestion. For this, label the oligonucleotide with [γ-^{32}P]ATP using polynucleotide kinase (2).
7. The transformation efficiency for the ssDNA obtained after subtraction can be increased by synthesizing second-strand using a T3 or T7 primer (depending on the polarity) and Klenow DNA polymerase.

8. The efficiency of subtraction should be checked against a mock control where biotinylated RNA is omitted. If the constitutive cDNA sequences have been subtracted from the library, the number of blue colonies (on X-Gal, IPTG plates), which contain no insert, will be dramatically increased.
9. The unannealed retinal ssDNA (obtained after passing the hybridization mixture through Vectrex–avidin) can be subjected to further rounds of hybridization with biotinylated RNA to enrich for tissue-specific genes expressed at low levels.
10. The amount of biotinylated RNA can vary between experiments, and will depend on the subtraction requirements.
11. Vectrex-avidin can be replaced by streptavidin magnetic beads (Dyna-beads M-280 Streptavidin, Dynal Inc., Great Neck, NY).
12. The yield and specificity of subtraction can be further improved by preannealing the ssDNA from retina cDNA library with a complementary oligonucleotide for the multiple cloning site region of the Bluescript plasmid (Dr. M. Coca-Prados, personal communication). For preannealing to (−) strand of ssDNA [derived from KS (−) plasmid], the complementary (+) strand oligonucleotide (25-30mer) in the region of KpnI to HindIII restriction sites should be used.

Summary

We have generated size-selected directional cDNA libraries from several human tissues and cell lines, including retina from a single adult donor and eyes from three fetuses at 11 weeks of gestation (A. Swaroop and J. Xu, unpublished data). cDNA libraries in two size ranges were constructed. The number of independent plaques for adult retinal libraries was 1×10^6 for the 0.4–1.2 kb range library and 2×10^6 for the over 1.2 kb library. Both fetal eye libraries (0.4–1.2 kb and >1.2 kb) had at least 3×10^6 independent phage plaques. A number of novel genes have been isolated from adult retina (9–11) and fetal eye libraries (11–13).

Subtraction cloning is a method for the removal of DNA sequences that are common between the two cDNA pools or libraries. The method (4) described here offers several advantages over previously published protocols (14–19). Because of the use of directional and single-stranded hybridizing species, the subtraction is efficient in removing cDNA sequences that are common between any two libraries. In addition, after the subtraction step the single-stranded circular DNA molecules can be directly used for transformation. The analysis of over 50 cDNA clones randomly isolated from the subtracted retinal library shows that more than 70% of these are not expressed in JY cDNA library. One of the random clones, AS321, showed a neural–

retina-specific expression and encoded a leucine zipper-containing protein (10).

Subtraction methods have been useful for the identification of genes for two mouse retinal degeneration mutants, namely, rd (20) and rds (21). The purpose of subtracting retina library against JY lymphoblastoid cell line (described in the example here) is only to reduce the complexity by removing most of the abundant constitutively-expressed housekeeping genes; the enriched retinal library (after one round of subtraction) is then used for selecting X-chromosome-encoded cDNAs (Yan *et al.*, manuscript in preparation). Undoubtedly, it will be valuable to generate human retinal libraries subtracted with a brain library, or a retinal cell library enriched by subtraction against the library of another cell type. The subtraction procedure can also be used for isolating specific genes expressed at a particular developmental stage. This technique becomes even more powerful when combined with differential hybridization screening using subtracted probes. Characterization of the novel retinal genes should enhance our understanding of retinal development and visual function and may provide candidate genes for inherited and congenital eye diseases (22).

Acknowledgments

The research in my laboratory is supported by grants from National Eye Institute (EY 07961), National Retinitis Pigmentosa Foundation, Inc., and the George Gund Foundation. I thank Drs. Peter Hitchcock and Debra Thompson for helpful comments and Ms. Dorothy Giebel for timely preparation of the manuscript.

References

1. A. Swaroop and S. M. Weissman, *Nucleic Acids Res.* **16**, 8739 (1988).
2. J. Sambrook, E. F. Fritsch, and T. Maniatis, "Molecular Cloning: A Laboratory Manual," 2nd Ed. Cold Spring Harbor Laboratory, Cold Spring Harbor, New York, 1988.
3. P. Chomczynski and N. Sacchi, *Anal. Biochem.* **262**, 156 (1978).
4. A. Swaroop, J. Xu, N. Agarwal, and S. M. Weissman, *Nucleic Acids Res.* **19**, 1954 (1991).
5. Bluescript instruction manual, Stratagene, La Jolla, California.
6. cDNA synthesis system, instruction manual, Bethesda Research Laboratories, Gaithersburg, Maryland.
7. T. V. Huynh, R. A. Young, and R. W. Davis, *in* "DNA Cloning" (D. M. Glover, ed.), Vol. 1, p. 49. IRL Press, Oxford, 1985.
8. U. Gubler and B. J. Hoffman, *Gene* **25**, 263 (1983).

9. N. Agarwal, C. L. Hsieh, D. Sills, M. Swaroop, B. Desai, U. Francke, and A. Swaroop, *Exp. Eye Res.* **52**, 549 (1991).

10. A. Swaroop, J. Xu, H. Pawar, A. Jackson, C. Skolnick, and N. Agarwal, *Proc. Natl. Acad. Sci. U.S.A.* **89**, 266 (1992).

11. A. Swaroop, N. Agarwal, J. R. Gruen, D. Bick, and S. M. Weissman, *Nucleic Acids Res.* **19**, 4725 (1991).

12. H. Shukla, A. Swaroop, R. Srivastava, and S. M. Weissman, *Nucleic Acids Res.* **18**, 2198 (1990).

13. C. T. Ton, H. Hirvonen, M. Hiroshi, M. Weil, P. Monaghan, V. van Heyningen, N. D. Hastie, H. Meijers-Heijboer, M. Drechsler, B. Royer-Pokora, F. Collins, A. Swaroop, L. C. Strong, and G. F. Saunders, *Cell (Cambridge, Mass.)* **67**, 1059 (1991).

14. J. R. Duguid, R. G. Rohwer, and B. Seed, *Proc. Natl. Acad. Sci. U.S.A.* **85**, 5738 (1988).

15. H. L. Sive and T. St. John, *Nucleic Acids Res.* **16**, 10937 (1988).

16. M. J. Palazzolo, D. R. Hyde, K. VijayRaghavan, K. Mecklenburg, S. Benzer, and E. Meyerowitz, *Neuron* **3**, 527 (1989).

17. C. Timblin, J. Battey, and W. M. Kuehl, *Nucleic Acids Res.* **18**, 1587 (1990).

18. J. L. R. Rubenstein, A. E. J. Brice, R. D. Ciaranello, D. Denney, M. H. Porteus, and T. B. Usdin, *Nucleic Acids Res.* **18**, 4833 (1990).

19. S. W. Lee, C. Tomasetto, and R. Sager, *Proc. Natl. Acad. Sci. U.S.A.* **88**, 2825 (1991).

20. C. Bowes, M. Danciger, C. A. Kozak, and D. B. Farber, *Proc. Natl. Acad. Sci. U.S.A.* **86**, 9722 (1989).

21. G. H. Travis, M. B. Brennan, P. E. Danielson, C. A. Kozak, and J. G. Sutcliffe, *Nature (London)* **338**, 70 (1989).

22. A. U. Jackson, K. Zheng, T. L. Yang-Feng, and A. Swaroop, *in* "Retinal Degeneration: Clinical and Laboratory Applications" (J. Hollyfield, ed.), Plenum Press, New York, (1993). In press.

[21] Expression of Opsin Genes in COS Cells

Daniel D. Oprian

Introduction

The ready availability of genes for the visual pigments and other membrane receptors makes the use of heterologous expression systems attractive as a source for the proteins. We have found that the African green monkey kidney cell line COS (1) is ideal for the expression of visual pigment genes (2). The COS cell expression system is transient, meaning that a permanent cell line is not established. Instead the cells are harvested 3 days after transfection, obviating the need for clonal selection of a cell line that has stably integrated the exogenous DNA into the genome.

This chapter describes procedures currently in use in our laboratory for expression of exogenous proteins in COS cells (2). The transfection procedure was developed for high-level expression of rhodopsin. No consideration was given to adverse effects of this procedure on COS cell physiology; the only criterion was to maximize the mass of rhodopsin obtained from each culture dish. Typically the yield is 3 to 4 μg of rhodopsin from each 100-mm culture dish, and it is straightforward to prepare 100 plates of transfected cells. The use of COS cells for expression of rhodopsin is made easy by the fact that the apoprotein opsin is stable in the cells. Thus, the tissue culture procedures may be performed under conditions of normal room lighting, and the protein may be combined with 11-*cis*-retinal chromophore during purification.

We have used three different expression vectors with essentially identical results: p91023B (3), pMT2 (4), and CDM8 (5). The salient features that all the vectors have in common are an SV40 origin of replication, a strong promoter, a splice site, and a polyadenylation signal.

In addition to transfection of the COS cells, this chapter also describes an immunoaffinity procedure for purification of rhodopsin using a monoclonal antibody, rho 1D4 (6), which recognizes the carboxy-terminal 8 amino acids of rhodopsin (7). The bound COS cell rhodopsin can be eluted from the immunoaffinity matrix under gentle conditions by means of competition with a synthetic peptide, Peptide I, corresponding to the carboxy-terminal 18 amino acids of rhodopsin (DEASTTVSKTETSQVAPA). This is a one-step purification that we have used with several different membrane receptors by splicing the 1D4 epitope into their sequence (2, 8).

Methods in Neurosciences, Volume 15

Routine Growth of COS Cells

COS cells are grown in monolayer on 100-mm diameter plastic culture dishes in a CO_2 incubator at 37°C and under an atmosphere containing 5% CO_2. The growth medium, medium A, is Dulbecco's modified Eagle's medium containing D-glucose (4.5 g/liter), streptomycin (100 mg/ml), penicillin (100 mg/ml), a supplement of 2 mM L-glutamine, and 10% (v/v) heat-inactivated calf serum (56°C for 30 min). For routine growth and propagation of the cells, 10 ml of medium A is used per plate, and fresh medium is provided every 2 days. As the cells multiply and the plates become confluent, it is necessary to replate the cells to ensure continued growth. A routine schedule that works well in our laboratory is to plate cells at a density of 5×10^5 cells per plate on Mondays, provide fresh medium A on Wednesdays, and replate at a density of 1×10^6 cells per plate on Fridays.

COS cells grow attached to the surface of the plate and must be removed physically before replating. This is generally accomplished by treatment with trypsin–EDTA solution (GIBCO, Grand Island, NY) as follows. The medium from a confluent plate of COS cells is removed by aspiration, and the cells are washed twice with 10 ml each time of phosphate-buffered saline (PBS; 10 mM sodium phosphate buffer, pH 7.0, containing 150 mM NaCl) while still attached to the plate. The cells are then treated with 2 ml of $1\times$ strength trypsin–EDTA solution for 3 min at room temperature and dislodged from the plate by jarring several times against an immovable surface. The cells come off the plate in sheets that are visible to the naked eye. The sheets must be broken up into single cells before replating. This is accomplished by pipetting the cell suspension up and down about 10 times in a 5-ml sterile pipette, transferring the solution to 8 ml of medium A (serum contains a trypsin inhibitor), and then pipetting up and down in a 10-ml pipette 10 times. About 1 ml of this suspension is added to 9 ml of medium A in a 100-mm culture dish, and the cells are dispersed evenly in the solution and then placed in a CO_2 incubator. The cells require about 1 hr to adhere to the plate and should be uniformly distributed.

It is important to break up the sheets of cells in this procedure to get evenly growing monolayers. However, too long an exposure to the trypsin–EDTA solution will result in cell death.

Transfection of COS Cells

Four days before transfection, cells are plated at a density of about 1×10^6 cells per plate. Typically, 10 plates are used for a single preparation of rhodopsin. At confluence (~1×10^7 cells per plate), the cells are washed twice with 5 ml of medium B (same as medium A but containing no calf serum) and then treated with 5 ml of a transfection cocktail composed of 10 μg of plasmid DNA, 5 ml of 1 M Tris buffer (pH 7.0), 35 ml medium B, 5 ml of a DEAE-dextran stock solution (2.5 mg/ml in medium B), and 5 ml of 1 mM chloroquine (recipe is for 10 plates). After addition of the transfection cocktail to the plates, the cells are incubated in a CO_2 incubator for 6 hr at 37°C. The transfection cocktail is then removed by aspiration, and the cells are washed with 5 ml of medium B.

The cells are then treated with dimethyl sulfoxide (DMSO). Two milliliters of a solution of 10% DMSO in 21 mM HEPES buffer (pH 7) containing 137 mM NaCl, 5 mM KCl, 0.7 mM Na_2HPO_4, and 5.5 mM dextrose (the 10% DMSO solution may be sterilized by filtration through a 0.2-μm Nalgene nylon membrane) is applied to each plate and incubated for 3 min at room temperature. It is essential that this treatment proceed no longer than 3 min. The DMSO treatment is harsh on the cells, and prolonged exposure will result in high cell mortality and low yield of protein.

Following the 3-min exposure to DMSO, the solution is removed by aspiration, and 5 ml of medium A containing 0.1 mM chloroquine is added to each plate. The cells are then incubated for 2 hr at 37°C in the CO_2 incubator. Note that the cells are not washed between the "DMSO shock" and application of the chloroquine solution. After 2 hr of incubation the chloroquine solution is removed, and the cells are washed twice with 5 ml of medium B. Ten milliliters of medium A is added to each plate, and the cells are incubated in a CO_2 incubator overnight. The next day the medium is removed by aspiration and 10 ml of fresh medium A added to each plate. The cells are then returned to the incubator, where they remain until harvested 48 hr later.

Harvesting of COS Cells

Transfected COS cells are harvested 72 hr after the initial treatment with DNA. Beyond this time the cells begin to die, and prolonged incubation times result in lower yield of protein. To harvest, the medium is removed from the plates, and the cells are washed twice with 5 ml of PBS. After aspiration of the final wash solution, 1 ml of PBS is added to each plate, and the cells are removed by scraping with a rubber policeman. The 1-ml suspension from each plate is collected with a Pasteur pipette and transferred to a 15-ml conical centrifuge tube. The combined cells are collected by centrifugation in a clinical centrifuge (1000 g for 5 min), washed twice by resuspending in 10 ml of PBS, and then repelleted. At this point the cell pellet may be frozen and stored at -70°C until use. The cell pellets are used either for purification of the protein or for the preparation of COS cell membranes containing the protein.

Purification of Rhodopsin

Reconstitution with 11-cis-Retinal

COS cell opsin is combined with 11-*cis*-retinal chromophore while the protein is in the membranes of unbroken cells. This and all subsequent procedures are performed at 4°C under dim red illumination [15-W bulb with a Kodak (Rochester, NY) safelight No. 2 filter]. The retinal stock solution is prepared in ethanol. It is important to use relatively concentrated stock solutions (~10 mM in retinal) so as to avoid exposing the protein to greater than 1% ethanol during the reconstitution procedure.

Frozen cell pellets are thawed on ice and resuspended in 5 ml of PBS. An additional 5 ml of PBS containing 40 μM 11-*cis*-retinal is added and the cells incubated with agitation for 30 min to allow the chromophore to combine with the protein. The cells are then collected by centrifugation in a clinical centrifuge (1000 g for 5 min) and the supernatant solution decanted.

Solubilization and Purification of Rhodopsin

The solubilization and purification of rhodopsin from COS cells may be effected with a variety of different detergents, depending on the particular needs of the investigator. The following procedure uses dodecyl-β-D-maltoside (Calbiochem, San Diego, CA) because of the high thermal stability of rhodopsin in this detergent. One of the few drawbacks with the use of dodecyl maltoside is its high cost.

The cell pellet is resuspended in 5 ml PBS containing 0.2 mg/ml PMSF (phenylmethylsulfonyl fluoride; prepared fresh daily as an ethanol stock solution). The cells are solubilized by addition of 5 ml PBS containing 2.0% (w/v) dodecyl maltoside and subsequent incubation for 30 min on ice. The use of nonionic detergents such as dodecyl maltoside, digitonin, and CHAPS in this procedure results in solubilization of most cellular membranes, but not the nuclear envelope. The nuclei are removed from the suspension by centrifugation in a clinical centrifuge (1000 g for 5 min), and the supernatant solution is decanted to a fresh 15-ml conical polypropylene centrifuge tube.

To the detergent extract is added 0.3 ml of a suspension containing 0.2 ml of packed rho 1D4–Sepharose 2B immunoaffinity matrix (1.4 mg of rho 1D4 per milliliter packed gel; see Ref. 2 for preparation of the matrix) in PBS containing 1% dodecyl maltoside. The rhodopsin is allowed to bind to the immunoaffinity matrix for 2 hr at 4°C with constant mixing. The matrix is then separated from the detergent extract by centrifugation in a clinical centrifuge (1000 g for 5 min) and transferred to a 1-ml polypropylene syringe containing a glass wool plug in the luer tip. The syringe is placed in a 15-ml conical polypropylene centrifuge tube so that washing and elution of the column can be accomplished by spinning in the clinical centrifuge (1000 g for 3 min). The column is washed 8 times with 1 ml of 0.1% dodecyl maltoside in PBS. The bottom of the syringe is then sealed with Parafilm, 0.15 ml of a solution of 50 μM Peptide I in PBS containing 0.1% dodecyl maltoside added, and the top of the syringe is sealed with Parafilm. Rhodopsin dissociates from the matrix during a subsequent 30-min incubation, and the eluant is collected by centrifugation. The column is washed with another 150-μl aliquot of the peptide solution, and the two fractions are combined. After recording the absorption spectrum, the sample may be stored at $-70°C$ for future use.

Isolation of COS Cell Membranes

For certain purposes (e.g., transducin assays) it is more convenient to use COS cell membranes containing rhodopsin rather than the purified pigment. The membranes are prepared in the absence of added chromophore, and the pigment is reconstituted immediately prior to use.

The COS cell pellet is resuspended in 15 ml of 10 mM Tris buffer (pH 7.4) containing 0.1 mg/ml PMSF. The cells are then broken by forcing the suspension through a 25-gauge needle 4 times using a 20-ml polypropylene syringe. The resulting extract is then layered onto an ice-cold 20-ml cushion of 37% (w/v) sucrose in 10 mM Tris buffer (pH 7.4), 150 mM NaCl, 1 mM MgCl$_2$, 1 mM CaCl$_2$, and 0.1 mM EDTA contained in a polyallomar centrifuge tube. The sample is spun in a Beckman (Fullerton, CA) SW 28.1 rotor at 15,000 rpm (33,000 g_{av}) for 20 min at 4°C, and the membranes, which collect as a cloudy layer at the interface of the two solutions, are collected through the side of the tube with the aid of a syringe equipped with an 18-gauge needle. The membranes are diluted at least 10-fold with 10 mM Tris buffer (pH 7.4) and collected by centrifugation in a Beckman 50.2 Ti rotor at 33,000 rpm (100,000 g_{av}) for 45 min at 4°C. The supernatant solution is discarded and the pellet resuspended in 1.0 ml of 10 mM Tris buffer (pH 7.4) containing 150 mM NaCl, 1 mM MgCl$_2$, 1 mM CaCl$_2$, and 0.1 mM EDTA to give a final protein concentration of about 3 mg/ml. This suspension may be stored at $-70°C$ for future use.

General Strategy for Purification of Expressed Proteins

Human Color Vision Pigments

We have expressed the genes for the three human color vision pigments in COS cells, reconstituted the pigments with 11-*cis*-retinal chromophore, and purified them using the same immunoaffinity procedure outlined above for rhodopsin (8). This was accomplished by extending the wild-type amino acid sequence of each protein by an additional 8 amino acids from the carboxyl terminus of rhodopsin, which is the epitope for the rho 1D4 antibody. That this is a general approach for the purification of heterologous proteins containing the rho 1D4 epitope is demonstrated by the fact that we have used this for the purification of functional β_2-adrenergic receptor from transfected COS cells (J. McPhee and D. D. Oprian, unpublished results), and that the epitope also works when placed on the amino terminus of rhodopsin (P. R. Robinson and D. D. Oprian, unpublished results).

Acknowledgments

I thank Peter Sorter and Hoffman-LaRoche for the generous gift of 11-*cis*-retinal, Randy Kaufman for the vectors p91023B and pMT2, Brian Seed for CDM8, Roland Franke for advice on the preparation of COS cell membranes, and Paul Katz and Steve Goldstein for comments on the manuscript. I also thank members of my laboratory for advice during the preparation of this chapter, in particular Phyllis Robinson, George Cohen, Ana Asenjo, Ning Lee, and Sandra Pelletier. This work was supported by National Institutes of Health Grant EY07965.

References

1. Y. Gluzman, *Cell (Cambridge, Mass.)* **23,** 175 (1981).
2. D. D. Oprian, R. S. Molday, R. J. Kaufman, and H. G. Khorana, *Proc. Natl. Acad. Sci. U.S.A.* **84,** 8874 (1987).
3. G. G. Wong, J. S. Witek, P. A. Temple, K. M. Wilkens, A. C. Leary, D. P. Luxenberg, S. S. Jones, E. L. Brown, R. M. Kay, E. C. Orr, C. Shoemaker, D. W. Golde, R. J. Kaufman, R. M. Hewick, E. A. Wang, and S. C. Clark, *Science* **228,** 810 (1985).
4. R. J. Kaufman, M. V. Davies, V. K. Pathak, and J. W. B. Hershey, *Mol. Cell. Biol.* **9,** 946 (1989).
5. B. Seed, *Nature (London)* **329,** 840 (1987).
6. R. S. Molday and D. MacKenzie, *Biochemistry* **22,** 653 (1983).
7. D. MacKenzie, A. Arendt, P. Hargrave, J. H. McDowell, and R. S. Molday, *Biochemistry* **23,** 6544 (1984).
8. D. D. Oprian, A. B. Asenjo, N. Lee, and S. L. Pelletier, *Biochemistry* **30,** 11367 (1991).

[22] *In Vitro* Synthesis of Bovine Rhodopsin Using Recombinant Baculovirus

Lieveke L. J. DeCaluwé, Jenny VanOostrum, Jacques J. M. Janssen, and Willem J. DeGrip

Introduction

Rhodopsin is the visual pigment of the rod photoreceptor cell in the vertebrate retina. It consists of an integral membrane protein, opsin, and a chromosphore, 11-*cis*-retinal. Bovine rhodopsin has a visible absorbance band with λ_{max} at 498 nm. Absorption of a photon triggers isomerization of the chromophore to all-trans. The resulting conformational changes (photolytic cascade) lead to signal site exposure, G protein (transducin) binding, and subsequent desensitization by the specific rhodopsin kinase and a 45-kDa protein (S-antigen or arrestin). In the photolytic cascade several intermediate steps can be distinguished. The first and the only light-dependent transition (rhodopsin to photorhodopsin) occurs within femtoseconds (1). The next intermediate, bathorhodopsin, is generated in picoseconds. Metarhodopsin II, the active form which triggers the signal transduction pathway, is generated in microseconds and decays slowly (half-life of several minutes) into metarhodopsin III (2).

Rhodopsin contains seven transmembrane helices, which harbor the chromophore 11-*cis*-retinal covalently linked to Lys-296 via a protonated Schiff base (3). The amino terminus is glycosylated (4) and is of structural importance, together with the three intradisk loops and the disulfide bridge between Cys-110 and Cys-187 (5, 6). Two cytoplasmic loops are supposed to play a role in signal transduction (7) together with an additional surface loop generated by palmitoylation and membrane anchoring at Cys-322 and Cys-323 (8).

Evidently, rhodopsin is a complex integral membrane protein that requires intermittent membrane translocation and several posttranslational modifications (glycosylation, palmitoylation, disulfide bridge formation, recombination with 11-*cis*-retinal) in order to fulfill all its structural and functional properties. *In vitro* expression allows exploration of properties like wavelength regulation, receptor mechanism, biosynthesis, and lipid–protein interactions in much detail through labeling and (site-specific) mutagenesis. For this purpose we have selected the recombinant *Autographa californica* nuclear polyhedrosis virus (AcNPV) baculovirus system, as this is an eukaryotic expression system that performs all common eukaryotic posttranslational modifications and has been used successfully for the high-level expression of foreign genes (for review, see Refs. 9 and 10). Baculoviruses are rather host-specific insect viruses (11), although recently a host range expansion by recombinant viruses of *Bombyx mori* nuclear polyhedrosis virus (BmNPV) and AcNPV has been reported (12). Still, the most commonly used host cell lines are Sf21 and Sf9, which originate from the oviduct of *Spodoptera frugiperda,* the fall army worm.

Nuclear polyhedrosis baculoviruses like AcNPV have the unique property of producing a protein matrix in which progeny virions are embedded at a late stage of infection (nuclear occlusion bodies) to protect virions on subsequent cell lysis. The strong promoter of the abundantly expressed matrix protein (polyhedrin) is generally used for the expression of heterologous protein (9, 10). Recombinant virus is obtained by homologous recombination after cotransfection of host cells with viral DNA (128 kb circular genome) and a transfer vector, which contains viral sequences of about 3 kb flanking the polyhedrin promoter and the cDNA insert. Several transfer vectors have been developed, which differ in the 5' and 3' region of the polyhedrin gene. For rapid identification of recombinant virus, transfer vectors containing an additional reporter gene, such as *LacZ,* have been constructed. Depending on the transfer vector used, recombinant virus can be isolated either via immunohistochemical/morphological screening (13, 14) or by chromogenic/morphological screening using constitutively expressed β-galactosidase (15).

In this chapter we elaborate on *in vitro* synthesis of bovine rhodopsin using recombinant AcNPV baculovirus.

Expression and Purification

Expression Level

Baculovirus-based expression systems produce very high levels of soluble proteins [5–10% of total cell protein (9, 10)] but generally much lower yields of membrane proteins [0.01–1% of total protein (16)]. Since a higher yield is much more efficient productionwise and reduces relative cost and purification losses, we have evaluated several factors in order to achieve maximal production of functional opsin. For quantitative determination of opsin the enzyme-linked immunosorbent assay (ELISA) described previously (17) was slightly adapted.

Enzyme-Linked Immunosorbent Assay of Opsin

The polystyrene wells of a 96-well microtiter plate are coated with 150 μl of a suspension of bovine rod outer segments (ROS) containing 20 pmol of rhodopsin per milliliter of phosphate-buffered saline (PBS; pH 7.4). For calibration bovine rhodopsin is used in the concentration range 0.02–10 pmol/well. Unknown samples are diluted to between 4×10^2 and 2×10^5 infected cells. The primary antiserum CERNJS858 (18) is used in a final dilution of 1 : 4000. Reaction with secondary antibody, horseradish peroxidase (HPO) assay, and computation are performed as described (17). Total protein is determined in parallel samples using Bio-Rad (Richmond, CA) and/or Pierce (Rockford, IL) protein assay kits with bovine serum albumin (BSA) as a standard.

Cell Culture

Baculovirus propagation, transfection, isolation of recombinant virus and insect cell culture are principally performed as described (19, 20). The *Spodoptera frugiperda* cell line IPLB-Sf9 is maintained at 27°C, either in TNM-FH medium plus 10% (v/v) fetal calf serum (FCS), 50 μg/ml streptomycin, and 50 units/ml penicillin, or in the serum-free medium Ex-Cell400 (Seralab, Crawley Down, U.K.). Cells are cultured in monolayer or suspension culture. Viral infections are performed in one-third of the final volume during 1–2 hr and then are supplemented with medium without FCS to a final cell density of 2×10^6 cells/ml. Large-scale production of recombinant protein can be achieved in suspension culture (21), but insect cells are very sensitive to mechanical shear. Addition of a cell protective agent like Pluronic F-68 is reported to improve cell viability (22). Inclusion of 0.3% Pluronic F-68 (Fluka, Buchs, Switzerland) in a suspension culture of Sf9 cells increases the opsin production after 3 days by about 50% (Fig. 1A, bar 1 versus 2). Hence, 0.3% Pluronic F-68 is used in all subsequent experiments employing suspension culture. The additional increase in production by approximately 30% on culturing the cells in the serum-free medium Ex-Cell400 (Fig. 1A, bar 3) is only marginal as compared to the about 5-fold higher levels reported for soluble proteins under the same conditions (23).

Rate of Production

Because the polyhedrin promoter is activated late in the infection cycle, we follow the opsin production in Sf9 cells at 1, 2, and 3 days postinfection (dpi) (Fig. 1C). Later stages are not appropriate since cell lysis starts as of 4 dpi and results in variable losses in yield of cellular membranes (not shown). As expected, peak levels are obtained after 3 dpi but are somewhat dependent on the infection conditions. At a multiplicity of infection (MOI) of 2, lower levels are usually obtained than at an MOI of 10 (Fig. 1C, bar 3 versus 4). Consequently, subsequent results are all based on infection at an MOI of 10 and cell harvest at 3 dpi.

Variation in 5' Noncoding Region of cDNA Insert

Bovine opsin cDNA (24) is cloned in three different transfer vectors (20): pAc373 (25), pAcRP23 (26), and pAcDZ1 (15). Only on reduction of the

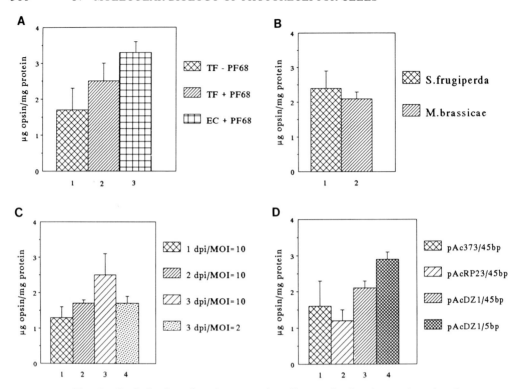

FIG. 1   Optimization of opsin expression. Expression levels are given in micrograms opsin per milligram protein ($n = 3$). Opsin levels were assayed at 3 dpi (A, B, D) or at 1, 2, and 3 dpi (C). Suspension culture was performed in spinner bottles (Bellco, Vineland, NJ, 1967-00250). In A, B, and C 100 ml suspension cultures of Sf9 cells ($\sim 2 \times 10^6$ cells/ml) or Mb cells ($\sim 1 \times 10^6$ cells/ml; B, bar 2) were infected with recombinant virus AcNPVRP23.ops (MOI = 10). (A) Effect of medium and Pluronic F-68 (0.1% during cell growth and 0.3% during infection): bar 1, TNM-FH (TF − PF68); bar 2, TNM-FH plus Pluronic F-68 (TF + PF68); bar 3, Ex-Cell400 plus Pluronic F-68 (EC + PF68). (B) Effect of cell type: Sf9 (bar 1) versus Mb (bar 2) cells. (C) Rate of opsin production at 1, 2, and 3 dpi, and effect of an MOI of 10 versus 2. (D) Variation in 5′ leader sequence. Monolayer cultures of Sf9 cells in 6-well petri dishes were infected with recombinant viruses (MOI = 10) obtained from the corresponding transfer vectors containing the opsin cDNA (ops; 45-bp leader sequence) or the 5′ truncated opsin cDNA (l-ops; 5-bp leader sequence): bar 1, AcNPV373.ops (pAc373/45bp); bar 2, AcNPVRP23.ops (pAcRP23/45p); bar 3, AcNPVDZ1.ops (pAcDZ1/45bp); bar 4, AcNPVDZ1.l-ops (pAcDZ1/5bp).

opsin 5' leader from 45 to 5 bases is a significant increase in opsin production observed (Fig. 1D). This is probably due to the fact that the opsin leader is GC-rich, whereas that of polyhedrin is AT-rich (27) to ensure high transcription levels (28).

Cell Type

A *Mamestra brassicae*-derived cell line (Mb) is reported to produce 2- to 3-fold higher levels of recombinant protein than Sf21 cells (29). We find similar yields of total protein, however, for Mb and Sf9 cells (454 ± 6 versus 499 ± 6 μg/10^6 cells) and similar expression levels for opsin (Fig. 1B). Sf9 cells are more easy to grow in suspension culture and have been used in the experiments reported in this chapter.

Conclusion

Under the various conditions described above, the functionality of the opsin produced (glycosylation, targeting, capacity to regenerate into rhodopsin on addition of 11-*cis* retinal; see following section) did not vary significantly. Hence, the highest expression level of functional opsin is achieved on using recombinant virus with 5' truncated opsin cDNA, a high infection density (MOI = 10), addition of 0.3% Pluronic F-68 to stabilize the cells, and a production time of 3 days. Under these conditions levels of 50 pmol opsin/10^6 cells (~4 μg opsin/mg protein; ~4 mg opsin/liter culture) are reproducibly achieved. This is a reasonably high level for a complex transmembrane protein (16), comparable in fact to the production rate of a bovine rod photoreceptor cell (15–25 pmol/day)!

Biosynthesis

Membrane Insertion

Immunofluorescent analysis shows that opsin produced in Sf9 cells is targeted to the plasma membrane (Fig. 2). To examine whether correct membrane translocation of the complex opsin sequence had been achieved, infected Sf9 cells are probed with monoclonal antibodies directed against epitopes distributed over the opsin sequence (30). Intact cells react with antibodies against the N-terminal domain (R2–12N) and the IV–V loop (T13–34L). In a correctly folded opsin structure both sequences are indeed located extracellularly. Intact cells are not immunoreactive with antibodies against the C-terminal domain [1D4 (31)] or the V–VI loop (K42–41L), sequences which should be located intracellularly. Only after permeabilization of the cells by fixation do the latter epitopes become accessible to antibodies (not

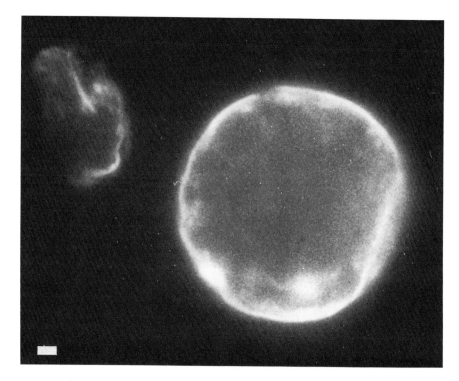

FIG. 2   Immunohistochemical analysis of opsin biosynthesis in Sf9 cells. Sf9 cells were cultured on a cover glass, infected with recombinant virus AcNPVRP23.ops, and fixed at 2 dpi by methanol (30 sec) and acetone (60 sec). Opsin was localized with the polyclonal antiserum CERNJS858 (dilution 1 : 500) elicited against bovine rhodopsin (18). Immunoreactivity was detected by reaction with fluorescein conjugated goat anti-rabbit immunoglobulin G (IgG) (DAKO Als, Glostrup, Denmark, dilution 1 : 25). Bar, 1 μm.

shown). We conclude that Sf9 cells accomplish correct membrane insertion and targeting of the opsin sequence.

Glycosylation

Immunoblot analysis shows that v-ops (opsin produced in insect cells by recombinant virus) migrates with the same apparent molecular weight as fully processed bovine opsin (Fig. 3, lanes 1 and 5). A positive immunoreaction with monoclonal antibodies against the N terminus and the C terminus indicates that the full-length protein is produced (20). Such data suggest that v-ops is glycosylated as well. This is confirmed by adding the N-glycosylation inhibitor tunicamycin on infection of Sf9 cells with recombinant virus. The

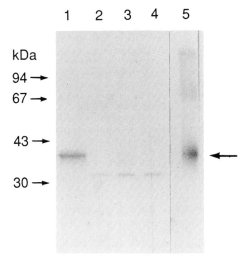

FIG. 3 Immunoblot analysis of Sf9 cells infected with recombinant virus AcNP-VRP23.ops (MOI = 10) in the absence (lane 1) or presence of increasing concentrations of tunicamycin, namely, 5 (lane 2), 10 (lane 3), and 25 μg/ml (lane 4). Lane 5 presents bovine ROS membranes as a control. The position of bovine opsin is indicated by the arrow at right. Lanes 1 to 4 represent approximately 5×10^4 cells. Total cell extracts (4 dpi) were separated on a 12% polyacrylamide gel and blotted onto nitrocellulose following standard procedures. Opsin was identified by incubation with antiserum 858 (dilution 1:500) followed by standard incubation with HPO-labeled antibodies and assay for HPO activity (20).

resulting immunopositive product now still contains the complete opsin sequence (20), but migrates with a lower apparent molecular weight (Fig. 3, lanes 2–4), which in fact corresponds to that of native nonglycosylated rhodopsin. Because insect cells are able to produce truncated high-mannose type glycomoieties throughout infection (32), the size of the sugar chains is probably very similar in native bovine opsin and v-ops. We have not investigated whether the v-ops moieties contain N-acetylglucosamine, since this complex type of N-glycosylation is apparently limited to the early stages of infection (32). As monoglycosylated bovine opsin migrates in between nonglycosylated and native bovine opsin, we tentatively conclude that v-ops is glycosylated at both glycosylation sites [Asn-2 and Asn-15 (4)].

Palmitoylation

Because insect cells are able to sustain thiopalmitoylation (33), we also decided to examine whether v-ops is palmitoylated. Hereto, Sf9 cells are incubated with [^{14}C]palmitic acid during infection with recombinant virus. After immunoprecipitation and polyacrylamide gel electrophoresis (PAGE) separation, the opsin band indeed contains radioactivity (not shown).

Regeneration and Spectral Properties

For functional analysis it is essential that the produced opsin be regenerated with the chromophore 11-*cis*-retinal into a photosensitive pigment. Regeneration can be accomplished in total cellular membrane preparations, a purified membrane fraction (see below), or a detergent extract using 5 mM dodecyl maltoside (DoM) (34). The extent of regeneration varies between the various fractions (see below), but maximal regeneration always requires a 20- to 40-fold molar excess of 11-*cis*-retinal over v-ops. The resulting photopigment is fully light sensitive, and the corresponding difference spectrum with λ_{max} at 498 nm is identical to that of native bovine rhodopsin (35). Hence, the photopigment derived from v-ops will be designated v-rho.

Purification

To study the functional and structural properties of the pigment obtained through *in vitro* expression, it is essential to purify the protein and reconstitute it into proper lipids. After extensive investigation, the scheme described in Fig. 4A proved to give reliable results. A density separation is required to separate membrane fractions of higher density, containing v-ops with low regeneration capacity, from a lower density fraction with high regeneration capacity. The latter fraction, which represents 40–50% of the total opsin produced, shows a comfortable 70–80% regeneration, compared to only 20–30% in the initial total cellular membrane preparation. Some further enrichment in v-rho is achieved on subsequent detergent solubilization using 10 mM DoM. The resulting supernatant contains 8–10 μg v-ops/mg protein, 70–80% of which is present as v-rho. Exploiting the fact that v-rho is mannoglycosylated, 20- to 40-fold purification can be accomplished by the simple and inexpensive technique of affinity chromatography over concanavalin A (ConA)–Sepharose. The resulting preparation (Fig. 4B, spectrum 1) contains 15–25% v-rho on a protein weight basis, with major contaminants originating from viral glycoproteins of 37 and 64 kDa (11, 14). Overall v-ops recovery is then 25–30%. Any residual retinal yields an additional absorbance peak around 360 nm (Fig. 4B, spectrum 1) but can be effectively removed by washing the column with 50 mM glucose before elution of v-rho.

Additional 2- to 3-fold purification can be achieved by immunoaffinity

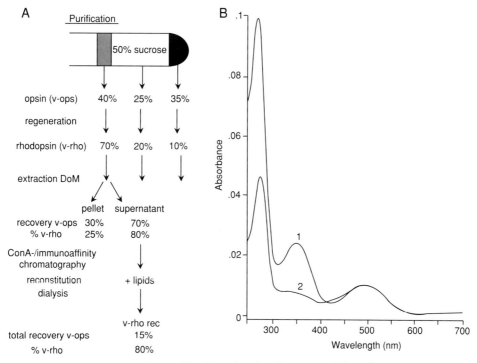

FIG. 4   (A) Scheme for purification of v-rho. Recovery is based on v-ops content. The percentage v-ops present as v-rho is given as % v-rho. (B) Typical absorbance spectra of v-rho after purification over ConA–Sepharose (spectrum 1) and immunoaffinity chromatography over immobilized 1D4 (spectrum 2). The residual retinal peak around 360 nm in spectrum 1 can be largely eliminated by washing the column before elution with 50 mM glucose.

chromatography over the immobilized monoclonal antibody 1D4 (31) using the corresponding epitope peptide 338–348 for elution of bound v-rho. This rather expensive procedure yields a preparation that contains at least 50% v-rho on a protein weight basis (Fig. 4B, spectrum 2) and is suitable for most functional analyses. Because reconstitution into proteoliposomes (see next section) by itself affords at least 3-fold purification, we usually strike a compromise between yield and purity by using ConA–Sepharose-purified preparations directly for reconstitution.

Procedures

Sf9 cells are harvested at 3 dpi, lysed, and homogenized in a Potter–Elvehjem tube in 1 ml buffer A/10^8 cells (buffer A is 5 mM PIPES; 10 mM EDTA, pH

6.5) with addition of 10 μg/ml leupeptin and 5 mM 1,4-dithioerythritol (DTE). The homogenate is layered on a 50% (w/v) sucrose cushion in buffer A and centrifuged for 1.5 hr at 70,000 g and 9°C. The band at the interface is collected, resuspended in buffer A, and centrifuged (30 min, 9°C, 100,000 g). The precipitate is resuspended in 0.5 ml/10^8 cells of buffer B (buffer B is 20 mM PIPES; 130 mM NaCl; 5 mM KCl; 2 mM MgCl$_2$; 2 mM CaCl$_2$; 0.1 mM EDTA; 5 mM DTE; pH 6.5) with addition of 10 μg/ml leupeptin and 0.5 mM DoM. The suspension is incubated while rotating with 11-cis-retinaldehyde [added as a dimethylformamide (DMF) solution; 20-fold molar excess over v-ops; final DMF concentration <2%] for 2–4 hr at room temperature. Then a 200 mM DoM solution is added to a final DoM concentration of 10 mM, and the suspension is rotated overnight at 4°C.

The DoM extract is freed from unsoluble material by centrifugation (20 min, 4°C, 2000 g), and applied to a column of ConA–Sepharose (Pharmacia, Uppsala, Sweden) (10 ml gel/10^9 cells) at a flow rate of 1 ml/hr. Unbound material is eluted with buffer C (10 volumes) (buffer C is buffer B with addition of 20 mM nonylglucose) followed by 50 mM glucose in buffer C (5 volumes). During these washing steps the detergent is exchanged for 20 mM nonylglucose (34). The v-rho is then eluted with buffer C containing 200 mM α-methylmannose. Reconstitution of v-rho is achieved by addition of a 150-fold molar excess of egg phosphatidylcholine (PC) dissolved in 20 mM nonylglucose, followed by dialysis 3 times against 50 volumes of buffer B (24–48 hr, 4°C). The resulting proteoliposomes are collected by centrifugation (16 hr, 4°C, 100,000 g).

For immunoaffinity chromatography the DoM extract is applied to a column of 1D4 immobilized onto Affi-Gel Hz (Bio-Rad) according to the manufacturer's instructions. The final gel contained approximately 3 mg antibody per milliliter of gel and 0.1 ml gel is used per initial 10^8 cells. Unbound material is eluted with 10 volumes of buffer C, and bound v-rho is subsequently eluted with buffer C containing 100 μM of peptide 338–348.

Conclusion

The recombinant baculovirus system affords relatively high yields of *in vitro* expressed opsin with correct folding, posttranslational modification, and targeting. The relatively low overall regeneration capacity remains unexplained, but it may be related to "structural stress" caused by a relative high packing density of this heterologous membrane protein in an unusual lipid environment. Relatively low ligand-binding capacity has also been reported for other membrane receptors expressed in this system (16). By the same reasoning the relatively low yield as compared to soluble proteins can be explained as well as the low response to changes in the 5′ noncoding region, which strongly affect expression levels of soluble proteins. Our purification scheme leads to preparations of at least 80% purity with 10–15% recovery of v-ops. This yield compares favorably with those obtained in mammalian expression systems (36, 37). In addition, bioreactors are being developed for insect cell culture, which will allow suspension cultures of 10–30 liters in the near future (21). Under these conditions sufficient material can be produced to permit studies by powerful but rather insensitive biophysical techniques like solid-state nuclear magnetic resonance (NMR) spectroscopy.

Functional Analysis

Photolysis

Reconstitution
To create a more native environment the purified v-rho is reconstituted into suitable lipids (egg PC or retina extract). Lipids are added in a molar ratio to v-ops of 150 : 1, and proteoliposomes are generated by removal of detergent through dialysis. This accomplishes at least 3-fold further purification but simultaneously results in about 50% loss of v-ops. Hence, about 15% of the initial v-ops is recovered in proteoliposomes and is accessible to functional analyses, which require a membrane environment.

Photolytic Cascade
Membrane films of reconstituted v-rho display the normal pattern of late photointermediates (Fig. 5). Metarhodopsin II (λ_{max} at 380 nm) decays at room temperature with a half-time of 4 ± 1 min into opsin and metarhodopsin III (λ_{max} at 455 nm). As in the case of native rhodopsin, only the photoproducts are unstable toward 50 mM hydroxylamine. The conformational transitions occurring during the rhodopsin to bathorhodopsin and rhodopsin to metarhodopsin II transitions of v-rho are probed by Fourier transform infrared (FTIR) spectroscopy. Both transition spectra are identical to those of native bovine ROS, in further confirmation of the identical nature of the expressed and the native protein (Bousché, G. L. J. DeCaluwé, K. J. Rothschild, and W. J. DeGrip, 1992, unpublished).

Transduction Cascade
When supplied with a soluble protein extract of bovine rod outer segments, v-rho is able to sustain the phototransduction cascade, and desensitization by ATP is observed as well (W. A. H. M. VanGroningen, J. J. M. Janssen, P. H. M. Bovee, and W. J. DeGrip, 1992, unpublished). This is established using the proton-release assay for activated cGMP phosphodiesterase, developed by Liebman and Evanczuk (38).

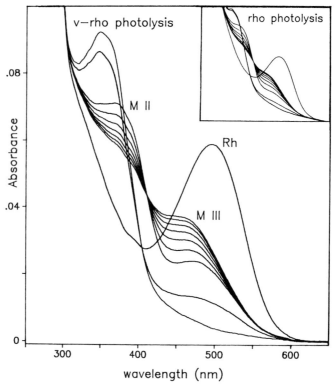

FIG. 5 Photolytic reactions of reconstituted v-rho deposited as a membrane film (39) on cellulose acetate (0.9 nmol v-rho). The absorbance bands of rhodopsin (Rh; maximum at 498 nm), metarhodopsin II (M II; 380 nm), and metarhodopsin III (M III; 455 nm) are indicated. (*Inset*) Photolysis of reconstituted bovine rhodopsin under similar conditions (3 nmol rhodopsin). After 15 sec of illumination, the spectra were taken at 3-min intervals.

Site-Specific Mutagenesis

Site-specific mutagenesis is a powerful tool to probe structural and/or functional roles of protein residues. We first addressed the highly conserved membrane-bound carboxyl residues Asp-83, Glu-113, Glu-122, and Glu-134, since they might play a role in wavelength regulation and/or photoconformational changes in visual pigments (39, 40). Point mutations are introduced using the approach developed by Kunkel (41) incorporated into the Bio-Rad Mutagene kit. This is based on growing M13 phage containing the cDNA insert in an *Escherichia coli* dut$^-$ ung$^-$ strain (inactivated dUTPase and uracil-*N*-glycosidase), isolation, and mutagenesis of uracil-containing single-stranded DNA using oligonucleotides with the desired mutation for strand duplication. On subsequent transformation in a wild-type *E. coli* strain, the original uracil-containing strand will be destroyed, and the mutant will predominantly replicate.

Mutation of Asp-83 or Glu-122 does not markedly affect biosynthesis of opsin or spectral properties of the resulting rhodopsin (20, 35), in agreement with other reports (42–44). Mutation of Glu-134 and/or Arg-135, however, results in impaired biosynthesis. In addition to a normal 38-kDa product, which produces a normal photopigment, a nonglycosylated and structurally abnormal 31-kDa product is obtained (20). We have postulated that the charge pair Glu-134/Arg-135, which is conserved throughout the G-protein-coupled receptor family, is part of a stop-transfer signal, alteration of which would increase the chance of incorrect membrane translocation and protein folding. Mutation of Glu-113 significantly affects the spectral properties of rhodopsin by interfering with the endogenous protonation of the Schiff base linkage between opsin and 11-*cis*-retinal, insofar that it now becomes dependent on the external pH or anion concentration (42, 45, 46). This explains our original observation of little change in spectral properties, which was obtained in isotonic conditions at relatively low pH (35). Whether Glu-113 directly protonates the Schiff base is still a matter of debate (20, 47). The remarkably nonspecific anion dependency (46) would also indicate a more indirect role. Evidence is accumulating that wavelength modulation (spectral shift of the 440 nm peak of an unperturbed protonated retinylidene Schiff base by the specific influence of a protein) does not depend on a small number of residues, but rather on the presence/absence of hydroxy residues at key positions (48, 49). This would agree with the extended hydrogen bond network proposed before on the basis of FTIR data (39).

Exciting material for mutagenesis studies has recently originated from genomic analysis of patients with autosomal-dominant retinitis pigmentosa. Already over 24 point mutations or small deletions in the rod rhodopsin gene have been described in families carrying this disease (50, 51). Identification of the structural or functional defect introduced by such mutations will undoubtedly contribute to elucidation of signal sequences relevant for biosynthesis and routing and of structure–function relationships in visual pigments. It might also lead to better insight into the relation between defective protein processing and cell degeneration. For instance, mutations near position Arg-135 have been shown to impair protein routing and regeneration on expression in a human kidney cell line (51) and glycosylation, protein folding, and regeneration on expression in the Sf9 insect cell line (20). This strongly suggests that changes at this position impair protein processing, which eventually evokes photoreceptor cell degeneration.

Acknowledgments

We acknowledge generous gifts of opsin cDNA (D. Hogness), monoclonal antibodies against rhodopsin (P. Hargrave and G. Adamus), the hybridoma cell line 1D4 (R. Molday and L. Molday), the *Mamestra brassicae* cell line (L. King), and transfer vector pAcDZ1 (D. Zuidema).

References

1. R. W. Schoenlein, L. A. Peteanu, R. A. Mathies, and C. V. Shank, *Science* **254,** 412 (1991).
2. L. Stryer, *J. Biol. Chem.* **266,** 10711 (1991).
3. P. A. Hargrave, J. H. McDowell, D. R. Curtis, J. K. Wang, E. Juszczak, S. L. Fong, J. K. M. Rao, and P. Argos, *Biophys. Struct. Mech.* **9,** 235 (1983).
4. P. A. Hargrave, *Biochim. Biophys. Acta* **492,** 83 (1977).
5. S. Al-Saleh, M. Gore, and M. Akhtar, *Biochem. J.* **246,** 131 (1987).
6. S. S. Karnik and H. G. Khorana, *J. Biol. Chem.* **265,** 17520 (1990).
7. B. König, A. Arendt, J. H. McDowell, M. Kahlert, P. A. Hargrave, and K. P. Hofmann, *Proc. Natl. Acad. Sci. U.S.A.* **86,** 6878 (1989).
8. Y. A. Ovchinnikov, N. G. Abdulaev, and A. S. Bogachuk, *FEBS Lett.* **230,** 1 (1988).
9. V. A. Luckow and M. D. Summers, *Bio Technology* **6,** 47 (1988).
10. V. A. Luckow, *in* Recombinant DNA Technology and Applications (A. Prokop, R. K. Bajpal, and C. S. Ho, eds.), p. 97. McGraw-Hill, New York, 1991.
11. R. R. Granados and B. A. Federici, "The Biology of Baculoviruses," Vol. 1. CRC Press, Boca Raton, Florida, 1986.
12. A. Kondo and S. Maeda, *J. Virol.* **65,** 3625 (1991).
13. J. J. M. Janssen, W. J. M. VanDeVen, W. A. H. M. VanGroningen-Luyben, J. Roosien, J. M. Vlak, and W. J. DeGrip, *Mol. Biol. Rep.* **13,** 65 (1988).
14. J. J. M. Janssen, Thesis, University of Nijmegen, The Netherlands (1991).
15. D. Zuidema, A. Schouten, M. Usmany, A. J. Maule, G. J. Belsham, J. Roosien, E. C. Klingeroode, J. W. M. VanLent, and J. M. Vlak, *J. Gen. Virol.* **71,** 2201 (1990).
16. E. M. Parker, K. Kameyama, H. Tsutomu, and E. M. Ross, *J. Biol. Chem.* **266,** 519 (1991).
17. J. J. Schalken and W. J. De Grip, *Exp. Eye Res.* **43,** 431 (1986).
18. W. J. De Grip, *Prog. Retinal Res.* **4,** 137 (1985).
19. M. D. Summers and G. E. Smith, A Manual of Methods for Baculovirus Vectors and Insect Culture Procedures, Texas Exp. Station Bulletin no. 1555, 1987.
20. J. J. M. Janssen, W. R. Mulder, G. L. J. DeCaluwé, J. M. Vlak, and W. J. DeGrip, *Biochim. Biophys. Acta* **1089,** 68 (1991).
21. J. Q. Wu, G. King, A. J. Daugulis, P. Faulkner, D. H. Bone, and M. F. A. Goosen, *Appl. Microbiol. Biotechnol.* **32,** 249 (1989).
22. A. W. Caron, J. Archambault, and B. Massie, *Biotechnol. Bioeng.* **36,** 1133 (1990).

23. G. Godwin, *In Vitro Cell Dev. Biol.* **24,** 19A (1989).

24. J. Nathans and D. S. Hogness, *Cell (Cambridge, Mass.)* **34,** 807 (1983).

25. G. E. Smith, B. L. Ericson, J. Moschera, H.-W. Lahm, R. Chizzonite, and M. D. Summers, *Proc. Natl. Acad. Sci. U.S.A.* **82,** 8404 (1985).

26. R. D. Possee and S. C. Howard, *Nucleic Acids Res.* **15,** 10233 (1987).

27. Y. Matsuura, R. D. Possee, H. A. Overton, and H. L. Bishop, *J. Gen. Virol.* **68,** 1233 (1987).

28. L. K. Miller, *Annu. Rev. Microbiol.* **42,** 177 (1988).

29. L. A. King, S. G. Mann, A. M. Lawrie, and S. H. Mulshaw, *Virus Res.* **19,** 93 (1991).

30. G. Adamus, Z. S. Zam, A. Arendt, K. Palczewski, J. H. McDowell, and P. A. Hargrave, *Vision Res.* **31,** 17 (1991).

31. R. S. Molday and D. MacKenzie, *Biochemistry* **22,** 653 (1983).

32. D. J. Davidson and F. J. Castellino, *Biochemistry* **30,** 6167 (1991).

33. M. Kloc, B. Reddy, S. Crawford, and L. D. Etkin, *J. Biol. Chem.* **266,** 8206 (1991).

34. W. J. DeGrip and P. H. M. Bovee-Geurts, *Chem. Phys. Lipids* **23,** 321 (1979).

35. J. J. M. Janssen, G. L. J. DeCaluwé, and W. J. DeGrip, *FEBS Lett.* **260,** 113 (1990).

36. D. D. Oprian, R. S. Molday, R. J. Kaufman, and H. G. Khorana, *Proc. Natl. Acad. Sci. U.S.A.* **84,** 8874 (1987).

37. J. Nathans, C. J. Weitz, N. Agarwal, I. Nir, and D. S. Papermaster, *Vision Res.* **29,** 907 (1989).

38. P. A. Liebman and A. T. Evanczuk, in "Methods in Enzymology" (L. Packer, ed.), Vol. 81, p. 532. Academic Press, New York, 1982.

39. W. J. DeGrip, J. Gillespie, and K. J. Rothschild, *Biochim. Biophys. Acta* **809,** 97 (1985).

40. K. Kakitani, *Proc. Yamada Conf.* **21,** 31 (1988).

41. T. A. Kunkel, *Proc. Natl. Acad. Sci. U.S.A.* **82,** 488 (1985).

42. E. A. Zhukovsky and D. D. Oprian, *Science* **246,** 928 (1989).

43. J. Nathans, *Biochemistry* **29,** 937 (1990).

44. T. P. Sakmar, R. R. Franke, and H. G. Khorana, *Proc. Natl. Acad. Sci. U.S.A.* **86,** 8309 (1989).

45. J. Nathans, *Biochemistry* **29,** 9746 (1990).

46. T. P. Sakmar, R. R. Franke, and H. G. Khorana, *Proc. Natl. Acad. Sci. U.S.A.* **88,** 3079 (1991).

47. S. O. Smith, J. M. L. Courtin, H. DeGroot, R. Gebhard, and J. Lugtenburg, *Biochemistry* **30,** 7409 (1991).

48. M. Neitz, J. Neitz, and G. H. Jacobs, *Science* **252,** 971 (1991).

49. T. A. Nakayama and H. G. Khorana, *J. Biol. Chem.* **266,** 4629 (1991).

50. T. P. Dryja, T. L. McGee, L. B. Hahn, G. S. Cowly, J. E. Olsson, E. Reichel, M. A. Sandberg, and E. L. Berson, *N. Engl. J. Med.* **323,** 1302 (1990).

51. C. H. Sung, B. G. Schneider, N. Agarwal, D. S. Papermaster, and J. Nathans, *Proc. Natl. Acad. Sci. U.S.A.* **88,** 8840 (1991).

[23] Transfection of Retinoblastoma Cells: Localization of Cis-Acting Elements for Human Interstitial Retinoid-Binding Protein Gene

Shao-Ling Fong, T. Allen Morris, Chao-Hung Lee,
Larry A. Donoso, and Wei-Bao Fong

Introduction

Since the 1980s there has been an enormous expansion in our knowledge concerning gene regulation from many different biological systems. Transient expression systems have played a major role in defining cis-acting elements. Usually, the 5' upstream region from the transcription initiation site of the structural gene is inserted into the 5' upstream region of the reporter gene in an expression vector (1). The recombinant plasmid is then introduced into a cell line, and the transient expression of the reporter gene is quantified. When a series of mutations is generated by deleting the nucleotides from the far end of the 5'-flanking fragment toward the reporter gene, the reporter gene activities driven by these deletion constructs can be used to define the DNA sequences that are responsible for the physiological functions (2).

In general, a stretch of several hundred nucleotides 5' upstream from the transcription initiation site is called a promoter region (3, 4). A promoter may contain several cis-acting DNA motifs and drives weak expression but will respond strongly to an enhancer element. An enhancer is a fragment of DNA that stimulates transcription in a manner independent of distance and orientation when it is positioned 5' upstream of the promoter or 3' downstream of the reporter gene (3–5).

Only limited information is available in the literature related to the regulation of gene expression in photoreceptor cells (6–8), because no representative cell lines are available for study. Fortunately, many photoreceptor-specific proteins are expressed in retinoblastoma cells (9–11), the most common primary intraocular tumor of childhood. We are currently using a retinoblastoma cell line, WERI-RB1, to dissect the regulatory sequences that are responsible for the expression of human interstitial (or interphotoreceptor) retinoid-binding protein (IRBP) *in vivo*.

IRBP is a large and elongated glycoprotein (12–15) that is universally distributed throughout the vertebrates (16). It is synthesized by the photore-

Methods in Neurosciences, Volume 15

ceptor cells in the retina and is secreted into the interphotoreceptor matrix. The major function of IRBP is believed to be the transport of 11-*cis*- and all-*trans*-retinoids between the neural retina and the retinal pigment epithelium. Human IRBP has been purified and characterized at both the biochemical and molecular levels. The gene has been localized to human chromosome 10, and the complete cDNA and genomic sequences have been published (17–20).

In this chapter, we report a 2.1-kb (kilobase) 5′ upstream sequence from the transcription initiation sites of the human IRBP gene, describe optimal conditions for the transfection of one of the pIRBP–CAT constructs (derived from a commercial vector, pCAT-Basic, Promega Co., Madison, WI) containing this 2.1 kb regulatory sequence into retinoblastoma cells (WERI-RB1), and compare chloramphenicol acetyltransferase (CAT) activities for four nested mutations.

Transfection Procedures

Construction of pIRBP–CAT Plasmids

An *Sst*I fragment containing the 5′ flanking sequence of the human IRBP gene is subcloned into M13mp19. Two clones, HGL3.S10 and HGL3.S18, represent the two orientations of the insert in M13. They are used for sequencing by the dideoxy chain-termination method (21) using the procedure of Dale *et al.* (22). One of the nested clones, HGL3.S10.22 (Fig. 1), generated by the Cyclone system (International Biotechnologies, Inc., New Haven, CT) contains a 3′ end which is located between the transcription and translation initiation sites, and this clone is used as the source for plasmid constructions. Clone HGL3.S10.22 contains 2131 base pairs (bp) of 5′ flanking sequences from the first cap site (position +1), an additional 68 bp of the first exon of the human IRBP gene, and a stretch of 13 G residues produced by the Cyclone system. The insert can be removed from the clone HGL3.S10.22 by *Sst*I and *Eco*RI digestions. In addition to this *Sst*I–*Eco*RI fragment, three shorter fragments, namely, *Acc*I–*Eco*RI (1074 bp), *Pst*I–*Eco*RI (958 bp), and *Hgi*AI–*Eco*RI (287 bp), are produced and blunt-ended with Klenow DNA polymerase I. After ligating to the expression vector pCAT-Basic that has been digested with *Sal*I and blunt-ended with Klenow, four plasmids containing inserts in physiological orientation (5′ to 3′), namely, pIRBP2131a-CAT (2212 bp insert), pIRBP993a-CAT (1074 bp insert), pIRBP877a-CAT (958 bp insert), and pIRBP206a-CAT (287 bp insert), and one in opposite orientation (3′ to 5′), namely, pIRBP2131b-CAT (2212 bp insert), are generated. The latter plasmid is used as a negative control. Plasmid DNAs used

```
                                    ▼ Sst I
        -2136 GAGCTCTCGGCTTTCACTCTGGGGACTTACCCAGAACATATTCTCCTCATGAGCTA
-2080 AGGAGGCTGGCTGCCATCTTCCTACATCCCCCCACGGCCTGGGGGCAAGGACACCCTGGCCCCCTGGAGTCTGGAGAACT
-2000 CTGAGGACAGAACTTGCTCTTCCACCTGCTTGGGCCTTACCCACAGGAGAAGCACTGCTTCTCTACCCATGCCCCATCCA
-1920 ACTCAGGCACCCCAGGGACTTGCAACAGTCTGATTTTTTCTCACGTCCTTCTTAAGGCTCTGGGCTAGCCACACAAATCA
-1840 AATCCCAGTGATAGGTCCAGACAATCCTATCCTGAAACTACATCTTAGTAAGACTCCAGGGAATCCTTTCCCCAAAGACA
-1760 GTCTTACTCCTGTTCTCCCCCAAGCCCTTTCTGGGCCAGAAGCTTTGCCTGGACTCAAGCAATGGCAGACAAGTGCCCTC
-1680 TGAGGACACGGAAGTGCATGCTCAGAACTGTGATTCTCCAAGTGGAGGCAGAGGAGAAGGCCCAGGCTTCCCAGCAGGGC
-1600 TAAGGATATGCAAGGAGTGCATTCATCCGGAGGTGTTGGCAGCATCCCAGCCCCACCCCATTCTCATCGTAAATCAGGCT
-1520 CACTTCCATTGGCTGCATACGGTGGAGTGATGTGACCATATGTCACTTGAGCATTACACAAATCCTAATGAGCTAAAAAT
-1440 ATGTTTGTTTTAGCTAATTGACCTCTTTGGCCTTCATAAAGCAGTTGGTAAACATCCTCAGATAATGATTTCCAAAGAGC
-1360 AGATTGTGGGTCTCAGCTGTGCAGAGAAAGCCCACGTCCCTGAGACCACCTTCTCCAGCTGCCTACTGAGGCACACAGGG
-1280 GCGCCTGCCTGCTGCCCGCTCAGCCAAGGCGGTGTTGCTGGAGCCAGCTTGGGACAGCTCTCCCAACGCTCTGCCCTGGC
-1200 CTTGCGACCCACTCTCTGGGCCGTAGTTGTCTGTCTGTTAAGTGAGGAAAGTGCCCATCTCCAGAGGCATTCAGCGGCAA
-1120 AGCAGGGCTTCCAGGTTCCGACCCCATAGCAGGACTTCTTGGATTTCTACAGCCAGTCAGTTGCAAGCAGCACCCATATT
                                                  ▼ Acc I
-1040 ATTTCTATAAGAAGTGGCAGGAGCTGGGATCTGAAGAGTTCAGCAGTCTACCTTTCCCTGTTTCTTGTGCTTTATGCAGT
 -960 CAGGAGGAATGATCTGGATTCCATGTGAAGCCTGGGACCACGGAGACCCAAGACTTCCTGCTTGATTCTCCCTGCGAACT
               ▼ Pst I
 -880 GCAGGCTGTGGGCTGAGCCTTCAAGAAGCAGGAGTCCCCTCTAGCCATTAACTCTCAGAGCTAACCTCATTTGAATGGGA
 -800 ACACTAGTCCTGTGATGTCTGGAAGGTGGGCGCCTCTACACTCCACACCCTACATGGTGGTCCAGACACATCATTCCCAG
 -720 CATTAGAAAGCTGTAGGGGGACCCGTTCTGTTCCCTGGAGGCATTAAAGGGACATAGAAATAAATCTCAAGCTCTGAGGC
 -640 TGATGCCAGCCTCAGACTCAGCCTCTGCACTGTATGGGCCAATTGTAGCCCCAAGGACTTCTTCTTGCTGCACCCCCTAT
 -560 CTGTCCACACCTAAAACGATGGGCTTCTATTAGTTACAGAACTCTCTGGCCTGTTTTGTTTTGCTTTGCTTTGTTTTGTT
 -480 TTGTTTTTTTGTTTTTTTGTTTTTTAGCTATGAAACAGAGGTAATATCTAATACAGATAACTTACCAGTAATGAGTGCTT
 -400 CCTACTTACTGGGTACTGGGAAGAAGTGCTTTACACATATTTTCTCATTTAATCTACACAATAAGTAATTAAGACATTTC
 -320 CCTGAGGCCACGGGAGAGACAGTGGCAGAACAGTTCTCCAAGGAGGACTTGCAAGTTAATAACTGGACTTTGCAAGGCTC
                                            ▼ HgiA I
 -240 TGGTGGAAACTGTCAGCTTGTAAAGGATGGAGCACAGTGTCTGGCATGTAGCAGGAACTAAAATAATGGCAGTGATTAAT
 -160 GTTATGATATGCAGACACAACACAGCAAGATAAGATGCAATGTACCTTCTGGGTCAAACCACCCTGGCCACTCCTCCCCG
  -80 ATACCCAGGGTTGATGTGCTTGAATTAGACAGGATTAAAGGCTTACTGGAGCTGGAAGCCTTGCCCCAACTCAGGAGTTT
        ┌→    ┌→   ┌→        ┌→
    1 AGCCCCAGACCTTCTGTCCACCAGCTGAGAAGGACAAGGGCGGAAGGCAGCTGCACAGAGCAGGGCCAGGGGGGGGGGGG
          ▼ EcoR I
   81 GGAATTC
```

FIG. 1 Nucleotide sequence of clone HGL3.S10.22. Three transcription initiation sites were detected at positions +1, +7, and +15 (20). The 5' flanking sequence of the human IRBP gene is indicated by negative numbers. The restriction endonuclease cleavage sites are underlined, and the cleavage points are indicated by arrowheads. A stretch of G residues produced by the Cyclone system is overlined.

for transfection are extracted by the alkali procedure and purified two times by cesium chloride equilibrium gradient centrifugation (23).

Cell Maintenance

The retinoblastoma cell line WERI-RB1 is grown in suspension in a culture medium made up of RPMI 1640 supplemented with 10% (v/v) fetal bovine serum, 2 mg/ml sodium bicarbonate, 0.29 mg/ml L-glutamine, 100 units/ml penicillin, and 100 μg/ml streptomycin at 37°C and 5% CO_2. Tissue culture reagents are purchased from GIBCO BRL (Gaithersburg, MD).

Transfection

Cells used for transfection are centrifuged at 190 g for 5 min and washed twice with Opti-Mem reduced serum medium (GIBCO BRL). During the second wash, an aliquot of cells suspended in Opti-Mem is counted.

Transfections are carried out by the method of Felgner *et al.* (24) using the cationic liposome Lipofectin (GIBCO BRL) with some modifications. For each transfection, 3.3×10^6 WERI-RB1 cells in Opti-Mem are pelleted in a polystyrene centrifuge tube. The DNA construct and Lipofectin are each diluted with 0.5 ml of Opti-Mem in polystyrene tubes just before the transfection. They are then mixed and immediately added to the cell pellet. The retinoblastoma cells, resuspended in this mixture, are plated out in a 35-mm well. After an overnight incubation, 1 ml of culture medium with 20% fetal bovine serum is added. The next day, the transfected cells are collected by centrifugation, resuspended in 1.7 ml of normal culture medium, and plated out in a new well. The cells are grown for 2 more days before being harvested.

Harvest and Lysis of Transfected Cells

After transfection, the WERI-RB1 cells are collected into 1.5-ml microcentrifuge tubes by centrifugation at 190 g for 5 min and then resuspended in 50 μl of 0.25 M Tris, pH 7.5. Cells are lysed in this buffer by a series of freeze–thaws. The tubes containing cells are immersed in a dry ice/ethanol slurry for 5 min and then immediately transferred to a 37° water bath for another 5 min. This procedure is repeated 2 more times. The cell lysate is collected after spinning the cell debris down in a microcentrifuge at the maximum speed for 5 min at 4°C. The lysate is weighed and stored at -20°C.

Chloramphenicol Acetyltransferase Assay

For determination of CAT enzyme activity in the cell extracts, we use ^{14}C-labeled chloramphenicol and nonradioactive acetyl-coenzyme A and then separate the acetylated chloramphenicol from the unacetylated chloramphenicol by thin-layer chromatography (1). In each CAT assay, one-half of the cell extract is brought up to a volume of 33 μl with 0.25 M Tris, pH 7.5, and is heat-inactivated at 65°C for 10 min. The following assay components are then added: 4.25 μl of 1 M Tris, pH 7.5; 1.75 μl of 40 mM acetyl-CoA (Sigma, St. Louis, MO); 4 μl (0.1 μCi) ^{14}C]chloramphenicol (55 mCi/mmol; Amersham, Arlington Heights, IL); and 7 μl water to bring the total assay volume to 50 μl. After incubating at 37°C for 1 hr, the acetylated and unacetylated chloramphenicol are extracted from the aqueous solution with 0.5 ml of ethyl acetate. The organic phase is evaporated in a SpeedVac concentrator and the residue resuspended in 30 μl ethyl acetate for loading onto thin-layer chromatography (TLC) sheets (silica gel with fluorescent indicator; Kodak, Rochester, NY). A chromatography tank is equilibrated with 200 ml of chloroform–methanol (190 : 10, v/v), and the solvent is allowed to progress three-quarters of the way to the top of the sheet. The amount of unacetylated and acetylated ^{14}C]chloramphenicol is determined by a two-dimensional β-scanner (Ambis, San Diego, CA), and the percent conversion is calculated.

Optimization of WERI-RB1 Transfections

The conditions required for optimal transfection will vary depending on each individual cell line (25). The amounts of the plasmid construct and the liposome used for transfection need to be adjusted so that the transfected cells will produce a maximal CAT enzyme activity for a given promoter. For the WERI-RB1 cells, we varied the amount of DNA, pIRBP2131a-CAT, from 8 to 24 μg and the amount of Lipofectin from 5 to 20 μg (1 μg/μl of total lipid) in order to determine the optimal conditions for transfection.

The results of this matrix optimization are illustrated in Fig. 2. It is apparent that higher amounts of Lipofectin, 15 or 20 μg, gave lower CAT expression as compared to 5 or 10 μg Lipofectin. Using 5 μg Lipofectin, the CAT expression appears to level off above 16 μg of DNA. At this point 25% of ^{14}C]chloramphenicol was converted to its derivatives. However, when 10 μg of Lipofectin was used, 24 μg of DNA gave the maximum CAT activity (33% conversion). This combination has been chosen as the optimum condition for transfection of WERI-RB1 cells.

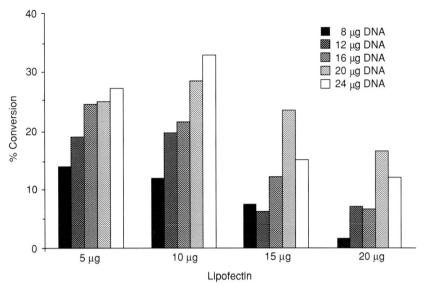

FIG. 2   Transfection of WERI-RB1 cells with Lipofectin. Lipofectin was varied from 5 to 20 μg, and DNA (plasmid pIRBP2131a-CAT) was varied from 8 to 24 μg. The CAT activities were measured as the percentage of conversion of [^{14}C]chloramphenicol to acetylated chloramphenicol.

Localization of Cis-Acting Elements by Transfecting pIRBP–CAT Plasmids into WERI-RB1 Cells

To determine the location of the cis-acting elements in the 5'-flanking regions, four pIRBP–CAT constructs differing in the length of the 5'-flanking sequence upstream of the CAT coding sequence were used for WERI-RB1 transfection. We used 10 μg of Lipofectin and 16 μg of a pIRBP–CAT construct for the transfection. The reason 16 μg of pIRBP–CAT construct was chosen instead of 24 μg is that we plan to add 8 μg of internal standard such as pRSV.Luc (with the luciferase gene used as a reporter gene) for the evaluation of the transfection efficiency.

   The levels of CAT expression driven by these constructs are compared as shown in Fig. 3. The deletion from −2131 to −993 results in a 69% drop in CAT activity (Fig. 3, lanes 1 and 2). Three constructs, namely, pIRBP993a-CAT, pIRBP877a-CAT, and pIRBP206a-CAT, showed comparable levels of CAT activities (Figs. 3, lanes 2, 3, and 4). The construct pIRBP206a-CAT contains sufficient information for the constitutive CAT expression in WERI-

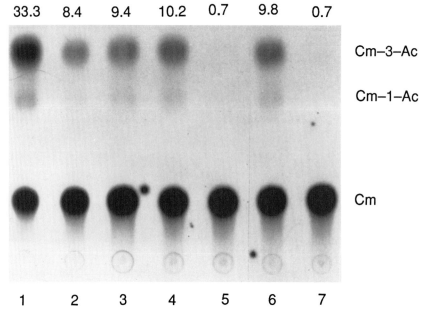

FIG. 3   CAT activities of pIRBP–CAT constructs. The conversion of [^{14}C]chloramphenicol (Cm) to 1-acetylated and 3-acetylated forms (Cm-1-Ac and Cm-3-Ac, respectively) was detected by autoradiography. Ten micrograms of Lipofectin and 16 μg of DNA were used for each transfection. The constructs used for lanes 1 through 7 are pIRBP2131a-CAT, pIRBP993a-CAT, pIRBP877a-CAT, pIRBP206a-CAT, pIRBP213lb-CAT, pCAT-Control, and pCAT-Basic, respectively. The CAT activities measured by the percent conversion are shown at top.

RB1 cells. The same observation has been reported in studies using transgenic mice (7). The plasmid pIRBP2131b-CAT, containing a reverse oriented insert, showed the same background expression as that of the vector pCAT-Basic (Fig. 3, lanes 5 and 7). The plasmid pCAT-Control (Promega) containing both the SV40 promoter and enhancer showed the same level of CAT expression as pIRBP206a-CAT in WERI-RB1 cells (Fig. 3, lanes 6 and 4). This indicates that two regions of the 5′-flanking sequence of the human IRBP gene, between -2131 and -993 and between -206 and $+68$, contain the regulatory elements. We are in the process of further refining those regions by producing deleted mutations with exo III/S1 nucleases, polymerase chain reaction (PCR), and synthetic oligonucleotides.

Conclusions

A transient expression system has been developed that is suitable for the study of gene expression of IRBP. It should be generally applicable for the gene expression studies of photoreceptor-specific proteins in retinoblastoma cells.

Acknowledgments

This project was supported in part by the Project Development Program, Research and Sponsored Programs, Indiana University at Indianapolis, and in part by a Developmental Grant from Research to Prevent Blindness Inc.

References

1. C. M. Gorman, L. F. Moffat, and B. H. Howard, *Mol. Cell. Biol.* **2,** 1044 (1982).
2. M. D. Walker, T. Edlund, A. M. Boulet, and W. J. Rutter, *Nature (London)* **306,** 557 (1983).
3. M. M. Muller, T. Gerster, and W. Schaffner, *Eur. J. Biochem.* **176,** 485 (1988).
4. W. S. Dynan, *Cell (Cambridge, Mass.)* **58,** 1 (1989).
5. M. L. Atchison, *Annu. Rev. Cell Biol.* **4,** 127 (1988).
6. G. I. Liou, L. Geng, M. R. Al-Ubaidi, S. Matragoon, G. Hanten, W. Baehr, and P. A. Overbeek, *J. Biol. Chem.* **265,** 8373 (1990).
7. G. L. Liou, S. Matragoon, J. Yang, L. Geng, P. A. Overbeek, and D.-P. Ma, *Biochem. Biophys. Res. Commun.* **181,** 159 (1991).
8. M. A. Morabito, X. Yu, and C. J. Barnstable, *J. Biol. Chem.* **266,** 9667 (1991).
9. S.-L. Fong, H. Balakier, M. Canton, C. D. B. Bridges, and B. Gallie, *Cancer Res.* **48,** 1124 (1988).
10. L. A. Donoso, N. T. Felberg, J. J. Angsburger, and J. A. Shields, *Invest. Ophthalmol. Visual Sci.* **26,** 568 (1985).
11. E. Bogenmann, M. A. Lochrie, and M. I. Simon, *Science* **240,** 76 (1988).
12. S.-L. Fong, G. I. Liou, R. A. Landers, R. A. Alvarez, and C. D. B. Bridges, *J. Biol. Chem.* **259,** 6534 (1984).
13. A. J. Adler, C. D. Evans, and W. F. Stafford III, *J. Biol. Chem.* **260,** 4850 (1985).
14. J. C. Saari, D. C. Teller, J. W. Crabb, and L. Bredberg, *J. Biol. Chem.* **260,** 195 (1985).
15. T. M. Redmond, B. Wiggert, F. A. Robey, N. Y. Nguyen, M. S. Lewis, L. Lee, and G. J. Chader, *Biochemistry* **24,** 787 (1985).
16. C. D. B. Bridges, G. I. Liou, R. A. Alvarez, R. A. Landers, A. M. Landry, Jr., and S.-L. Fong, *J. Exp. Zool.* **239,** 335 (1986).

17. S.-L. Fong, G. I. Liou, R. A. Landers, R. A. Alvarez, F. Gonzalez-Fernandez, P. A. Glazebrook, D. M. K. Lam, and C. D. B. Bridges, *J. Neurochem.* **42,** 1667 (1984).
18. G. I. Liou, S.-L. Fong, J. Gosden, P. van Tuinen, D. H. Ledbetter, S. Christie, D. Rout, S. Bhattacharya, R. G. Cook, Y. Li, C. Wang, and C. D. B. Bridges, *Somatic Cell Mol. Genet.* **13,** 315 (1987).
19. S.-L. Fong and C. D. B. Bridges, *J. Biol. Chem.* **263,** 15330 (1988).
20. S.-L. Fong, W.-B. Fong, T. A. Morris, K. M. Kedzie, and C. D. B. Bridges, *J. Biol. Chem.* **265,** 3648 (1990).
21. F. Sanger, S. Nicklen, and A. R. Coulson, *Proc. Natl. Acad. Sci. U.S.A.* **74,** 5463 (1977).
22. R. M. K. Dale, B. A. McClure, and J. P. Houchins, *Plasmid* **13,** 31 (1985).
23. F. M. Ausubel, R. Brent, R. E. Kingstone, D. D. Moore, J. G. Seidman, J. A. Smith, and K. Struhl, "Current Protocols in Molecular Biology," Green Publ. and Wiley (Interscience), New York, 1989.
24. F. Felgner, T. R. Gadek, M. Holm, R. Roman, H. W. Chan, M. Wenz, J. P. Northrop, G. N. Ringold, and M. Danielsen, *Proc. Natl. Acad. Sci. U.S.A.* **84,** 7413 (1987).
25. M. A. Whitt, L. Buonocore, J. K. Rose, V. Ciccarone, A. Chytil, and G. Gebeyehu, *Focus* **13,** 8 (1991).

[24] Use of Transgenic Mice to Study Retinal Gene Expression

Donald J. Zack

Introduction

Gene expression in the retina, as in all other tissues, is primarily controlled by the interplay of cis-acting DNA regulatory regions and trans-acting protein factors. The cellular diversity of gene expression patterns reflects a complex regulatory system which involves a combinatorial array of these DNA elements and transcription factors. In recent years there have been significant advances in identifying some of the cis-acting DNA elements responsible for the tissue-specific regulation of a number of retinal and other ocular genes. Most of these studies have relied on the introduction of reporter–fusion constructs into mice and the analysis of the expression patterns of the reporter genes in the resulting transgenic mice. This chapter briefly reviews these results and then focuses on the methods involved in using transgenic mice to study the regulation of retinal gene expression. Other potential applications of transgenic and embryonic stem cell technologies to the study of retinal biology are also briefly mentioned. Owing to the ready availability of a number of excellent discussions of the methods involved in the actual generation of transgenic mice (1, 2), these methods are not covered here.

The analysis of hybrid (or fusion) genes is the most common approach to defining cis-acting DNA regulatory regions (3). First a hybrid gene is generated by ligating a segment of DNA containing putative regulatory elements to a "reporter gene." The reporter gene codes for an enzyme or other molecule that is easily measured quantitatively and serves to "report on" the level of gene expression directed by the putative regulatory elements. The hybrid gene is then introduced into a suitable assay system, such as a cell line, and its level of expression is measured. If, for example, the DNA segment introduced into the fusion construct contains sufficient information to direct high-level transcription in the particular assay system being used, then high levels of the reporter activity will be detected. Once a DNA segment of interest is identified, the DNA regulatory elements within it can be further defined by deletion and mutation analysis.

Commonly employed assay systems are cell lines, primary cell cultures, and transgenic mice. The best choice of an assay system depends on the question being asked. Cell lines are useful for the initial characterization of

Methods in Neurosciences, Volume 15

promoters and enhancers. The advantages of studies with cell lines are that they are relatively easy, rapid, and inexpensive. The disadvantages of cell lines are as follows: (1) some cell lines are difficult to transfect; (2) tissue specificity is difficult to study since cell lines at best only approximate the differentiated phenotype; (3) developmental regulation of expression can only be studied with a few inducible systems; (4) spatial (topographical) patterns of expression across a tissue can not be studied; and (5) there are several examples in which essential regulatory elements identified with cell lines have been found to be nonessential in transgenic studies (4–6), probably because of greater regulatory redundancy in the *in vivo* situation. In addition, for those specifically interested in the retina this approach is further limited by the paucity of retinal cell lines. Transgenic mice have the advantage that the hybrid gene (in this case the transgene) is analyzed in the context of a whole, normal, functioning organism. Thus, the transgenic approach is well suited to studies of developmental, tissue-specific, and topological patterns of gene expression. The disadvantages of transgenic studies are that they are slow, labor intensive, and costly. The advantages and disadvantages of primary cell cultures as assay systems are intermediate between those of cell lines and transgenic mice.

An additional issue which must be considered with transgenic studies is the influence of position effects (7). Position effects refer to the effects of the site of integration on the expression of a transgene. Specific regulatory elements near the integration site, which can be either positively or negatively acting, as well as more generalized factors such as local chromatin structure can affect both the tissue specificity and level of expression of a transgene. Because the site of integration of a particular transgene is largely random, analysis of a number of lines tends to average out the effects of the environment. It is thus important to analyze several independent lines of mice carrying the same construct before drawing any general conclusions. Copy number, which is the number of copies of a transgene that have integrated, can also affect expression levels. In a few cases, most notably the β-globin locus control region (LCR), dominant regulatory elements have been identified that make transgene expression independent of integration site (8).

Transgenic mice provide a good choice of assay system for retinal studies because of the importance in retinal studies of such issues as cell-type specificity, developmental regulation, and spatial expression gradients. With this in mind, a number of groups have begun to use transgenic mice to define the cis-acting retinal regulatory elements. We have studied the sequences required for the photoreceptor-specific expression of rhodopsin by introducing hybrid constructs containing bovine rhodopsin upstream sequences ligated to the reporter gene *lacZ*, which codes for the *Escherichia coli* enzyme β-galactosidase (9). We have also used the same approach to study the topography of expression across the retina, a study that could not be performed without transgenic mice. Lem *et al.* have performed similar experiments with murine rhodopsin upstream sequences (10). Al-Ubaidi *et al.* have demonstrated retinal degeneration in mice carrying a murine upstream rhodopsin–SV40 T antigen fusion gene, an observation consistent with photoreceptor expression (11). There has been a recent report that fragments upstream of the human blue opsin gene can direct cone-specific expression of β-galactosidase (12). Liou *et al.* (13) and Borst *et al.* (14) have shown that 1.3 and 1.8 kb fragments, respectively, upstream of the human interphotoreceptor retinoid-binding protein (IRBP) gene can direct retinal expression of the reporter gene chloramphenicol acetyltransferase (CAT). More recent work suggests that a 218-bp fragment may be sufficient (15). Photoreceptor cell expression of CAT under the control of a 1.3-kb fragment upstream of mouse S-antigen has been reported (16). Retinal bipolar cell and cerebellar Purkinje cell-specific expression has been demonstrated using a *lacZ* reporter attached to murine L7 gene upstream sequences (17). Sequences from the human gene for phenylethanolamine *N*-methyltransferase, an enzyme involved in epinephrine synthesis, have been shown to direct synthesis to retinal amacrine and adrenal medullary cells (18).

Methods

Choice of Reporter Gene

The two most commonly used reporter genes are the *E. coli* genes for β-galactosidase (*lacZ*) and for chloramphenicol acetyltransferase (CAT). Some workers like CAT because mouse tissue has essentially no background activity, the enzymatic reaction is sensitive, and the reaction is easily quantified. However, for study of tissues such as the retina which contain multiple morphologically distinct cell types and for which distinction of expression patterns is important, we strongly prefer *lacZ*. The cleavage of the chromogenic substrate 5-bromo-4-chloro-3-indolyl-β-D-galactoside (X-Gal) by β-galactosidase produces an insoluble indigo with brilliant blue color. β-Galactosidase cleaves X-Gal at the β-galactoside bond, and then the resulting indoxyl nonenzymatically oxidizes and dimerizes to form chlorbromindigo. The histochemical reaction of β-galactosidase with X-Gal in retinal frozen sections easily provides resolution at the single cell level. The reduced sensitivity of β-galactosidase compared to CAT is usually not an issue since for most promoters β-galactosidase is more than sensitive enough. Mammalian tissues do contain low levels of endogenous β-galactosidases, but these are usually not a problem because the endogenous enzymes have optimal activity at acid pH and staining reactions are usually carried out at pH 7.5–8.0. We have stained control retinal sections for greater than 48 hr at 37°C and have not seen any evidence of background activity.

Good monoclonal and polyclonal anti-β-galactosidase antibodies are also available for immunohistochemical studies of β-galactosidase. More recently, good commercial anti-CAT reagents have reportedly become available, but they are still not as good as the anti-β-galactosidase reagents. Because of this author's preference and greater experience with *lacZ,* this review concentrates on its use.

We have had good experience using the plasmid placF (kindly provided by Dr. Jacques Peschon, Immunex Corp., Seattle, WA) as a source of a *lacZ* cassette. The placF plasmid contains a *lacZ* gene that has been modified so as to include an intron, a poly(A) addition site, and a eukaryotic consensus ribosome binding site. These changes tend to lead to greater expression of the transgene.

Once an appropriate reporter gene is chosen, it is ligated to the test sequence of interest and cloned, and the DNA is purified by one of several standard molecular biology techniques. Because of the finding that plasmid sequences can sometimes interfere with transgene expression, it is advisable to purify the insert away from contaminating plasmid sequences (19). The purified insert is microinjected into 1-cell embryos, which are then implanted into pseudopregnant mothers by standard techniques (1, 2). For retinal studies it is desirable that the embryos not carry any genes affecting retinal development, such as the retinal degeneration (*rd*) gene.

Screening Animals

Putative transgenic animals can be screened for transgene incorporation by Southern blotting, dot/slot blotting, or the use of the polymerase chain reaction (PCR). We prefer PCR because it is quicker and easier. However, because of the extreme sensitivity of PCR, one must be very careful with all manipulations, or contamination can become a serious problem. Both positive and negative controls must always be included. A number of protocols for template preparation have been published. Our current protocol is as follows. After suitable anesthesia, mice are ear punched for identification, and then an approximately 5-mm tail specimen is cut with a fresh razor blade and placed in a 1.5-ml microcentrifuge tube containing 0.1 ml of tail digest buffer (10 m*M* Tris-HCl, pH 7.5, 100 m*M* NaCl, 20 m*M* EDTA, 2% Triton X-100, and 0.1 mg proteinase K/0.1 ml). The proteinase K is added just before use from a 20 mg/ml stock that is stored at −20°C. The tail in digest buffer is then incubated at 55°C for 3–4 hr, until there is complete digestion of the tail. Frequent vortexing (every 15–30 min) speeds the digestion process. Following digestion, the tubes are incubated for 5 min in a boiling water bath to inactivate the proteinase K. Then 0.8 ml of TE (10 mM Tris, pH 7.5, 1 mM EDTA) is added to each tube to dilute the Triton X-100. One microliter from this mixture can then be used directly as template in a standard 25- to 50-μl PCR reaction. The conditions for the PCR amplification depend on the specific primers being used.

For studies utilizing placF we have designed three PCR primers that allow simultaneous amplification of an endogenous sequence that serves as an internal control for the PCR reaction and amplification of a specific sequence that is unique to placF (9). The three primers are 5'-GCGAGATGCTCTTGAAGTCTG-3', 5'-AGCGCCGGTCGCTACCATTAC-3', and 5'-CTCCTGATGCCAAAGCCCTGC-3'. These primers direct amplification of a 0.6-kb endogenous protamine control sequence and a 0.4-kb transgene-specific *lac*Z–protamine fusion sequence. In a typical reaction we now add 1 μl of template prepared as just described to 25 μl of reaction mix [0.5 μM each primer, 125 μM each deoxynucleoside triphosphate (dNTP), 50 mM KCl, 10 mM Tris, pH 8.3, 1.5 mM MgCl$_2$, 0.1% (w/v) gelatin, and 0.1 μl AmpliTaq (Perkin-Elmer Cetus, Norwalk, CT)]. Amplification is carried out in a Perkin-Elmer 9600 thermocycler as follows: 94°C for 5 min; 25 cycles of 62°C for 30 sec, 72°C for 30 sec, and 94°C for 60 sec; 62°C for 2 min; and 72°C for 5 min. (With a different thermocycler, amplification conditions may need to be adjusted.) PCR products are then analyzed by agarose gel electrophoresis.

Analysis of Transgenics

Once transgene-positive animals are obtained, one commonly wishes to answer the following questions: Is the transgene expressed? In which tissues and which cell types is it expressed? What is the developmental pattern of expression? What is the spatial (topographical) pattern of expression? What is the quantitative level of expression? How do genetic and environmental factors affect the level of expression? With *lacZ* fusion constructs these questions can be answered with a combined use of histochemical analysis and quantitative solution assay.

Histochemical and Immunocytochemical Assays

Eyes are enucleated from either sacrificed or appropriately anesthetized animals. If one is interested in the spatial pattern of expression across the retina, then the orientation of the eye must be marked prior to enucleation. Although the extraocular muscles of the mouse eye are asymmetrically arranged and theoretically could be used as markers, in reality the muscles are so small that they are difficult to use as markers. A number of methods for orientation have been tried including sutures, retinal tacts, and various dyes. We have found that the simplest and most reliable method is to use a microsurgical cautery unit. A light burn is placed at 12 o'clock on the cornea near the limbus (see Fig. 1). Care is taken to ensure that the burn is not full thickness because the resulting softness of the eye leads to distortion and makes it difficult to enucleate the eye. In addition, excess heat causes scleral contraction and secondary distortion.

Frozen sectioning with X-Gal staining is the best method for examining *lacZ* expression at the cellular level. Figure 2 is an example of the specificity that can be obtained. It demonstrates photoreceptor cell-specific expression of β-galactosidase activity in a frozen section from a transgenic mouse carrying a fusion construct consisting of bovine rhodopsin upstream regulatory sequences ligated to a modified *lacZ* gene reporter gene. Good results with frozen sectioning can be obtained either (1) with the whole eye frozen intact or (2) with the posterior segment (retina, choroid, sclera, and vitreous body) first dissected away from the anterior segment (cornea, iris, lens, etc.) and then frozen. The former method is better at maintaining spatial relationships and obviously makes possible the study of both anterior and posterior structures in the same section. The latter method gives slightly better histological preservation.

The whole eye or dissected posterior segment is fixed in 0.5% glutaraldehyde in phosphate-buffered saline (PBS) for 1 hr. (If desired, for improved histological preservation, the live animal can be first cardiac perfused with PBS and then fixative, but for most light microscopic studies this is unnecessary.) The specimen is then cryoprotected for 6–18 hr (until the specimen sinks) in 30% sucrose in PBS at 4°C. Using standard techniques, the eye or posterior segment is quick-frozen in 2-methylbutane in liquid nitrogen, mounted in OCT medium (Miles, Elkhart, IN), and sectioned at 5–20 μm in a cryostat at -16 to -22°C. Subbed slides should be used because retina does not stick well to untreated slides. A variety of protocols have been suggested. We have had the best results using chrome alum. (Dissolve gelatin at 5 g/liter in boiling water, cool, add chromium potassium sulfate to 0.5 g/liter, filter, dip clean slides in the solution, and either air-dry slides overnight or place in a 37–40°C oven.) Mounted sections are then rinsed in PBS, postfixed for 3 min in 0.5% glutaraldehyde in PBS, and stained at 37°C in X-Gal staining solution. X-Gal staining solution consists of 1 mg/ml X-Gal, 5 mM K$_3$Fe(CN)$_6$, 5 mM K$_4$Fe(CN)$_6 \cdot$ 3H$_2$O, and 1 mM MgCl$_2$ in PBS. X-Gal is insoluble in water and should be made up as a 2–4% stock solution in

N,N-dimethylformamide. The concentration of the ferrous and ferric salts can be varied between 5 and 40 mM with resulting changes in the speed of formation and size of the chlorbromindigo crystals.

As an alternative method to marking eyes prior to enucleation to maintain orientation, one can perform whole head sections. Because other head structures are present on the final section, this method maintains eye orientation unequivocally. Following decapitation, appropriately trimmed heads are immersed directly in liquid nitrogen. The heads can then be mounted in OCT, and 20-μm sections can be cut and treated as above. This method works best with mice under 1 month of age, when the cranial bones are still relatively soft. Standard cryostat blades can be used, but they need to be sharp and require frequent resharpening. Tungsten–carbide blades can also be used to cut through bone. The quality of whole head sections is not quite equal to that of enucleated eyes, but with practice decent sections can be obtained (see Fig. 3).

To analyze spatial expression patterns across the retina it is possible to generate three-dimensional reconstructions from serial frozen sections. However, such reconstructions can be tedious. Other histological preparations such as eye and retinal whole mounts are more suitable for analyzing the topography of transgene expression across the retina. For eye whole mounts, the sclera and choroid are gently peeled away from the retina, leaving the retina and cornea intact. If the cornea is marked by cautery as described above, the orientation of the retina can be maintained. Scleral and choroidal dissection is begun at the optic nerve using Dumont No. 55 superfine tweezers (Biomedical Research Instruments, Rockville, MD, or equivalent). Dissection is advanced on all sides toward the limbus. When the limbus is reached the dissected tissue is cut off using a spring-action microsurgical scissors such as a Vannas or equivalent. The remaining tissue is then fixed at room temperature for 5 min in 0.5% glutaraldehyde in PBS, washed in PBS, and then stained in X-Gal staining solution. For retina whole mounts, the cornea, lens, and iris are removed from eye whole mounts prepared as above. Alternatively, retinas can be first dissected free of adjoining tissue and then fixed and stained as for eye whole mounts.

It is possible to combine X-Gal staining with immunocytochemistry. The addition of an immunological marker allows definition of cellular subtypes that are not morphologically distinguishable. Our best experience has been with the eye whole mount technique, although the protocol should work with the other preparations as well. After peeling off the sclera and choroid, the retina and associated tissue is placed in 4% paraformaldehyde in PBS for 30 to 60 min at room temperature. (Paraformaldehyde fixation yields weaker X-Gal staining than glutaraldehyde fixation but is preferable for antibody staining because many epitopes are better preserved with paraformaldehyde.) The specimen is then washed in PBS containing 2 mM MgCl$_2$ and stained in X-Gal staining solution as described above. The tissue is postfixed in 4% paraformaldehyde in PBS at 4°C overnight, cryoprotected, frozen, and sectioned as above. The sections are thawed in PBS/Triton (PBS containing 0.2% Triton X-100) and blocked in PBS containing 10% normal goat serum (NGS) for 30–60 min at room temperature.

The primary antibody at the appropriate concentration (usually 1/100 to 1/10,000) in PBS is then added, and the sections are incubated for approximately 1 hr at room temperature. (Depending on the antibody, it is sometimes advisable to use an affinity-purified reagent.) The sections are washed 3–5 times at room temperature in PBS/Triton with or without 0.5% bovine serum albumin (BSA) and then reacted with the secondary antibody of choice. We have used the avidin–biotin–peroxidase complex (ABC Elite) kit from Vector Laboratories (Burlingame, CA) according to the manufacturer's recommendations. The biotin-conjugated goat anti-rabbit secondary antibody is used at a 1 : 200 dilution for 2 hr at room temperature. The sections are washed

---

FIG. 1   Whole-mount preparation from a 2-month-old transgenic animal carrying a rhodopsin promoter–*lacZ* fusion transgene. Prior to enucleation, the 12 o'clock position in the cornea was marked with light microsurgical cautery. The position of the burn is indicated by the arrow. After peeling off the sclera and choroid, the cornea, iris, and lens were removed. The remaining tissue was then fixed and stained with X-Gal as described in the text. Note that the staining across the retina is nonhomogeneous. [Reprinted with permission from D. J. Zack *et al.*, *Neuron* **6,** 187–199 (1991), copyright Cell Press.]

FIG. 2   (A) Retinal frozen section (16 μm thick) from a 1-month-old transgenic animal carrying a rhodopsin promoter–*lacZ* fusion transgene. The section was fixed and stained for 30 min with X-Gal as described in the text. Note that staining is present only in the photoreceptor cell layer. (B) Section similar to that shown in (A) stained with hematoxylin and eosin to demonstrate the retinal layers. NFL, Nerve fiber layer; GCL, ganglion cell layer; IPL, inner plexiform layer; INL, inner nuclear layer; OPL, outer plexiform layer; ONL, outer nuclear layer; IS, inner segments; OS, outer segments; RPE, retinal pigment epithelium. The choroid and sclera are also shown but are not labeled. [Reprinted with permission from *Neuron* **6,** 187–199 (1991), copyright Cell Press.]

FIG. 3   Whole head frozen section (20 μm thick) from a 1-month-old transgenic animal carrying a rhodopsin promoter–*lacZ* fusion transgene. This type of section shows the orientation of the eyes relative to the other structures in the head. The section was fixed and stained with X-Gal as described in the text.

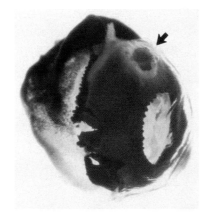

FIG. 1

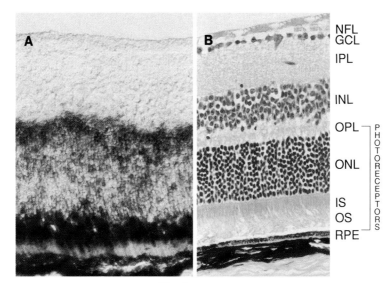

NFL
GCL
IPL

INL

OPL
ONL
IS
OS
RPE

PHOTORECEPTORS

FIG. 2

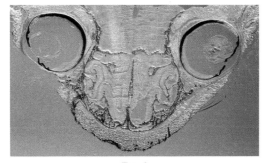

FIG. 3

3 times in PBS/Triton. The avidin–biotin–peroxidase complex (prepared by mixing Vector solutions A and B, usually at a dilution of 1 : 100, and allowing them to incubate for 30 min) is then added and allowed to bind for 1 hr at room temperature. The sections are washed 3 times, 15 min each time, in PBS/Triton. The peroxidase reaction is carried out in PBS, 0.015% H_2O_2, and 0.5 mg/ml diaminobenzidine. After appropriate development, usually 30 sec to 15 min, the reaction is stopped by washing with PBS. Coverslips are then applied to the sections using 50% glycerol in PBS and sealed using nail polish. Owing to variation between different epitopes and different antibodies, some of the detailed steps, particularly the fixation steps and the concentration of detergent, may need to be altered to give maximal staining. It is also desirable to use minimal X-Gal staining so the blue precipitate does not obscure the peroxidase staining.

Quantitative Solution Assay

The tissue of interest is obtained from the appropriate age animal. For studies of retinal gene expression in which the transgene is known not to be expressed elsewhere in the eye, β-galactosidase activity is most easily measured per whole eye. Eyes are enucleated and placed in 1 ml of reaction buffer containing 100 mM phosphate buffer, pH 7.0, 10 mM potassium chloride, 1 mM magnesium sulfate, and 35 mM 2-mercaptoethanol (2-ME). (The 2-ME is added freshly on the day of use.) Generally one eye per reaction tube is sufficient, but if the level of transgene expression is low it is possible to homogenize up to three eyes in 1 ml of reaction buffer. The eye(s) is homogenized in a Brinkman (Westbury, NY) Polytron or equivalent instrument at a setting of 5 for 30 sec. The homogenate is transferred to a 1.5-ml microcentrifuge tube and centrifuged at approximately 14,000 rpm for 1 min, and the supernatant is transferred to a fresh tube. A 300-μl aliquot of the supernatant is prewarmed to 37°C, and then the enzymatic reaction is begun by mixing the prewarmed supernatant with 60 μl of the substrate (o-nitrophenyl-β-D-galactopyranoside at 2 mg/ml).

The reaction is monitored in a spectrophotometer at 420 nm using a water-jacketed cuvette set at 37°C. It is convenient to use a kinetics program which takes readings every 15 sec for 5–10 min. A plot of time versus optical density (OD) should be linear. If the amount of enzyme activity in the 300 μl of supernatant is too large, then the supernatant can be diluted with reaction buffer to stay in the linear range. A negative control eye should be included to determine the background activity. In our experience, background readings are in the range between -0.005 and 0.005 OD_{420} units per minute. It is also advisable to use an aliquot of commercial β-galactosidase

(Sigma, St. Louis, MO, or equivalent) as an internal positive control so results from one day can be confidently compared with those from another. It is best to make many aliquots, store them at $-70°C$, and use a fresh aliquot each day.

Future Prospects

The use of transgenic mice to analyze cis-acting elements responsible for the expression of retinal genes is in its relative infancy. So far most emphasis has been on a limited number of genes expressed in photoreceptor cells. Future studies are likely not only to further define the photoreceptor regulatory elements but also expand to define the elements specific for the variety of other retinal cell types. Efforts are underway and probably eventually will be successful at developing cell type-specific inducible promoters. Once cell-specific promoters and enhancers are available for all the major retinal cell types, it will be possible to express heterologous and mutant proteins in the cell type of choice. Several laboratories are already in the process of directing the expression of mutant rhodopsin molecules responsible for human autosomal-dominant retinitis pigmentosa to mouse photoreceptors (20). Through the use of hybrid genes carrying toxins such as diphtheria toxin it will be possible to ablate individual cell lineages. Mice lacking photoreceptors have already been engineered (10).

The developments in the use of embryonic stem (ES) cells will provide investigators with additional control in manipulating the mammalian retina. With traditional transgenic techniques the investigator has no control of integration site or copy number. When mutations are introduced, the wild-type or preexisting allele remains. Thus, only dominant and codominant mutations can be studied. With ES cells and homologous recombination it is possible to actually replace one allele with another (21). If the introduced mutation is in the germ line, then through breeding and selection homozygous offspring carrying the mutation can be obtained. This allows the study of recessive mutations. As more genes responsible for human retinal diseases are identified, this will make possible the generation of animal models that have not been previously available. In addition, these studies may also have implications for future efforts toward human retinal gene therapy.

Acknowledgments

The author gratefully acknowledges the intellectual and other support provided by Dr. Jeremy Nathans, in whose laboratory the rhodopsin transgenic studies referred to above were initiated, and thanks Ms. Yanshu Wang who improved the technique for combining X-Gal staining and immunohistochemistry. The author also gratefully acknowledges support from the National Eye Institute (Physician Scientist Award EY20097) and from the Johns Hopkins University School of Medicine (Career Development Award).

References

1. B. Hogan, F. Constantini, and E. Lacy, "Manipulating the Mouse Genome: A Laboratory Manual." Cold Spring Harbor Laboratory, Cold Spring Harbor, New York, 1986.
2. K. A. Kelley, in "Gene Probes" (P. M. Conn, ed.), Vol. 1, p. 392. Academic Press, San Diego, 1989.
3. J. H. Kelly and G. J. Darlington, *Annu. Rev. Genet.* **19**, 273 (1985).
4. J. Dente, U. Ruther, M. Tripodi, E. F. Wagner, and R. Cortese, *Genes Dev.* **2**, 259 (1988).
5. K. Zimmerman, E. Legouy, V. Stewart, R. Depinho, and F. W. Alt, *Mol. Cell. Biol.* **10**, 2096 (1990).
6. C. M. Sax, D. M. Donovan, and Piatigorsky, *Invest. Ophthalmol. Visual. Sci.* **32**, 781 (1991).
7. C. Wilson, H. J. Bellen, and W. J. Gehring, *Annu. Rev. Cell Biol.* **6**, 679 (1990).
8. F. Grosveld, G. B. van Assendelft, D. R. Greaves, and G. Kollias, *Cell (Cambridge, Mass.)* **51**, 975 (1987).
9. D. J. Zack, J. Bennett, Y. Wang, C. Davenport, B. Klaunberg, J. Gearhart, and J. Nathans, *Neuron* **6**, 187 (1991).
10. J. Lem, M. L. Applebury, J. D. Falk, J. G. Flannery, and M. I. Simon, *Neuron* **6**, 201 (1991).
11. M. Al-Ubaidi, P. Overbeek, M. Naash, and W. Baehr, *Invest. Ophthalmol. Visual Sci.* **31**, 298 (1990).
12. C. L. Tucker, D. Hinton, and E. Bogenmann, *J. Cell Biol.* **115** (Part 2), 312a (1991).
13. G. I. Liou, L. Geng, M. Al-Ubaidi, S. Matragoon, G. Hanten, W. Baehr, and P. A. Overbeek, *J. Biol. Chem.* **265**, 8373 (1990).
14. D. E. Borst, J.-S. Si, and J. M. Nickerson, *J. Cell Biol.* **115** (Part 2), 312a (1991).
15. G. I. Liou, S. Matragoon, D. P. Ma, and P. A. Overbeek, *Invest. Ophthalmol. Visual Sci.* **32**, 1251 (1991).
16. T. Kikuchi, M. Breitman, and T. Shinohara, *Invest. Ophthalmol. Visual Sci.* **32**, 1007 (1991).
17. J. Oberdick, R. J. Smeyne, J. R. Mann, S. Zackson, and J. I. Morgan, *Science* **248**, 223 (1990).
18. E. E. Baetge, R. R. Behringer, A. Messing, R. L. Brinster, and R. D. Palmiter, *Proc. Natl. Acad. Sci. U.S.A.* **85**, 3648 (1988).
19. K. Chada, J. Magram, K. Raphael, G. Radice, E. Lacy, and F. Constantini, *Nature (London)* **314**, 377 (1985).
20. J. E. Olsson, J. W. Gordon, B. S. Pawlyk, D. Roof, A. Hayes, R. S. Molday, S. Mukai, G. S. Cowley, E. L. Berson, and T. P. Dryja, *Neuron* **9**, 815 (1992).
21. E. J. Robertson, *Biol. Reprod.* **44**, 238 (1991).

[25] Transgenic Rescue of the Photoreceptor Dysplasia and Degeneration in Retinal Degeneration Slow (*rds*) Mutant Mice

Gabriel H. Travis and Dean Bok

Introduction

Historically, important lessons have been learned about the function of specific brain structures by studying the neurological deficits that result from their loss. For example, much has been learned about the functional organization of the cerebral cortex by correlating the destruction of discrete cortical areas with the resulting neurobehavioral deficits. This same model is applicable on the molecular level. Clues about the function of a previously unknown protein may be gained by correlating its primary structure with the phenotype that results from its functional loss in a recessive mutation. The potential for gaining this type of mechanistic information is an important reason to undertake cloning the gene for an inherited disorder of the mammalian visual system. This type of analysis is likely to be informative even if the product of the gene for a mutation turns out to be a previously identified protein. There are few proteins whose functions are so clearly understood that nothing would be learned by studying the results of their absence in a recessive mutant. In cases where the gene for a mutation is later shown to encode a protein of known function, the phenotype is often surprising. An example of this in vision science is the recent demonstration that the gene for a subset of autosomal-dominant retinitis pigmentosa (ADRP), an inherited retinal degenerative disease of humans, encodes the visual pigment protein rhodopsin (1).

An important component in the molecular characterization of a mutation is to demonstrate convincingly that the correct gene has been identified. Functional complementation of the phenotype *in vivo* provides compelling genetic evidence that the gene for the mutation has been cloned. With mutations of the mammalian retina, this is best accomplished by a transgenic approach, since no satisfactory tissue culture systems exist. An advantage of this approach is that the rescue takes place in an entirely native cellular environment. This eliminates many variables of *in vitro* approaches and greatly simplifies interpretation of the results.

Methods in Neurosciences, Volume 15

The Retinal Degeneration Slow Mutation

Retinal degeneration slow (*rds*) is a neurological mutation of mice that is characterized phenotypically by abnormal development of rod and cone photoreceptors, followed by their slow degeneration. No other cell types in the retina or the central nervous system (CNS) are affected. In *rds/rds* homozygotes, the retina undergoes entirely normal development and differentiation of cells until the first postnatal week, the time at which photoreceptor outer segments normally appear. While other retinal cells continue their normal development, the photoreceptors fail to elaborate outer segments and rarely form outer segment disks (2). The photoreceptor inner segments, however, including the ciliary processes, are morphologically normal. The synaptic termini of photoreceptors with second-order retinal neurons also appear normal in these mutants.

The process of photoreceptor degeneration in *rds/rds* mice is first detectable histologically during the third postnatal week. The rate of loss of photoreceptors is greatest during the following few weeks and then becomes more gradual. Virtually all are gone by 1 year. Rods and cones are affected equally. Although the *rds* mutation was originally described as autosomal recessive, *rds*/+ heterozygotes are phenotypically somewhat abnormal. In contrast to homozygotes, heterozygotes do form outer segments. However, these are reduced in length and contain irregularly arranged disks that appear swollen and vacuolated. Very slow degeneration of photoreceptors is seen in *rds*/+ heterozygotes (3).

Cloning the *rds* Messenger RNA and Gene

Prior to the work described below, nothing was known about the underlying biochemical defect in *rds*. The *rds* gene had been assigned to mouse chromosome 17 by classic linkage analysis (4). The strategy that we used to clone the *rds* gene was based on two observations: (i) photoreceptors are the only cell type affected in *rds* mutant retina; and (ii) patchy dysplasia and degeneration of photoreceptors were seen in the retinas of *rds/rds* ↔ +/+ and *rds*/+ ↔ +/+ tetraparental mice (5, 6), suggesting a cell autonomous process. We therefore assumed that, in normal mouse retina, the *rds* gene is expressed exclusively in photoreceptor cells. The first step was to clone a collection of complementary DNAs (cDNAs) representing photoreceptor-specific messenger RNAs (mRNAs). To this end, we took advantage of the unrelated mouse mutant, retinal degeneration (*rd*) to isolate photoreceptor-specific mRNAs. Mice with this mutation show rapid photoreceptor degeneration. By 4 weeks, an *rd/rd* retina is virtually devoid of photoreceptors, while all other retinal cells are spared (7). An mRNA present in wild-type but absent from *rd/rd* retina therefore would be photoreceptor-specific. We used subtractive cDNA cloning (8) to isolate a collection of several hundred photoreceptor-specific mRNAs. Matrix hybridization analysis revealed that this set contained twelve distinct mRNAs. The photoreceptor specificity of each clone was confirmed by Northern blotting (9).

The next step was to determine the chromosome assignment for the genes encoding these photoreceptor-specific mRNAs. This was done by using each clone to probe a panel of mouse × hamster hybrid cell line DNAs. Clone B9A mapped to mouse chromosome 17 with 100% concordance, and it thus became a candidate for the *rds* mRNA.

Northern blot analysis was performed on retinal RNA from 2-month-old (predegenerate) *rds/rds* and wild-type mice, using clone B9A as a probe. In the wild-type lane, two bands at 1.6 and 2.7 kb were detected. In the *rds/rds* lane, these species were not detected, but a doublet band at approximately 12 kb was visualized. These results suggested that B9A was a clone of *rds*, and that a significant disruption of the gene had occurred.

To define the mutation at the level of the gene, genomic libraries were prepared from *rds/rds* and wild-type mice, and phage λ clones of the *rds* locus were isolated. Fine structure analysis of these clones revealed that the mutation was due to the insertion of an approximately 10-kb mouse repetitive element into a protein-coding exon in the *rds* gene (9). This inserted element is contained within the mutant transcript and is responsible for its increased molecular weight relative to the wild-type mRNA.

Sequence analysis of B9A revealed a clone of 2632 bp followed by a poly(A) tail. Examination of the sequence revealed a second potential poly-adenylation signal at position 1627, suggesting an explanation for the 1.6-kb mRNA seen on the Northern blot. Rescreening of the mouse retina library with clone B9A yielded clone D6 with a sequence identical to B9A except that it ended with a poly(A) tail 24 bp downstream of the second polyadenyla-tion site. Thus, the two *rds* transcripts detected in wild-type retina are due to alternative polyadenylation; both are encoded by the same gene, and both encode the identical protein product.

The *rds* Protein

The cDNA clone contained a single long open reading frame beginning at nucleotide 213 that encoded a putative protein of 346 amino acids. Computer database analysis showed no similarity to any known proteins. Hydropho-bicity analysis of the predicted protein showed four uncharged stretches of 23–26 residues, suggesting four membrane-spanning segments (Fig. 1). In

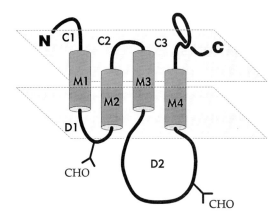

Fig. 1   Structural model for the *rds* protein within the disk membrane. The four putative membrane-spanning segments are labeled M1–M4. This orientation places the amino- and carboxy-terminal regions within the cytoplasm. The D1 and D2 loops, containing the sites for N-glycosylation (CHO), are located within the extracellular (intradiscal) space.

addition, there were two potential sites at residues 53 and 229 for N-linked glycosylation.

To begin a biochemical characterization of the *rds* protein, we raised antibodies against a synthetic peptide corresponding to residues 311–323 from near the carboxyl terminus (peptide J97). We also raised antibodies against a β-galactosidase–*rds* fusion protein, using the prokaryotic expression vector pUR292 (10). These were used for immunoblot analysis of retinal protein extracts from wild-type, *rd/rd*, and *rds/rds* mice. In wild-type mice these reagents reacted with a broad band of approximately 39 kDa (11). No reactivity was observed in fully degenerate *rd/rd* retinal extracts, consistent with the original observation that the *rds* mRNA is photoreceptor specific. Endoglycosidase F digestion of the retinal extract caused the immunoreactive band to shift downard by approximately 2 kDa, suggesting that the *rds* protein is normally glycosylated. When extracts were prepared in a nonreducing medium, the immunoreactive band migrated at approximately 78 kDa. This suggests that the native *rds* protein is covalently coupled to another protein, possibly itself as a homodimer. Extraction of proteins with Triton X-114 prior to immunoblotting showed that the *rds* protein was confined to the membrane-rich fraction. This confirmed that the *rds* protein was associated with outer segment membranes. No immunoreactivity was observed in retinal extracts from *rds/rds* mice with the antipeptide or the anti-fusion protein sera.

The distribution of the *rds* protein in photoreceptors was determined by immunocytochemistry using antisera against the J97 peptide and the β-galactosidase–*rds* fusion protein. Under the light microscope, the only cell type showing immunoreactivity was the photoreceptors. This confirmed our earlier observations that both the *rds* mRNA and protein were absent from fully degenerate *rd/rd* retina. Within photoreceptors, the immunoreactivity was confined to the outer segments, precisely the structure absent in *rds/rds* mutants. Under the electron microscope, the immunoreactive material appeared associated with the outer segment disks.

Molday and co-workers conducted independent studies on the biochemistry and distribution on the bovine homolog of the *rds* protein, which they named "peripherin/*rds*," with similar results (12). Thus, the normal product of *rds* appears to be a new outer segment disk membrane-associated glycoprotein of approximately 39 kDa. Based on the phenotype in *rds* heterozygote and homozygote mutants, the function of *rds* protein may be to stabilize or to assist in the folding of outer segment disks.

The Human *rds* Gene (*RDS*)

The phenotype in *rds/+* heterozygotes (13) is similar to the pathological picture of ADRP (14). To test the hypothesis that some patients with ADRP may have mutations in this gene, we cloned the human homolog of *rds* (*RDS*) (15). This was found to encode a protein that contained the same number of residues and was 91% identical to the mouse *rds* protein. Many of the predicted structural features, including the membrane-spanning segments and glycosylation sites, were conserved in the human protein. The *RDS* gene was found to map to proximal human chromosome 6p. The sequence of the *RDS* mRNA was used to define the intron–exon junctions in the *RDS* gene. Oligonucleotide primers were designed to amplify *RDS* exons in human DNA. In two studies on patients with ADRP, point mutations and small deletions were detected in the *RDS* gene, resulting in nonconservative single amino acid substitutions and deletions (16, 17) in the D2 loop and the third membrane-spanning segment. Thus, mutations in *RDS* are responsible for a subset of ADRP in humans.

Transgenic Rescue of *rds*: Generation of Transgenic Mice

We assembled a transgenic construct containing regulatory sequences upstream of the mouse opsin gene, transcriptionally fused to a wild-type *rds* minigene (Fig. 2). A fragment of SV40 containing the early splice and polyade-

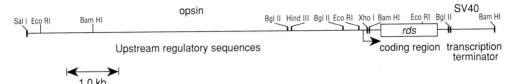

FIG. 2   Physical map of the opsin–*rds*–SV40 fusion transgene. A segment of the mouse opsin gene from nucleotides −6500 to +80 is followed by a central fragment of the cDNA clone, B9A, containing the complete wild-type *rds* coding block, followed by the SV40 t-antigen intron and polyadenylation signal. The opsin transcription initiation site [W. Baehr, J. D. Falk, K. Bugra, J. T. Triantafyllos, and J. F. McGinnis, *FEBS Lett.* **238**, 253 (1988)] is indicated by the arrow, and the *rds* coding block by the open box. Restriction sites are indicated by the labeled vertical lines.

nylation sites was included downstream as a transcription terminator. Insert DNA containing the construct, purified on a sucrose gradient, was injected into the pronuclei of fertilized eggs from (BALB/c × C57BL/6) hybrid mice that were heterozygous for *rds*. Eggs surviving micromanipulation were transferred to the oviducts of pseudopregnant foster mothers following established procedures (18). All mice were maintained on 12 hr light/dark cycles at low levels of illumination to minimize photic injury. A total of six transgenic lines were established. Three were chosen for study based on their breeding productivity. To move the transgene onto an *rds*/*rds* homozygous mutant background, F₁ mice from lines 96, 113, and 80 were mated with nontransgenic *rds*/*rds* homozygotes. The genotype of each F₂ mouse at *rds* was determined by following a *Bgl*II restriction fragment length polymorphism on Southern blots that results from an insertional mutation within the *rds* gene (9) (Fig. 3).

Expression of the Transgene

To quantify expression of the transgene in the three lines, RNA was prepared from the retinas of individual F₂ mice for Northern blot analysis, using SV40 DNA and a mouse *rds* cDNA as probes. The SV40 probe hybridized to a 2.6-kb band in the lanes containing retinal RNA from the transgenic mice, but not the nontransgenic control mice (Fig. 4A). This was the predicted size for the transcript from the opsin–*rds*–SV40 transgene (Fig. 2). The 2.6-kb transcript was abundant in RNA from lines 96 and 113, but rarer in RNA from line 80.

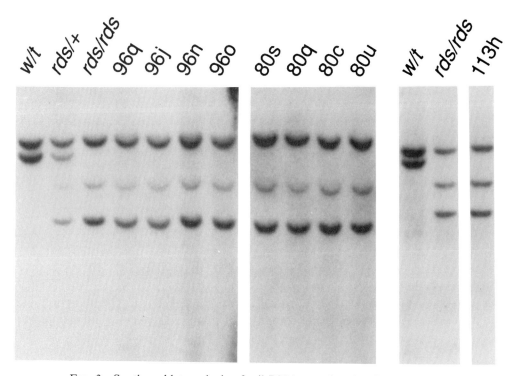

FIG. 3 Southern blot analysis of tail DNA samples showing the genotype at *rds*. Each sample was digested with restriction endonuclease *Bgl*II, and the blot was probed with DNA from clone B9A. Wild-type (w/t), *rds*/+ heterozygote, and *rds*/*rds* homozygote DNAs were included as genotype controls. The *Bgl*II polymorphic pattern for each of the test animals is identical to that of the *rds*/*rds* homozygote control.

FIG. 4 Northern blot analysis of retinal RNA showing expression of the transgene. **(A)** RNA from line 96, 113, and 80 transgenic (*TG*) and nontransgenic (*nTG*) mice probed with the transcription terminator fragment of SV40. RNA from nontransgenic C57BL/6 wild-type (w/t) and *rds*/*rds* homozygous mutant control retina were included as controls. **(B)** RNA from line 96 and 80 transgenic and nontransgenic mice probed with clone B9A. Samples of nontransgenic wild-type (w/t), *rds*/+ heterozygote, and *rds*/*rds* homozygote retinal RNA were included as controls. The insets labeled G3PDH show the autoradiographic signal after the blots were stripped and reprobed with a cDNA for glyceraldehyde-3-phosphate dehydrogenase as a control for equal loading of lanes.

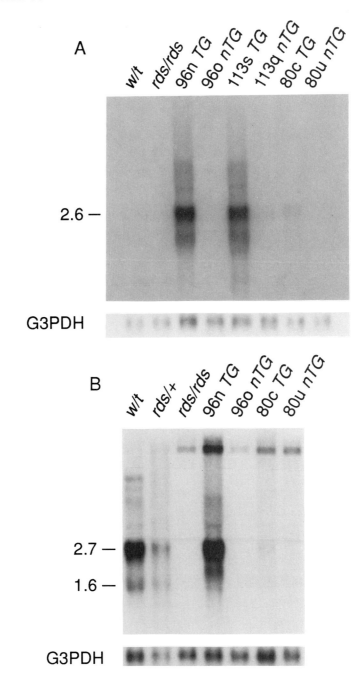

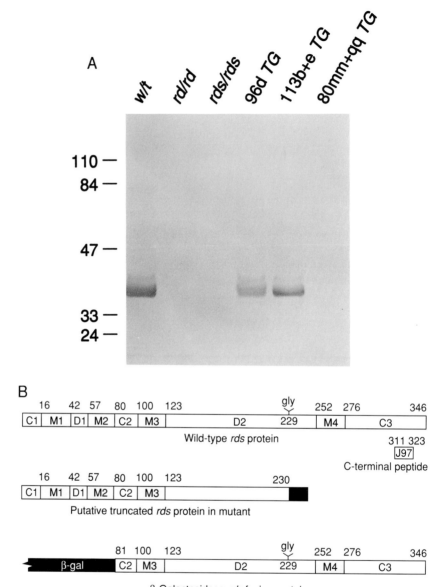

FIG. 5   Protein expression in *rds* transgenic mice. **(A)** Immunoblot analysis of retinal proteins showing expression of the transgene. Retinal extracts from line 96, 113, and 80 transgenic mice, each on an *rds/rds* genetic background, were reacted with an anti-β-galactosidase–*rds* fusion protein serum. Retinal extracts from nontransgenic C57BL/6 wild-type (w/t), fully degenerate *rd* (*rd/rd*), and predegenerate *rds* (*rds/*

The *rds* probe detected two mRNAs of 2.7 and 1.6 kb, arising from alternative polyadenylation (9), in wild-type retina and a doublet of mRNAs at approximately 12 kb in *rds/rds* mutant retina (Fig. 4B). As predicted, all four bands were detected in retinal RNA from *rds/+* heterozygotes. The 2.6-kb mRNA from the transgene was present in retina from lines 113, 96, and 80, but not in their nontransgenic littermate controls. The abundance of the 2.6-kb transgenic transcript in line 96 was approximately equal to that of the 2.7-kb transcript of the endogenous *rds* gene in wild-type retina. In line 80, the 2.6-kb transgenic transcript was only one-tenth as abundant as the 2.7-kb wild-type mRNA, based on autoradiograph signal intensity (Fig. 4B). The abundance of this 2.6-kb transcript in retina roughly correlated with the number of copies of the transgene detected by Southern blot analysis of DNA from each line. Lines 96 and 113 each had 10–20 copies per haploid genome, and line 80 had 2–4 copies.

The level of expression of the *rds* protein in the three transgenic lines was estimated by immunoblotting, using polyvalent antisera raised against a β-galactosidase–*rds* fusion protein. The antisera reacted with a protein species of approximately 39 kDa in retinal extracts from wild-type mice, but not with extracts from retinal degeneration (*rd/rd*) mutant mice, which virtually lack photoreceptors (7) (Fig. 5A). No immunoreactivity was observed in retinal extracts from predegenerate *rds/rds* mutant mice. Given that the gene is transcribed in *rds* mutants (Fig. 4B), the absence of immunoreactivity in extracts from these animals may be due either to instability of the mutant translation product or to exclusive reactivity of the anti-fusion protein sera against epitopes within the carboxy-terminal third of the normal protein, which is deleted in *rds* mutants (Fig. 5B) (9).

An immunoreactive band of 39 kDa was also present in lanes containing retinal extracts from the line 96 and 113 transgenic/*rds* mutants, but not in the nontransgenic littermate controls (Fig. 5A). This band was shifted downward by approximately 2 kDa after endoglycosidase F digestion, similar to the shift seen with the wild-type protein. Thus, an *rds*-immunoreactive glycoprotein of normal size is produced in the retinas of high-expressing transgenic lines 113 and 96. There was no detectable immunoreactivity in

---

rds) mice were included as controls. Positions of molecular mass size standards are shown at left in kilodaltons. **(B)** Schematic drawing of the different *rds* protein fragments. The top line shows the complete wild-type *rds* protein. The middle line shows the putative translation product of the mutant *rds* gene with an aberrant carboxyl terminus. The bottom line shows the β-galactosidase–*rds* fusion protein that was used to immunize rabbits for antisera. The C, M, and D designations refer to cytoplasmic, membrane-spanning, and intradiscal segments. The J97 C-terminal peptide, used in previous studies (11), is also shown.

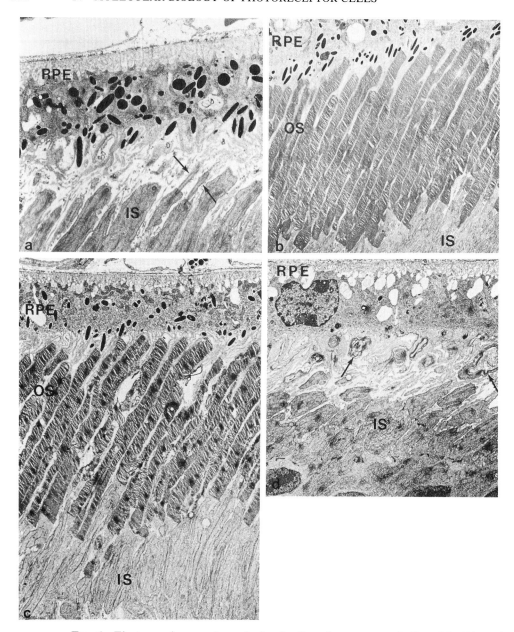

FIG. 6   Electron microscopic analysis of retinas from transgenic lines 96, 113, and 80 on an *rds/rds* mutant background. In all cases, the retinal pigment epithelium (RPE) is at the top. **(a)** Two-month-old, nontransgenic control mouse 96j. Rod inner segments **(IS)** and connecting cilia (arrows) are present, but outer segments are absent. Magnification ×3300. **(b)** Two-month-old transgenic mouse 96q (littermate

the lanes containing extracts from transgenic line 80. This was probably due to the low level of transgene expression in line 80.

Phenotype in Transgenic rds/rds Homozygous Mutants

Retinas from line 96, 113, and 80 transgenic mice on an *rds/rds* mutant background at 2 and 5 months of age were studied by electron microscopy. Nontransgenic littermates were used as controls. All features of the *rds* phenotype for animals at these ages were present in the controls, including absence of outer segments, partial degeneration of photoreceptor cell bodies, and vesicular debris in the subretinal space (19) (Fig. 6a). In contrast, retinas from transgenic lines 96 and 113 were indistinguishable from wild-type retinas, with normal outer segment morphology and no evidence of photoreceptor degeneration (Fig. 6b,c). A complete rescue of the *rds* phenotype was thus effected in rod cells from line 96 and 113 mice.

Interestingly, retina from transgenic line 80 had an appearance that was intermediate between those of wild-type mice and *rds/rds* mutants (Fig. 6d). There were fewer exracellular vesicles, and whorls of disorganized disks were present in the subretinal space, likely representing dysplastic outer segments. This pattern is similar to that seen in *rds/+* heterozygotes (13), except that in animals from line 80 the outer segment dysplasia was more severe. This difference in severity may be due to a dosage effect; in line 80, the level of the mRNA encoding the normal *rds* protein is only about 10% of wild-type levels, whereas in heterozygotes it is approximately 50% (Fig. 4B).

Further Reflections on Transgenic Rescue of rds

The opsin promoter was chosen to drive expression of the *rds* transgene because steady-state levels of the endogenous opsin mRNA are exceptionally high (9), suggesting that the opsin promoter is quite powerful in photoreceptors. The autologous promoter from the *rds* gene would have probably also

---

of 96j). Fully developed outer segments (**OS**) containing regularly arranged disk structures are visible between the retinal pigment epithelium (**RPE**) and inner segments (**IS**). Magnification ×2900. (**c**) Five-month-old transgenic mouse 113h. As with 96q, the outer segments (**OS**) appear morphologically normal, and there is no evidence of photoreceptor degeneration. Magnification ×3800. (**d**) Two-month-old, low-expressing transgenic mouse 80q. Partial development of outer segment disks is evident from the membranous whorls (arrows) between the retinal pigment epithelium (**RPE**) and inner segments (**IS**). Magnification: ×3800.

worked. On Northern blots, the endogenous *rds* mRNAs in wild-type retina are approximately one-tenth as abundant as the endogenous opsin mRNAs. However, in lines 96 and 113, the mRNA product of the transgene, driven by the opsin promoter, was approximately equally abundant to the endogenous wild-type *rds* transcript. This difference in abundance may be due to reduced stability of the *rds* transgene mRNA relative to the opsin mRNA, or to reduced strength of the opsin promoter in the context of the transgenic construct.

In normal mice, the *rds* gene is expressed in both rods and cones (20). If we assume that the *rds*-containing transgene, transcriptionally regulated by the opsin promoter, has the same pattern of expression as the endogenous opsin gene, then we would expect the *rds* phenotype to have been rescued in rod but not cone photoreceptors. We are currently unable to confirm rod-specific correction, however, since only 3% of photoreceptors in mice are cones (7), and since our oldest transgenic mice are only five months and hence only partially degenerate.

In two previous reports, where smaller upstream genomic segments of opsin were used to read a *lacZ* reporter gene, nonuniform patterns of expression of the *lacZ* product were observed in the retinas from several transgenic lines (21, 22). In the present study, rescue of the *rds* phenotype in photoreceptors was uniform across the retina in all three lines, with no patchy or gradient changes in the morphology of outer segments. Here, more uniform expression of the transgene may be due to our use of a larger opsin promoter segment.

We used a "minigene" derived from the cDNA for the wild-type *rds* coding sequence in our transgene construct. This offered several advantages. Assembly of the construct was simplified by the presence of multiple flanking cloning sites derived from the polylinker in the library vector. The entire coding region was contained within a *Bgl*II fragment of 1.1 kb. Had we used a genomic fragment of *rds*, the transgene construct would have been larger by at least 10 kb. Because we had chosen to use the 6.5-kb opsin promoter fragment, this construct would have been too large to clone in a plasmid, further complicating its assembly. Finally, in checking the construct prior to injection, it was useful to have no DNA within the coding region that had not been previously sequenced. Our use of a minigene seems to have caused no problems. Five of the six lines established expressed the transgene, three of these at high levels.

The *rds* mutation has been shown to result from the insertion of a 10-kb mouse genomic repetitive element into a protein-coding exon of the *rds* gene. This gene is transcribed in *rds* mutants, giving rise to a pair of mRNAs between 12 and 14 kb, each bearing the entire inserted element. It is not known if these mRNAs are translated. If so, the putative mutant protein is truncated and contains an abnormal carboxyl terminus (Fig. 5B). The last

116 residues of the normal *rds* protein, which includes a glycosylated portion of the D2 loop, the fourth membrane spanning segment, and the cytoplasmic carboxy-terminal C3 region (11), are deleted in this putative protein. In their place is an aberrant stretch of amino acids encoded by the inserted element, before the first in-frame stop codon.

There are two plausible mechanisms for the dysplastic phenotype in *rds*/+ heterozygotes consistent with these observations. One is a dominant-negative effect of the putative anomalous protein in outer segment disks, perhaps through displacement of the normal protein from its sites of interaction with other proteins. The second mechanism is haploinsufficiency, where a 50% reduction in wild-type gene dosage results in a critical loss of the normal *rds* protein. Our results are more consistent with the second mechanism. In lines 96 and 113, both the mRNA and protein products of the transgene were at levels similar to the levels in normal mice of the endogenous, wild-type *rds* mRNA and protein. Because the transgenic mice were on a background with two mutant alleles of *rds*, if a dominant-negative mechanism were operative we would not have expected a complete rescue, but rather a phenotype similar to that of the *rds*/+ heterozygote. Similarly, in the case of low-expressing line 80, if a dominant-negative mechanism were operative, the toxic product of both mutant alleles would have been expected to overwhelm the small amount of normal *rds* protein from the transgene, and no rescue of the phenotype would have been expected.

Summary

We have completely rescued the phenotype in *rds*/*rds* mutant mice by transgenic complementation. To this end we used a transcriptional fusion construct containing upstream regulatory sequences of the mouse opsin gene reading a wild-type *rds* minigene. SV40 was used as a transcriptional terminator. This result represents formal confirmation that we have identified the *rds* gene. The relationship between the levels of transgene expression and the retinal phenotype in the three lines studied suggests that *rds* is a simple loss-of-function mutation. This fact has ramifications for the eventual development of somatic gene therapy for the group of ADRP patients with mutations in the *RDS* gene.

Acknowledgments

We gratefully acknowledge Karen Groshan, Marcia Lloyd, and Orna Yaron for excellent technical assistance, and Jenny Price for skillful manipulation of mouse ooctyes. This work was supported by grants from the National Eye Institute and the National Retinitis Pigmentosa Foundation. G.H.T. is a John Merck Fund Scholar. D.B. is the Dolly Green Professor of Ophthalmology.

References

1. T. P. Dryja, T. L. McGee, E. Reichel, L. B. Hahn, G. S. Cowley, D. W. Yandell, M. A. Sandberg, and E. L. Berson, *Nature* (*London*) **343**, 364 (1990).
2. S. Sanyal, G. Chader, and G. Aguirre, *in* "Retinal Degeneration: Experimental and Clinical Studies," p. 239. Alan R. Liss, New York, 1985.
3. R. K. Hawkins, H. G. Jansen, and S. Sanyal, *Exp. Eye Res.* **41**, 701 (1985).
4. R. Van Nie, D. Ivanyi, and P. Demant, *Tissue Antigens* **12**, 106 (1978).
5. S. Sanyal and G. H. Zeilmaker, *Exp. Eye Res.* **39**, 231 (1984).
6. S. Sanyal, C. Dees, and G. H. Zeilmaker, *J. Embryol. Exp. Morphol.* **98**, 111 (1986).
7. L. D. Carter-Dawson, M. M. LaVail, and R. I. Sidman, *Invest. Ophthalmol. Visual Sci.* **17**, 489 (1978).
8. G. H. Travis and J. G. Sutcliffe, *Proc. Natl. Acad. Sci. U.S.A.* **85**, 1696 (1978).
9. G. H. Travis, M. B. Brennan, P. E. Danielson, C. A. Kozak, and J. G. Sutcliffe, *Nature* (*London*) **338**, 70 (1989).
10. U. Rüther and B. Müller-Hill, *EMBO J.* **2**, 1791 (1983).
11. G. H. Travis, J. G. Sutcliffe, and D. Bok, *Neuron* **6**, 61 (1991).
12. G. Connell, R. Bascom, L. Molday, D. Reid, R. R. McInnes, and R. S. Molday, *Proc. Natl. Acad. Sci. U.S.A.* **88**, 723 (1991).
13. R. K. Hawkins, H. G. Jansen, and S. Sanyal, *Exp. Eye Res.* **41**, 701 (1985).
14. J. G. Flannery, D. B. Farber, A. C. Bird, and D. Bok, *Invest. Ophthalmol. Visual Sci.* **30**, 191 (1989).
15. G. H. Travis, L. Christerson, P. E. Danielson, I. Klisak, R. S. Sparkes, L. B. Hahn, T. P. Dryja, and J. G. Sutcliffe, *Genomics* **10**, 733 (1991).
16. G. J. Farrar, P. Kenna, S. A. Jordan, R. Kumar-Singh, M. M. Humphries, E. M. Sharp, D. M. Shells, and P. Humphries, *Nature* (*London*) **354**, 478 (1991).
17. K. Kajiwara, L. Hahn, S. Mukai, G. H. Travis, E. L. Berson, and T. P. Dryja, *Nature* (*London*) **354**, 480 (1991).
18. B. Hogan, F. Costantini, and E. Lacy, "Manipulating the Mouse Embryo." Cold Spring Harbor Laboratory, Cold Spring Harbor, New York, 1986.
19. H. G. Jansen and S. Sanyal, *J. Comp. Neurol.* **224**, 71 (1984).
20. K. Arikawa, L. L. Molday, R. S. Molday, and D. S. Williams, *J. Cell Biol.* **116**, 659 (1992).
21. J. Lem, M. L. Applebury, J. D. Falk, J. G. Flannery, and M. I. Simon, *Neuron* **6**, 201 (1991).
22. D. J. Zack, J. Bennett, Y. Wang, C. Davenport, B. Klaunberg, J. Gearhart, and J. Nathans, *Neuron* **6**, 187 (1991).

[26] *In Situ* Hybridization of Retinal Messenger RNA Using Nonradioactive Synthetic Probes

John G. Flannery, William J. Dinehart, Chrissie Street, and William W. Hauswirth

Introduction

In situ hybridization is a tool for localizing cellular RNAs to tissue sections. Its primary advantage is that it maintains detail in the tissue while permitting the detection of RNA transcripts with high resolution and sensitivity. We have adapted this *in situ* technique to the retina and have been able to localize specific mRNAs to individual cells and quantify their expression.

We selected this technique because it bridges a gap between the more widely used molecular techniques. The traditional method to assess mRNA expression in tissues is Northern blotting. However, blotting preparations introduce an intrinsic disadvantage as the technique separates the mRNAs from the cells, thus sacrificing information on the position of the messenger RNA within the "host" tissue. In addition, acquisition of the mRNA from a tissue combines the characteristics of thousands or millions of cells of varying types. *In situ* hybridization offers the ability to examine regional changes in mRNA expression in a tissue, to determine the cell type expressing a specific mRNA, and to locate a specific mRNA in the cell. In this way, *in situ* hybridization becomes a very powerful complement to blotting techniques as well as morphological techniques for studies of gene expression and development.

In our studies, *in situ* hybridization provides the ability to monitor changes in the quantity of a particular mRNA in individual cells in the context of very small areas of the retina. This ability to examine small numbers of cells is expected to be of particular value in understanding retinal development. In earlier studies (1–3), we attempted to examine regional changes by dividing the retina surgically before biochemical or morphological examination, but we always found this approach to be severely limited. The physical size of the eye in most laboratory animals precludes this approach, and surgical dissection generally results in the homogenization of cells from a poorly defined region of the fundus and from many retinal layers. An alternative technique, the production of transgenic animals (3, 4), has proved useful for the study of gene expression in the retina and has allowed examination of some molecular aspects of cell differentiation, but it frequently does not reproduce normal development in the cell population containing the target molecules. We have found that regional changes in normal or transgene expression in different classes of retinal cells are better visualized by direct hybridization of DNA or RNA probes to tissue sections.

Background

In situ techniques for localizing specific sequences on chromosomes and detecting RNA transcripts in cells were initially described in the late 1960s (5–8). These techniques involved relatively long RNA and DNA probes that incorporated a radioactive label and required detection by autoradiography. Although widely used, positional resolution was limited by the fact that silver grains reside in the emulsion overlay and interact with β particles emitted at random angles from the hybridized probe. The random track of emitted particles results in a signal "scatter" that is compounded by the relative thickness of both the sample and emulsion.

The development of nonradioactive nucleic acid probes increases the effective resolution of *in situ* hybridization because visualization of the hybridized probe nucleic acid is achieved by recognition of tags on the probe itself. These tags may be directly visualized (fluorescent labels), detected by secondary antibodies against an antigenically marked probe (digoxigenin), or detected by avidin–biotin complexes. Secondary labels may be fluorescent-tagged antibodies, antibody–colloidal gold conjugates, or enzymes that lead to a chromogenic reaction. In this way, probe signal is restricted to the hybridization locale, resulting in high resolution of the target nucleic acids within tissue.

Confocal Microscopy

We have been able to further enhance the resolving power of this technique by use of a confocal laser scanning microscope. The blue-purple end product of the BCIP/NBT colorimetric reaction (described below) is readily imaged in the reflective mode of most confocal microscopes. (We have had success with both the Leitz, Heidelberg, Germany, and Bio-Rad, Richmond, CA, instruments.) Alternatively, oligonucleotide primers containing the common fluorophores Texas red, rhodamine, and fluorescein are available (Molecular Probes, Inc., Eugene, OR). All three of these molecules are excited by the laser lines emitted by most of the common confocal microscopes and fluoresce at wavelengths detected with high efficiency by the photomultipliers of these instruments.

Nonisotopic methods additionally benefit from the fact that time scale of the detection reaction is significantly shorter than for autoradiographic *in situ* hybridization. In addition, nonradioactive probes are not subject to radioactive decay; they are stable reagents that remain functional for long periods of time. Although the general technique is still in the developmental stage, it has already proved capable of detecting a few hundred copies of a sequence less than 1 kb in length. The ultimate sensitivity of this technique has yet to be ascertained, but the potential for enormous signal amplification through the use of localized polymerase chain reaction (PCR) and multistep reactions of antibiotin, biotinylated secondary antibody, and streptavidin–colloidal gold is clear. At the detection end, the rapid development of low-noise photomultipliers promises potential for rapid detection of single-copy sequences through the use of probe–fluorophore hybrids directly visualized in the laser scanning confocal microscope.

A great number of questions concerning gene expression in the retina could be answered using this technique, but to date surprisingly little has been published. In this chapter, we describe the use of nonisotopically labeled synthetic oligonucleotide probes to visualize photoreceptor specific mRNA in human and bovine retinal tissue sections.

Design of Oligonucleotide Probes

Probe design is critical to successful *in situ* analysis. Although a long DNA or RNA single-stranded probe can be more sensitive than a short, synthetic DNA probe, selecting a region of sequence to distinguish between closely related genes becomes increasingly difficult with length. Therefore, we have focused on the design and use of short, synthetic DNA oligonucleotide probes to distinguish among related sets of individual genes such as the rod and cone opsins.

Alignment of published gene sequences for the human opsins allowed us to design and synthesize 20-nucleotide DNA probes specific for one opsin gene, which would contain six or more mismatches with all other opsin genes. The human red opsin gene probe used as an example in Fig. 1 spans the 20 nucleotides from position 1315 to 1334 and contains six mismatches with the corresponding region of the human green opsin gene, the most closely related of the human opsins. Thus, at the hybridization stringency [37°C, 50% (v/v) formamide, $2\times$ SSC solution (standard saline–citrate; $2\times$ SSC is 0.3 M sodium chloride and 30 mM sodium citrate in distilled water (9)] and washing stringency (45–50°C, $0.1\times$ SSC) used, we only expected

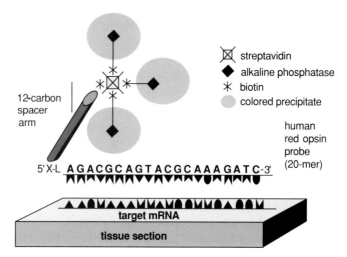

FIG. 1   Schematic diagram of the hybridization of a biotinylated oligonucleotide to the mRNA of a tissue section. The target mRNA is retained with the tissue section during fixation. In this example, a 20-mer oligonucleotide designed to detect human red opsin is hybridized to the target mRNA. A 12-carbon spacer arm extends from the 5′ end of the oligonucleotide, separating the biotin from the hybridization site. The biotin is visualized in this example by a posthybridization reaction with streptavidin conjugated to alkaline phosphatase. A colorimetric reaction (described in the text) is used to generate a blue-black precipitate.

cone red opsin mRNA to be detected. Other, more universal probe design features were also incorporated, including keeping the G/C content close to 50% and avoiding runs of G residues and self-complementary (palindromic) sequences.

Biotin Tagging of Oligonucleotide Probes

Oligonucleotide probes were produced by automated synthesis on an Applied Biosystems Model 380B synthesizer (ABI, Inc., Foster City, CA) using phosphoramidite chemistry. Biotin was incorporated into the probe by one of the following two methods.

Probe Incorporation during Oligonucleotide Synthesis

A biotin and incorporated spacer may be added during the automated synthesis of the probe as if it were another base in the oligonucleotide. This is accomplished by the use of a reagent containing the biotin moiety, a spacer of appropriate length (10 carbons), a diisopropyl group to facilitate coupling to the 5' end of the growing probe, and a dimethoxytrityl-protected hydroxyl group to allow multiple biotin additions (Glen Research, Inc., Sterling, VA.). We chose to incorporate the biotinylated spacer one nucleotide inside the 5' end because it allows the possibility of subsequent 5'-end-labeling using polyonucleotide kinase and it assures that the majority of the oligonucleotide will hybridize as expected. Therefore, a 20-nucleotide probe would contain the biotinylated residue at its 5' end and one more normal nucleotide following it. In such a design, all of the nucleotides would be expected to find complementary bases with the exception of the two 5' residues.

Probe Incorporation after Oligonucleotide Synthesis

Alternatively, the biotin can be added to the probe after synthesis. The probe is produced by conventional automated synthesis with one exception: a spacer capped with a primary amine (Amino link-2, ABI) is coupled as the 5' base of the sequence. An activated biotin-*N*-hydroxysuccinamide (biotin-NHS) ester will react efficiently with this primary amine under weakly alkaline conditions at room temperature. The oligonucleotide should be completely deprotected and then desalted by ethanol precipitation before the coupling reaction. Biotin is incorporated into the probe as follows.

1. Pipette a volume of probe calculated to give 3.0 OD units into a microcentrifuge tube and evaporate to dryness in a centrifugal evaporator.
2. Add 25 μl of freshly prepared 0.5 *M* NaHCO$_3$/Na$_2$CO$_3$, pH 9.0 buffer, vortex, centrifuge briefly, and place on ice.
3. Prepare a fresh 100 mg/ml solution of biotin-NHS in *anhydrous* dimethylformamide (DMF).
4. Add 7.5 μl of biotin/DMF to the oligonucleotide solution and gently mix by repipetting several times.
5. Incubate at room temperature overnight.

Purification of Tagged Oligonucleotides

High-quality synthetic oligonucleotides will not need to be purified prior to biotin labeling. Probes of uncertain quality should be checked by high-performance liquid chromatography (HPLC) or polyacrylamide gel electrophoresis and then purified if necessary. Biotin linked too closely to the target probe may cause steric hindrance when the tagged probe is later annealed to target DNA or RNA. Biotin derivative containing spacers of various types and sizes are available to alleviate such problems. We used a 6-atom amino-linked spacer and a 7-atom link for the biotin-NHS reagent for a total of 13 atoms between the oligonucleotide backbone and the biotin tag.

After reaction, the biotin-tagged probe needs to be separated from the unincorporated biotin-NHS and reaction by-products. This can be quickly accomplished by running the reaction mix over a fast protein liquid chromatography (FPLC) desalting column packed with Sephadex G-25sf (Pharmacia-LKB Biotechnology, Piscataway, NJ) (Fig. 2a). The reaction mix should be brought up to a final volume of 200 μl with 30% acetonitrile in 0.1 M TEAA (TEAA is tetraethylammonium acetate), pH 7.0, to ensure that the biotin–probe is completely solubilized. A column with an 8.0 ml Sephadex bed volume (10 mm × 10 cm) will give close to baseline resolution of product versus reactants (Fig. 2a). The column should be preequilibrated with at least three column volumes of 0.1 M TEAA, pH 7.0, flowing at 4.0 ml/min. The sample should be applied to the column with an initial mobile phase flow rate of 1.0 ml/min for 0.5 min, then the flow is increased to 4.0 ml/min and samples collected. The biotin–probe will be eluted with a retention time of about 1 min and the reaction by-products at about 2 min. The probe fractions (1 ml) should be evaporated to dryness, dissolved in 100 μl of double-distilled water, and dried again to remove all the TEAA before use.

The extent of the biotin coupling reaction and the subsequent separation step can be checked by FPLC reversed-phase chromatography (Fig. 2b). Aliquots of each peak from the above desalting column and a sample of the original oligonucleotide should be brought to a concentration of 0.5 OD units/ml in 200 μl of 0.1 M TEAA, pH 7.0, and run on a 2.0-ml Pharmacia ProRPC column. The column should run from 0 to 30% acetonitrile in 0.1 M TEAA, pH 7.0, in 20 min at a flow rate of 1.0 ml/min, with the detector set at 0.05 absorbance units full scale. Peak 2 from the desalting column is the unincorporated biotin reagent. This reagent will not be retained by the column and will elute with the void volume (Fig. 2b). Peak 1 from the desalting column is the biotin-tagged probe and will have a retention time 1–2 min longer than the nontagged oligonucleotide (Fig. 2b).

FIG. 2   Purification of the biotin-tagged oligonucleotide following synthesis. Initially, the probe is separated from the unincorporated biotin-NHS and reaction by-products with an FPLC desalting column packed with Sephadex G-25sf (Fig. 2a). Near baseline resolution of product versus reactants is obtained with a column of 8.0 ml bed volume. The biotin–probe elutes at 1 min (peak 1) and the reaction by-products at 2 min (peak 2). The extent of the biotin coupling reaction and the subsequent separation step are examined by FPLC reverse-phase chromatography (b). Aliquots of each peak from the above desalting column and a sample of the original oligonucleotide are separated with a 2.0-ml Pharmacia ProRPC column. Peak 2 from the desalting column is the unincorporated biotin reagent. This reagent will not be retained by the column and will elute with the void volume (b). Peak 1 from the desalting column is the biotin-tagged probe and will have a retention time 1–2 min longer than the nontagged oligonucleotide (b).

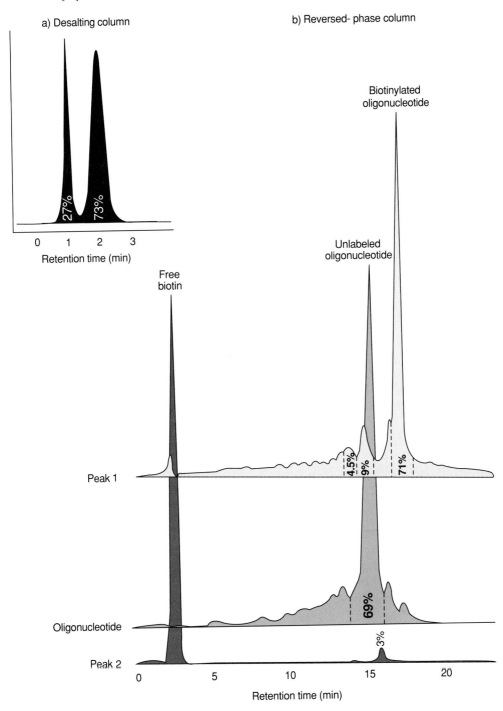

a) Desalting column

b) Reversed- phase column

Choice of Labeling Method

The choice between tagging the oligonucleotide probe with biotin during synthesis or after synthesis using an amino-linked reagent depends on several practical factors. We have found that either method yields probes that function equally well for *in situ* hybridization. Synthetic incorporation of biotin is more expensive (~$50 per probe) but assures 100% tagging, and the product usually requires no further purification. Coupling to an amino-linked oligonucleotide costs less (~$10 per probe) but requires the additional labor of purification as outlined above. Alternatively, commercial tagging is available, typically for $200–300 in addition to the cost of the oligonucleotide synthesis itself.

Specimen Collection, Processing, and Fixation

Tissue preparation for *in situ* hybridization requires somewhat different considerations than processing for conventional histology. The goal is to preserve the association of mRNAs with cellular structures. Fixation must be adequate to preserve the tissue architecture and prevent loss of nucleic acids by extraction during the subsequent dehydration and infiltration of the tissue. Conventional fixation protocols are optimized for light microscopy and can interfere with hybridization.

Glutaraldehyde exerts its primary fixative effect through formation of cross-links that bridge randomly spaced primary amino groups of cellular proteins. The extent and rate of cross-linking vary in cells, depending on the availability of these amino groups. Glutaraldehyde also reacts with tissue lipids containing free amino groups. Less information is available on the interaction of glutaraldehyde with nucleic acids in tissue. Osmium tetroxide, another common component of conventional fixation protocols, is primarily used for its ability to promote retention of lipids in tissues. Although these agents reduce cell component loss by extraction in the dehydration steps of tissue processing, they can also yield poor hybridization apparently by interfering with penetration of the probe to the target mRNA. Therefore, OsO_4 is avoided and glutaraldehyde kept to a minimum (low concentration and short time) in fixatives for *in situ* hybridization.

Formaldehyde, a monoaldehyde, is the fixative of choice for *in situ* hybridization. It is structurally the simplest of the aldehyde fixatives, its small size yielding rapid tissue penetration. Formaldehyde acts as a fixative by cross-linking peptide chains of proteins, but lipids are lost during dehydration of formaldehyde-fixed tissues. Formaldehyde is known to interact with nucleic acids and nucleoproteins, but generally it does not significantly interfere with the accessibility of probe molecules to the target mRNA. Penetration of the probe into the tissue is minimized by using short, synthetic oligonucleotide probes, and thus fixation with a greater degree of cross-linking and better preservation of tissue structure is possible. Achieving a balance between optimal tissue detail and detection of the mRNA signal always results in compromised morphology, however.

Interpretation of the *in situ* localization results is often simplified by having optimally preserved tissue available for detailed anatomic comparison. This should be carried out by conventional processing of a tissue sample from a region adjacent to the sample taken for *in situ* hybridization. The techniques described elsewhere in this volume (10) are suggested for these comparisons.

Although the fixation constraints do not result in optimal morphology in the tissue, they allow *in situ* hybridization and immunocytochemistry to be compatible techniques (11). Tissues preserved for *in situ* hybridization are appropriate for immunocytochemistry protocols and allow the use of the same tissue block for both investigations. Complex questions may require that these techniques be used on alternate serial sections or combined on the same tissue section by using colloidal gold markers of differing sizes (11).

Fixation and Processing of Retinal Tissue

The eye is removed from the animal, the anterior segment is cut away, and the vitreous humor carefully removed. Eyes from large animals are usually divided into hemispheres or quadrants prior to processing. The posterior segment of the eye is immersed in 4% formaldehyde (freshly made from paraformaldehyde) and 0.1% glutaraldehyde (pH 7.4) in 0.1% sodium phosphate buffer at 4°C for 1 hr. The posterior segment is then rinsed by immersion in 0.1% sodium phosphate buffer at 4°C for 30 min. Dehydration is by a graded series of 50, 70, 85, 95, and 100% methanol at 4°C, 30 min per step. Tissue is then infiltrated in Paraplast Plus (Fisher Scientific, Pittsburgh, PA) overnight. The following day the tissue is transferred to new Paraplast Plus in molds and hardened by slow cooling for several hours.

Tissue samples of corresponding or adjacent regions to those processed for ultrastructural analysis are processed for direct ultrastructural examination. The samples are fixed in 4% glutaraldehyde and 2% formaldehyde, postfixed in 4% OsO_4, dehydrated in ethanol, infiltrated in propylene oxide, and embedded in Araldite 502 epoxy resin (Ciba Products Co., Summit, NJ). This procedure yields the highest resolution of fine ultrastructural detail, but the OsO_4 postfixation and type of epoxy renders it unusable for *in situ* hybridization and immunocytochemical studies.

Tissue Sectioning and Mounting

Paraffin sections of 2 to 10 μm thickness are collected on subbed glass slides. We have found that the advance mechanisms in the latest generation of microtomes (such as the Reichert Biocut 2030, Buffalo, NY) offer a significant advantage in reproducibly cutting paraffin sections thinner than 5 μm. Sections are lifted from the knife edge and floated onto a water bath at 40°C with conventional histopathology technique. Sections are picked up from below with glass slides. Slides *must* be subbed before use to ensure adhesion of the sections to the glass surface in the later posthybridization washes (see below). Slides should also be frosted or marked with a diamond scribe to show the surface that has the section attached, as this will be less evident after removal of the paraffin embedment. It is important to reserve space around the perimeter of the section for application of a sealing compound. For large eyes, we recommend the substitution of wider (75 × 38 mm) slides (Corning, Corning, NY, 2947) for the conventional 3 × 1 inch histology slides. Steps should be taken to avoid touching surfaces that will contact the tissue, as RNase is present on the fingers. Filter sterilization of solutions for the water bath, etc., is recommended. Sections are then affixed to the slides at 55–60°C for 1 hr with a forced air slide drying cabinet (Lipshaw Model 218, Detroit, MI) or a conventional oven overnight.

Slide Subbing

It is not uncommon for tissue sections to come off the glass slides during hybridization procedures. The enzymatic tissue digestion and the stringent washes cause the tissue sections to detach from the glass. Silane coating the slides prior to use greatly improves the adhesion of the sections without interfering with hybridization procedures. The technique that we use is as follows.

1. Prepare a solution of 2% silane in acetone. (Silane is 3-aminopropyltriethoxysilane, Sigma, St. Louis, MO, A-3648).
2. Place slides in a rack and immerse in pure acetone solution for 5 min.
3. Remove slides from the solution, blotting the bottom edges. Dry at room temperature for 5 min.
4. Place in silane solution for 5 min.
5. Remove slides from the solution, blotting the bottom edges, and rinse in two changes of distilled water.
6. Dry in an oven overnight. This step can be reduced to 1 hr or less with the use of a forced air slide drying cabinet.
7. Slides can be prepared in advance and stored in closed boxes until needed.

Removal of Embedment

Prior to hybridization, sections are deparaffinized by immersion in toluene
or xylene, twice for 5 min each. Sections are then rehydrated by immersion
in 100% ethanol for two 5 min washes, 95% ethanol (twice, 5 min each), and
then in distilled water for two additional 5-min steps. Sections are then
subjected to proteolytic digestion with 0.1% pronase (Pronase E, Sigma) at
room temperature for 5 min to remove proteins from the tissue and expose
target sequences. Residual enzyme activity is removed by washing in water
twice for 5 min each. It is important to predigest the pronase solution at
37°C for 30 min to remove any trace of RNase before adding it to the
tissue sections.

Sections are washed twice for 5 min each in distilled water prior to application of the prehybridization solution. Also before application of the prehybridization solution, the slide is carefully blotted dry around the section with
an absorbent tissue, without contacting the section. The section is then
surrounded with a bead of rubber cement to form a retaining dam to contain
the hybridization mixtures. Cement is applied with a 50- to 100-ml syringe
with a large gauge blunted needle affixed. Care should be exercised to keep
the cement away from the section as the cement may spread before drying.
The dam should be dry prior to application of the prehybridization solution.

In Situ Hybridization

Prehybridization

Prehybridization consists of an application of the hybridization mixture (see
below) with the omission of the oligonucleotide probe and dextran sulfate
to the sections for 1 hr at 35°C. Dextran sulfate is an inert component of the
hybridization mix, which is included to maximize the local concentration of
the probe in the mixture, and therefore it is not required in the prehybridization mixture. Its presence increases the viscosity of the prehybridization
solution significantly, making it difficult to decant from the slide prior to
hybridization. After prehybridization, the prehybridization mixture is decanted, and an additional bead of cement is applied *outside* the original, dry
cement bead. A sealed chamber is then formed by the application of a baked,
RNase-free coverslip.

Preparation of Hybridization Mix

The oligonucleotide is resuspended in the following buffer to achieve a final
probe concentration in the range of 0.2 to 2 ng/μl. A dilution series is

recomended in this range. Add sufficient hybridization mix to cover the tissue (typically 200 μl). The hybridization mix is for 1 ml.

Component	Volume (μl)	Final concentration
50$\times$ Denhardt's[a]	20	1$\times$
Formamide	500	50%
NaCl (5 M stock)	120	0.6 M
EDTA (0.5 M stock)	2	1 mM
Tris-Cl, pH 7.5 (1 M stock)	100	100 mM
Salmon sperm DNA (5 mg/ml)	100	500 μg/ml
Diethyl pyrocarbonate-treated water	158	To make final volume of 1 ml

[a] 1$\times$ Denhardt's solution is 0.2% Ficoll, 0.2% bovine serum albumin, and 0.2% poly(vinylpyrrolidone and is supplemented with 10 mM dithiothreitol (DTT).

The slides containing the probe and hybridization mix are placed on a hot plate at 35°C for 12 hr. Subsequent to hybridization, slides are washed 3 times for 10 min each by immersing them in 2$\times$ SSC. Complete immersion is necessary to remove unbound probe that may have leaked to the back side of the slide.

Stringent Washing

The overall stringency of the hybridization is controlled by the following washing steps. Two factors are important. The degree of nonspecific background labeling increases with increasing concentration of SSC in the wash buffer, and the amount of background is reduced by increasing the temperature. An acceptable level of background to signal therefore must be established empirically for each tissue/fixation/embedment/probe combination. We have found that washing at 0.1$\times$ SSC for 30 min at 35°C is minimally necessary. Best signal-to-noise ratios are usually achieved by higher temperature 0.1$\times$ SSC washes (40–55°C), determined empirically.

Visualization of Probe–Target Hybrids

It has been difficult to predict the optimal hybridization temperature for *in situ* analysis by applying theoretical methods because the calculations were developed for liquid hybridization conditions, whereas the conditions of *in situ* hybridization are liquid–solid phase. We have found that the initial hybridization is best performed at a stringency of 35°C in 50% formamide. This temperature is well below the melting temperature (T_m) for the typical probe. Higher stringency is attained by increasing the washing temperature. After hybridization, sections are rinsed twice each with $2 \times$ SSC and $0.1 \times$ SSC at increasing temperatures up to 55°C. For the red opsin and rhodopsin probes shown, final washing at 50°C in $0.1 \times$ SSC was possible without significant loss of specific hybridization. Specific localization of an antisense oligonucleotide for rod opsin mRNA to the inner segment of a bovine rod photoreceptor is illustrated by Figs. 3 and 4. The colored reaction product is seen to be restricted to the inner segment of the rod photoreceptor cells, the cellular compartment in which mRNA is known to be concentrated.

Streptavidin is used as the link between the biotinylated probe and biotinylated reporter molecules of alkaline phosphatase. A colored reaction product is produced as a result of the hydrolysis of BCIP (5-bromo-4-chloro-3-indolyl phosphate) and the reduction of nitro blue tetrazolium (NBT) to yield a blue-purple chromogen. We have used the biotin visualization reagents provided by Dako Corporation (Carpinteria, CA). After the final $0.1 \times$ SSC wash, streptavidin is added as recommended for 30 min at room temperature, followed by a 5-min TBS wash at room temperature. Biotinylated alkaline phosphatase is then added as recommended for 30 min at room temperature followed by a 5-min wash in TBS and a 2-min wash in distilled water, also at room temperature. Finally, the alkaline phosphatase substrate solution is added as recommended at room temperature.

It is important not to process too many tissue sections to this point simultaneously because color development, once the substrate solution is added, will occur fairly rapidly over a peiod that may vary from 5 to 30 min depending on probe concentration in the tissue. We find that it is most efficient to store all sections in the final distilled water wash prior to substrate addition and add this final reagent to only three or four sections at a time.

After the substrate is on the sections, they are kept in the dark and briefly examined at regular intervals in the light microscope until the desired level of color has developed. At that point, which must be empirically determined for each probe, excess solution is shaken off, and the slides are immediately placed in a distilled water bath at room temperature to stop further color development. We find it best to stop development somewhat before the desired end point because alkaline phosphatase-catalyzed color generation continues for a short period in the stop bath. Generally, development times in excess of 30 min are undesirable because by this time nonspecific color has deposited throughout all layers of the retina.

a

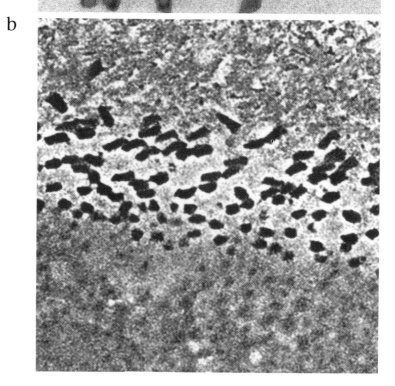

b

Colloidal Gold Labels

A 1 : 10 dilution of streptavidin conjugated to 30-nm colloidal gold may be used in place of the chromogen to allow counting of discrete probe–target pairs. The 30-nm gold particles can be directly visualized or enhanced using a silver-enhancement technique (Janssen Life Sciences, B-2340 Beerse, Belgium) for observation in the light microscope. We have found that these probes can be visualized at very high resolution at magnifications approaching electron microscopy by the use of the confocal laser scanning microscope.

Design of Oligonucleotide Probes as Controls

As controls to evaluate the hybridization accessibility with each new tissue sample, we utilize probes that specify an abundant transcript known to be restricted to a particular retinal cell type. We have synthesized biotinylated oligonucleotide probes for bovine rhodopsin and human red, green, and blue cone opsins for this purpose. Labeling over the retinal cells and background labeling over the choroidal and other nonretinal regions is estimated and compared. The use of these probes allows us to evaluate adjustments and modifications to the aforementioned protocols. As a control for the specificity of labeling to tissue mRNA, we use tissue sections hybridized with sense oligonucleotide probes to the bovine rhodopsin. Additionally, some sections are processed at very high stringency by heating to a temperature significantly above the T_m of the probe (usually 65°C). We observe no labeling above background in any of these preparations.

Quantitative Image Analysis

We currently use methods for quantitative analysis of *in situ* hybridization that are adapted from methods developed for quantitation of immunocyto-

FIG. 3   Confocal microscope images of the hybridization of synthetic oligonucleotide to adult bovine retina. The chromogenic reaction product is observed over the inner segments of the rod photoreceptors. (a) Transverse section of the photoreceptor layer shows the specific hybridization of antisense rod opsin probe to the rod inner segments. Magnification: ×1432. (b) Section cut slightly oblique to transverse demonstrates hybridization to the inner segment of rod photoreceptors, with no visible hybridization to the outer segment layer observed in the upper third of the section, nor to the more sclerad region of the photoreceptor layer below. A slight hybridization signal revealing a matrix pattern can be observed in the lower third of the section. Magnification: ×477.

a

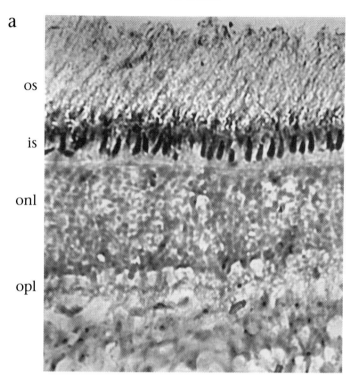

os

is

onl

opl

b

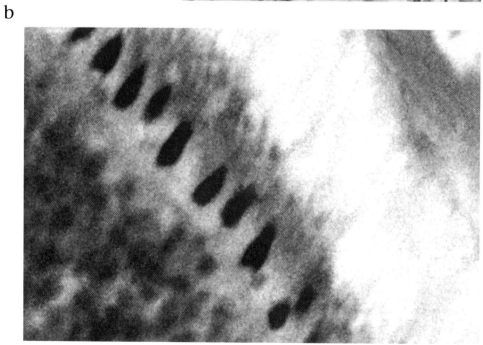

chemical labeling (12). To begin these tests, we begin by examining a minimum area of retina hybridized with each oligonucleotide probe. The minimum area to be studied is determined empirically. We define it as the area that will give a ratio of labeling density of the antisense probe to the sense probe which is statistically significant to the $p = .01$ level by t-test analysis. We use JMP statistical software (SAS Institute, Cary, NC) to obtain t-test and analysis of variance (ANOVA) comparisons of the labeling densities. We routinely perform pairwise t-tests between sense and antisense oligonucleotide probes, for each of the retinal cell classes we are interested in at each developmental stage to be examined. Sampling errors between each sample type can be minimized using the K-ratio t-test (13, 14) and the multiple range test (15) for analysis of the variance.

We have used three methods to acquire quantitative data from *in situ* hybridizations. A flatbed scanner (such as a Microtek 600zs, Microtek, Inc., Torrance, CA) can be used to digitize photographic prints and negatives if it supports a minimum of 75 dots per inch and 256 gray levels. Scanners which support only 4-bit (16 gray level) scans work poorly for image quantitation. The disadvantage of this method is that hybridized slides must be photographed and printed before analysis.

Direct video input from a light microscope does not require the time and expense of film and paper processing. It can be done with a frame grabber attachment and a personal computer such as the Data Technologies Quick-Capture (Data Translation, Inc., Marlboro, MA) or the Scion card (Scion Corp., Frederick, MD). This method also requires a high-quality video camera to acquire the image such as the Sierra Scientific MS-4030 (Sierra Scientific, Sunnyvale, CA) or the COHU Model 4815-5000 (COHU, Inc., San Diego, CA).

We have found that the method yielding the greatest resolution and control is to directly transfer images to disk from a confocal microscope. Confocal microscope images are digitized as they are acquired. The only requirement is to save them in a format that can be readily manipulated. Images that are saved in the "TIFF" file format can be easily transferred from the confocal microscope with floppy disks or other removable media and quantified on a Macintosh or IBM personal computer. These files can generate publication-quality images by transferring them to a typesetting program such as Pagemaker (Aldus Corp., Seattle, WA) and outputting to film or paper with an imagesetter such as the Linotronix 500.

FIG. 4 Hybridization of red opsin oligonucleotide to bovine cone inner segments. (a) os, Outer segment; is, inner segment; onl, outer nuclear layer; opl, outer plexiform layer. Magnification: ×620. (b) Section at higher magnification (×1860).

a

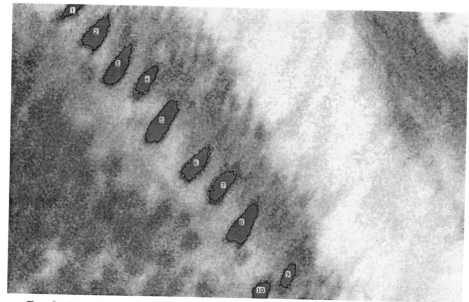

FIG. 5 Densitomentric scan of rod opsin hybridization as quantitated by the IMAGE software. (a) The area of hybridization is outlined and thresholded as the darkest segment of the gray scale in the confocal image (magnification: ×1432). This region is then measured and assigned a number. (b) Histogram of the results of analysis of the confocal image in (a). Area and density measurements for the hybridization of rod opsin oligonucleotide to individual inner segments are presented.

Thresholding is the technique used to segment an image into objects of interest and background for quantification of staining intensity. It is done on the basis of assigning a unique gray level to the specific staining product from the hybridization reaction. An example of this technique is shown in Fig. 5. This algorithm can be used to measure the area, average density, center of gravity, and angle of orientation of a staining reaction. When thresholding is performed, objects to be measured are displayed in black (or red), and the background remains white. Background pixels are ignored, and area and density measurements are made from the black pixels only. The computer scans across the image until it finds the boundary of an object, outlines the edge of the object, measures the object, and then redraws the object in a different gray level so that it becomes invisible to the scanning process. The amount of background labeling over extracellular space and peripheral to the tissue can be measured separately.

Quantitative image analysis can be performed with several software packages on many different computers. We use the IMAGE quantitation software provided at no cost by the Research Services Branch, National Institute of

b

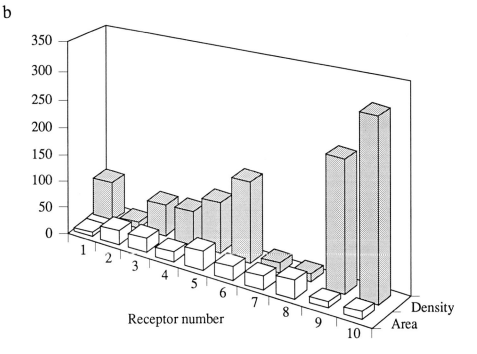

FIG. 5 *(continued)*

Mental Health, National Institutes of Health, on a Macintosh II computer. Several similar programs (NCSA Image, NCSA, Champaign, IL; Image Analyst, Automatrix, Billerica, MA) are supported on IBM and UNIX platforms.

References

1. D. Farber, J. G. Flannery, R. Lolley, and D. Bok, *Invest. Ophthalmol. Visual. Sci.* **20,** 24 (1981).
2. J. Flannery, D. B. Farber, A. C. Bird, and D. Bok, *Invest. Ophthalmol. Visual. Sci.* **30,** 191 (1989).
3. J. Lem, J. Flannery, T. Li, M. Applebury, D. Farber, and M. Simon, *Proc. Natl. Acad. Sci. U.S.A.* **89,** 4422 (1992).
4. G. Travis, K. Groshan, M. Lloyd, and D. Bok, *Invest. Ophthalmol. Visual. Sci.* **33,** 946 (1992).
5. J. G. Gall and M. L. Pardue, *Proc. Natl. Acad. Sci. U.S.A.* **63,** 378 (1969).
6. H. A. John, M. L. Birnstiel, and K. W. Jones, *Nature (London)* **223,** 582 (1969).

7. M. Buongiorno-Nardelli and F. Amaldi, *Nature (London)* **225,** 946 (1970).
8. H. Höfler, *Pathol. Res. Pract.* **182,** 421 (1987).
9. T. Maniatis, E. F. Fritsch, and J. Sambrook, "Molecular Cloning: A Laboratory Manual." Cold Spring Harbor Laboratory, Cold Spring Harbor, New York, 1982.
10. S. K. Fisher, D. H. Anderson, P. A. Erickson, C. J. Guérin, G. P. Lewis, and K. A. Linberg, this volume [1].
11. R. H. Singer, G. L. Langevin, and J. B. Lawrence, *J. Cell. Biol.* **108,** 2343 (1989).
12. A. C. Bird, J. G. Flannery, and D. Bok, *Invest. Ophthalmol. Visual. Sci.* **29,** 1028 (1988).
13. R. Waller and K. Kemp, *J. Stat. Computation Simul.* **75,** 169 (1976).
14. R. Waller and D. B. Duncan, *J. Am. Stat. Assoc.* **64,** 1484 (1969).
15. D. B. Duncan, *Biometrics* **31,** 339 (1975).

[27] Identification of Rhodopsin Gene Mutations Using GC-Clamped Denaturing Gradient Gel Electrophoresis

Edwin M. Stone, Kimberlie Vandenburgh, Brian E. Nichols, and Val C. Sheffield

Introduction

The primary linkage of the rhodopsin gene with autosomal-dominant retinitis pigmentosa (ADRP) (1) and the subsequent identification of rhodopsin coding sequence mutations in ADRP families (2, 3) were major advances toward understanding human retinal degenerations at the level of individual genes. However, the fact that multiple mutations within a gene can cause the same or a similar phenotype is a significant impediment to the development of practical assays for molecular diagnosis. For example, over 100 different mutations have been shown to cause β-thalassemia, and over 75 mutations are associated with cystic fibrosis. To date, over 30 mutations of the rhodopsin gene (see Table I and Fig. 1) have been associated with ADRP (2–11), and even more rhodopsin mutations are likely to be identified. It is thus necessary to have sensitive methods by which nearly all mutations in genes may be readily identified. Because most mutations are single base substitutions, these methods must be capable of detecting single base changes.

Several techniques have been developed which make it possible to detect single base changes in DNA. These techniques include allele-specific oligonucleotide (ASO) hybridization (12), RNase cleavage (13, 14), chemical cleavage (15, 16), single-stranded conformation polymorphism (SSCP) analysis (17–19), heteroduplex analysis (20, 21), and denaturing gradient gel electrophoresis (DGGE) (22–29). Some of these techniques are not suitable for screening DNA for mutations. For example, ASO hybridization is a useful technique for identifying single base substitutions only when the base substitution is already known. DGGE is a powerful technique capable of identifying single base changes and has been used by us and others to identify rhodopsin mutations (5, 9, 11). DGGE, as originally described, can be used to detect about 50% of all single base changes (22, 23). An improvement of this technique, known as GC-clamped DGGE, makes it possible to detect nearly 100% of single base changes in DNA fragments of about 500 bp in length (28, 29). In this chapter, we describe the use of GC-clamped DGGE for the

TABLE I   Rhodopsin Mutations

Exon	Codon	Sequence	Ref.
1	17	Thr → Met	5
1	23	Pro → His	2
1	23	Pro → Leu	6
1	45	Phe → Leu	7
1	51	Gly → Val	6
1	58	Thr → Arg	5
1	68	68–71 deletion	8
1	87	Val → Asp	7
1	89	Gly → Asp	7
1	106	Gly → Arg	9
1	106	Gly → Trp	7
2	125	Leu → Arg	6
2	135	Arg → Leu	7
2	135	Arg → Trp	7
2	167	Cys → Arg	6
2	171	Pro → Leu	6
3	178	Tyr → Cys	10
3	181	Glu → Lys	6
3	182	Gly → Ser	5
3	186	Ser → Pro	6
3	188	Gly → Arg	6
3	190	Asp → Tyr	11
3	190	Asp → Asn	8
3	190	Asp → Gly	7
3	211	His → Pro	8
4	255	Deletion	4
4	267	Pro → Leu	5
4	296	Lys → Glu	8
5	344	Gln → Stop	7
5	345	Val → Met	6
5	347	Pro → Ser	5
5	347	Pro → Leu	5

detection of rhodopsin coding sequence mutations. These methods are also applicable to the study of other candidate genes that may be involved in human retinal degenerations.

GC-Clamped Denaturing Gradient Gel Electrophoresis

DGGE can physically separate fragments differing by a single base substitution on the basis of a difference in melting temperature (T_m) of the two molecules (22). A single base change has been shown to change the T_m of a

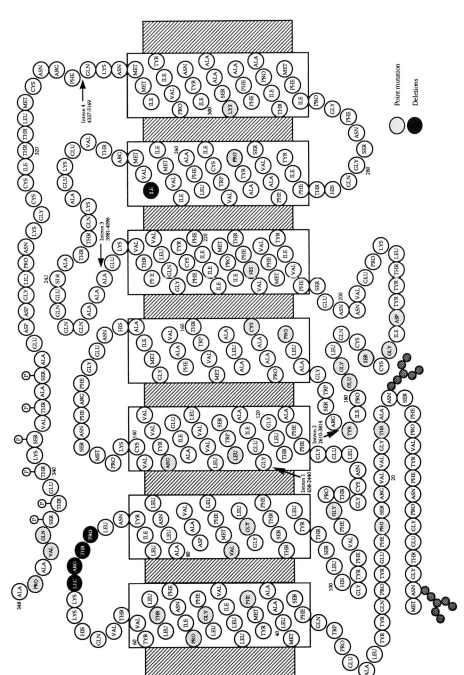

FIG. 1 Known mutations in the rhodopsin coding sequence associated with retinitis pigmentosa. The protein chain traverses the disk membrane (shaded zone) seven times. The intron positions as they map to the protein are shown with arrows. Known point mutations are shown by diagonal lines within a circle corresponding to an amino acid, whereas areas known to be deleted are shown as shaded circles.

given DNA melting domain by up to 2°C (22). Melting of a domain changes the conformation of the DNA molecule and thus affects its rate of migration through a polyacrylamide gel matrix.

The DGGE technique consists of electrophoresing the DNA molecule through a polyacrylamide gel containing a linear gradient of DNA denaturants (formamide and urea) which increase from top to bottom in the gel. These denaturants cause the DNA strands to separate (melt) just as they would with increased temperature. The DNA molecule migrates through the gel at a constant velocity until it reaches a concentration of denaturant where the domain with the lowest T_m becomes single-stranded. At this point, the DNA fragment undergoes a conformational change, forming a partly single-stranded and partly double-stranded molecule. The conformational change causes the molecule to migrate more slowly through the gel. Two molecules differing by a single base in one of their lower melting domains will undergo the conformational change and slow their rate of migration at slightly different points in the gel, and hence can be separated from each other. This technique can only detect about 50% of all single base changes within a given DNA molecule, however, because substitutions in the highest melting domain of a given fragment will not be detected.

The addition of a very high melting domain (a G + C-rich sequence) to a given DNA molecule will allow detection of nearly all base substitutions within the original molecule, by maintaining the molecule in a partially duplexed/partially single-stranded conformation even when the highest temperature melting domain of the original molecule has denatured (see Fig. 2) (26, 28, 29). This G + C-rich sequence is known as a GC clamp. We have found the attachment of a 40-bp GC clamp to one end of a DNA fragment up to 500 bp in length makes it possible to detect over 90% of all possible base changes in that fragment by DGGE (28). This fraction can be increased to nearly 100% by examining the heteroduplex DNA fragments that are formed between two DNA sequences that differ by a single base pair (Fig. 3). The heteroduplexes contain a single mismatch that destabilizes the molecule and greatly increases their separation on the gel.

Our original rhodopsin assays utilized 40-bp clamps (5), but we have recently synthesized some primers with shorter clamps (Table II) and found them to be just as sensitive as the former in the rhodopsin system. The length of the clamp required for the greatest possible assay sensitivity depends to a large extent on the GC content of the sequence to be tested. For fragments with a low GC content, a shorter clamp is sufficient to detect nearly all single-base changes within the fragment. The primary advantage of shorter clamps is the reduced cost of oligonucleotide synthesis.

The development of the polymerase chain reaction (PCR) (30) for amplifying specific DNA fragments from genomic DNA led to a simplified approach

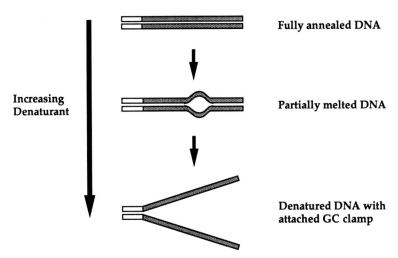

Fig. 2   Effect of a GC clamp on the denaturation of PCR products. PCR products are depicted as two thick bars. The white portions of each bar correspond to the GC-rich clamp at one end of the molecule. As this molecule migrates through the increasing concentration of denaturant, the molecule melts in specific domains determined by primary sequence. The GC clamp is so stable that it never melts, which enables most mutations to be detected even if they fall in the higher melting domains of the remainder of the molecule.

for using GC-clamped denaturing gradient gel electrophoresis. A GC clamp can be attached to PCR-amplified genomic DNA fragments by including a G + C sequence at the 5′ end of one of the oligonucleotide primers. This GC clamp then becomes incorporated into the amplified product. When heterozygous genomic DNA samples are amplified, the PCR product is comprised of both homoduplexes and heteroduplexes (30). The amplified DNA fragments are electrophoresed in a denaturing gradient gel, and the products are visualized by ethidium bromide staining of the gel. The large amplification of the fragment obviates the need for a radioactive probe and greatly reduces the amount of genomic DNA needed.

A 500-base DNA fragment can be completely screened for DNA sequence polymorphisms using GC-clamped denaturing gradient gel electrophoresis. Nearly all single base changes within the 500-bp DNA fragment will be detected by this approach. This has been demonstrated using human and mouse β-hemoglobin mutations (28) and p53 tumor suppressor gene mutations (31). We have also used this approach to identify polymorphisms within DNA probes that were not detectable using restriction enzyme digestion (32).

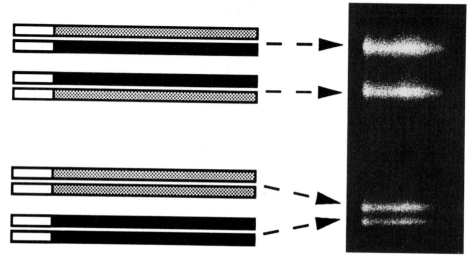

FIG. 3   Heteroduplex formation during PCR amplification of DNA from heterozygous individuals. PCR products from a wild-type gene are shown in black, whereas PCR products from a mutant gene are stippled. The white segments of each line correspond to the GC clamps. A PCR amplification from a heterozygote results in four possible DNA species: homoduplex wild type (all black), homoduplex affected (all stippled), and two heteroduplexes (one wild-type strand and one mutant strand annealed together). The heteroduplexes have a single base mismatch and melt at a lower denaturant concentration than the homoduplexes.

Methods

DNA is prepared from each blood sample using the protocol of Grimberg *et al.* (33). This protocol allows the isolation of purified DNA in only a few hours without the use of organic solvents. Briefly, whole blood is mixed with a 4-fold volume of cold CLB buffer (0.32 M sucrose, 10 mM Tris-HCl, pH 7.6, 5 mM MgCl$_2$, 1% Triton X-100). The resulting lysate is centrifuged to obtain a nuclear pellet. The pellet is redissolved in proteinase K buffer and digested for 2 hr at 65°C. The DNA concentration is then determined using spectrofluorometry with Hoechst 33258 dye. Approximately 500 ng of the DNA sample can then be used in a PCR amplification.

Following preparation of the DNA, the entire coding sequence of the rhodopsin gene is amplified by PCR in seven separate reactions using seven sets of primers (Table II). Two primer pairs per exon are used to amplify exons 1 and 5, whereas one primer pair is used to amplify each of the remaining four exons. Each pair of primers includes one primer with a 5′

TABLE II Primer Sequences

Exon and primer	Location	Size (bp)
1A		
fwd 5′ CGGGTCAGCCACAAGGGCCA 3′	270–289	269
rev 5′ CGCCCGCCCGGCGCCCGGCCCGCGCCCCGCCCCCGCCCGCCAGCTTCTTGTGCTGGACGGT 3′	478–500	
1B		
fwd 5′ TCTGCTGATCGTGCTGGGCTT 3′	429–449	390
rev 5′ GCCCCGCCCGGCGCCCGCGCCCCGCCCCCGCCGAGGGCTTTGGATAACATTG 3′	769–788	
2		
fwd 5′ CGCCCGCCCGGCGCCCGGCCCGCGCCCCGCCCCCGCCCGCCCCCGCCCGGCAGTGGGGTCTGTGCTGAC 3′	2397–2417	241
rev 5′ AGCCGGCGAGTGGGGTGCG 3′	2581–2600	
3		
fwd 5′ GGCAGCCACCTTGGCTGTTC 3′	3749–3768	303
rev 5′ GCCCCGCCCGGCGCCCGCGCCCCGCCCCCGCCCGCTGGACCCTCAGAGCCGTGA 3′	4003–4023	
4		
fwd 5′ GCCCCGCCCGGCGCCCGCGCCCCGCCCCCGCCCCCGCCCGAGGAGCCATGGTCTGGACC 3′	4056–4075	332
rev 5′ GGCCCTCCCACCCGCAGTA 3′	4340–4358	
5A		
fwd 5′ GCCCCGCCCGGCGCCCGCGCCCCGCCCCCGCCCCCGCCCTGACTCAAGCCTCTTGC 3′	5139–5160	273
rev 5′ ACTTCGTTCATTCTGCACAGGCG 3′	5364–5386	
5B		
fwd 5′ CGCCCGCCCGGCGCCCGCGCCCCGCCCCCGCCCGTCTGCTACCGTGTCCAAGAC 3′	5231–5250	117
rev 5′ TATAGTCGGGCCACAGAGTCC 3′	5289–5308	

GC clamp that becomes incorporated into the amplified fragment during the PCR amplification (Fig. 4).

PCR amplification using GC-clamped primers has been previously described (28). Briefly, primers are synthesized using phosphoramidite chemistry with an Applied Biosystems (Foster City, CA) Model 391 DNA synthesizer. Fifty-microliter amplification reactions contain the following: 5 μl of 10× PCR buffer (670 mM Tris, pH 8.8, 67 mM MgCl$_2$, 160 mM ammonium sulfate, 100 mM 2-mercaptoethanol), 10% dimethyl sulfoxide (DMSO), deoxynucleoside triphosphates (final concentration 1.25 mM each dNTP), 250 ng of genomic DNA, 25 pmol of each primer, and 0.75 units of Taq DNA polymerase. PCR is performed for 40 cycles in a Perkin-Elmer (Perkin-Elmer Cetus, Norwalk, CT) thermocycler using the following thermocycler conditions: 94°C for 30 sec, 58°C for 30 sec, and 72°C for 30 sec. Successful PCR amplification is confirmed by electrophoresing 5 μl of the product on a 1.5% agarose gel.

Fifteen microliters of each PCR-amplified product is then analyzed on a denaturing gradient gel as follows. An 8% polyacrylamide gel containing a linear gradient of DNA denaturants is prepared using a Hoefer (San Francisco, CA) Series SG gradient maker. The method for pouring the gradient has been described in detail elsewhere (14, 24, 29). The precise gradient

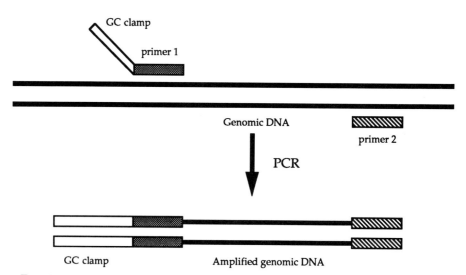

FIG. 4   Incorporation of a GC-clamp sequence into the amplified DNA fragment using PCR. Primer 1 contains a 5′ 30- to 40-nucleotide GC-rich sequence and 20 nucleotides of sequence homologous to rhodopsin. During the PCR amplification the GC-rich sequence becomes incorporated into the amplified DNA fragment.

varies slightly depending on the fragment being analyzed (see Table III). Samples are loaded onto the gel and electrophoresed at 150 V for 7 to 10 hr at 60°C constant temperature. The gel is then stained with ethidium bromide and photographed. Base substitutions are identified by the presence of one or more new bands or a shift in position of a band compared to control samples. Exons shown to contain a base substitution by DGGE can be further analyzed by direct sequencing of the PCR products (34) to identify the precise base change. Segregation of the mutation with the disease phenotype can be demonstrated by analyzing all available family members.

It should be noted that each individual can be screened for mutations anywhere in the rhodopsin gene coding sequence by performing seven PCR amplifications requiring a maximum of 3 μg of DNA and by utilizing seven lanes on denaturing gradient gels. This is a relatively simple and cost-effective approach compared to sequencing the entire coding portion of the gene. With the DGGE approach, only fragments known to contain a substitution need to be sequenced. The algorithm for identifying rhodopsin mutations is summarized in Fig. 5.

Results

Figures 6–11 are photographs of denaturing gradient gels containing PCR products from individuals affected with a variety of rhodopsin mutations. In most cases, a mutation causes four bands to be visible on the denaturing gradient gel: one from each homoduplex (wild type and mutant) and one band from each of the possible heteroduplexes. It is worth noting that the spacing of the bands is mutation specific, that is, no two mutations have exactly the same banding pattern when run side by side on the same gel.

TABLE III   Conditions for Denaturing
Gradient Gel Electrophoresis

Exon	Gradient (%)	Time (hr)
1A	50–80	7
1B	50–75	8
2	50–80	9
3	45–75	9
4	50–80	10
5A	50–80	8
5B	50 80	8

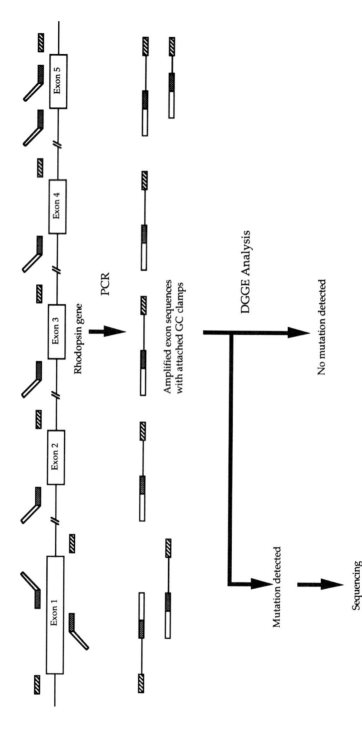

FIG. 5 Algorithm for the analysis of rhodopsin exon sequences using PCR and DGGE. Primer pairs are chosen that span all five exons, including two pairs each for exons 1 and 5. All primer pairs include one with a GC clamp. PCR amplification of genomic DNA results in amplified exon sequences with attached GC clamps. DGGE analysis reveals which exons contain single nucleotide changes. Sequencing of the exons that contain substitutions reveals the specific nucleotide changes.

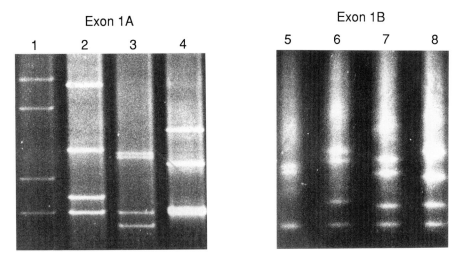

FIG. 6   Denaturing gradient gel electrophoresis analysis of PCR-amplified sequences from the 5′ portion of exon 1. The photograph is a positive image of an ethidium bromide-stained gel. Each lane contains DNA from a patient with a different rhodopsin mutation: lane 1, Thr17Met; lane 2, Pro23His; lane 3, Pro23Leu; lane 4, Thr58Arg. DNA from affected patients was kindly provided by Drs. Bhattacharya, Dryja, Fishman, Kimura, and Nathans (references to initial reports of mutations are given in Table I; the source of each individual sample is listed in the acknowledgments).

FIG. 7   Analysis of PCR-amplified sequences from the 3′ portion of exon 1 by DGGE. The photograph is a positive image of an ethidium bromide-stained gel. Each lane contains DNA from a patient with a different rhodopsin mutation: lane 5, Val87Asp; lane 6, Gly89Asp; lane 7, Gly106Arg; lane 8, Gly106Trp. DNA from affected patients was kindly provided by Drs. Bhattacharya, Dryja, Fishman, Kimura, and Nathans (references to initial reports of mutations are given in Table I; the source of each individual sample is listed in the acknowledgments).

All the known rhodopsin gene base substitutions examined by us to date have had a detectable electrophoretic abnormality using the denaturing gradient gel assay reported in this chapter.

Discussion

The ability to detect specific mutations within the rhodopsin gene is important for several reasons. First, it allows some cases of ADRP to be diagnosed accurately even when visual loss and clinical findings are minimal. Second, it allows counseling of patients with regard to the autosomal-dominant mode

Exon 2

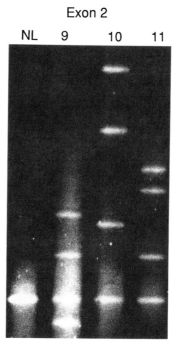

FIG. 8   Analysis of PCR-amplified sequences from exon 2 by DGGE. The photograph is a positive image of an ethidium bromide-stained gel. Each lane contains DNA from a patient with a different rhodopsin mutation: lane NL, normal; lane 9, Leu125-Arg; lane 10, Arg135Leu; lane 11, Arg135Trp. DNA from affected patients was kindly provided by Drs. Bhattacharya, Dryja, Fishman, Kimura, and Nathans (references to initial reports of mutations are given in Table I; the source of each individual sample is listed in the acknowledgments).

of inheritance even in the absence of a family history. Third, it makes possible the correlation of specific phenotypes with specific mutations, so that improved counseling with regard to visual prognosis can be offered to patients. Finally, it raises the possibility that correlation of mutations with phenotypes will offer clues to the pathogenesis of the disease. An ideal rhodopsin mutation assay needs to be accurate, sensitive, and relatively inexpensive. Since most of the rhodopsin mutations described to date are single base substitutions, the sensitivity of a rhodopsin mutation assay depends on the ability of the assay to detect single base changes. In this chapter, we describe a GC-clamped DGGE assay which meets the above criteria. The GC-clamped DGGE approach has been shown to be a sensitive technique for identifying single base substitutions in DNA molecules up to 500 bp in size. The rhodop-

Exon 3

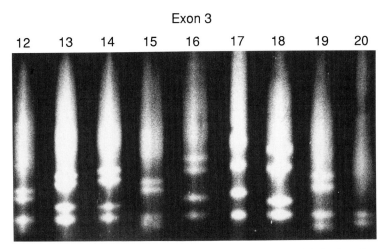

FIG. 9   Analysis of PCR-amplified sequences from exon 3 by DGGE. The photograph is a positive image of an ethidium bromide-stained gel. Each lane contains DNA from a patient with a different rhodopsin mutation: lane 12, Tyr178Cys; lane 13, Glu181Lys; lane 14, Gly182Ser; lane 15, Ser186Pro; lane 16, Gly188Arg; lane 17, Asp190Tyr; lane 18, Asp190Asn; lane 19, Asp190Gly; lane 20, His211Pro. DNA from affected patients was kindly provided by Drs. Bhattacharya, Dryja, Fishman, Kimura, and Nathans (references to initial reports of mutations are given in Table I; the source of each individual sample is listed in the acknowledgments).

sin gene is a favorable gene for the application of DGGE analysis because it has only five small exons, each of which can be analyzed using one or two GC-clamped primer pairs. In the assay described here, the entire coding region of the gene including splice junction sites can be screened for mutations by PCR amplification and DGGE of seven short DNA fragments. Using this assay, we have identified five novel rhodopsin mutations associated with ADRP (5, 9, 11). Furthermore, we have been able to detect all previously identified rhodopsin mutations provided to us by other investigators.

It is possible for a disease-causing rhodopsin mutation to be missed by the GC-clamp DGGE method. For example, 11 bp at the 3' end of exon 2 are not sampled by the assay reported here, because inclusion of that segment in the PCR product introduces enough low-melting domain to diminish the effectiveness of the primers for detecting mutations in the remainder of the exon. Similarly, mutations in the rhodopsin promoter sequences and mutations within introns that create cryptic splice sites would not be detected by the assay described here. It should be noted that no cryptic splice mutations have been detected for the rhodopsin gene using any assay method,

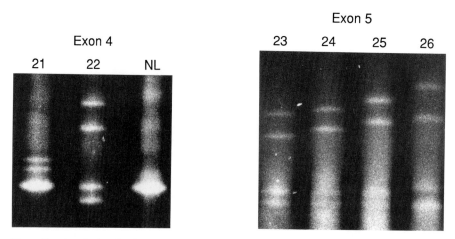

FIG. 10   Analysis of PCR-amplified sequences from exon 4 by DGGE. The photograph is a positive image of an ethidium bromide-stained gel. Each lane contains DNA from a patient with a different rhodopsin mutation: lane 21, Pro267Leu; lane 22, Lys296Glu; lane NL, normal. DNA from affected patients was kindly provided by Drs. Bhattacharya, Dryja, Fishman, Kimura, and Nathans (references to initial reports of mutations are given in Table I; the source of each individual sample is listed in the acknowledgments).

FIG. 11   Analysis of PCR-amplified sequences from exon 5 by DGGE. The photograph is a positive image of an ethidium bromide-stained gel. Each lane contains DNA from a patient with a different rhodopsin mutation: lane 23, Gln344Stop; lane 24, Val345Met; lane 25, Pro347Ser; lane 26, Pro347Leu. DNA from affected patients was kindly provided by Drs. Bhattacharya, Dryja, Fishman, Kimura, and Nathans (references to initial reports of mutations are given in Table I; the source of each individual sample is listed in the acknowledgments).

and that such mutations would also be missed by some other methods for detecting single base changes, including direct DNA sequencing of coding sequences. This point serves to emphasize that failure to detect a mutation in a gene is not equivalent to proving that no mutation is present. In families in which several affected individuals are available, rhodopsin can be excluded as the disease-causing gene with genetic linkage analysis. Linkage analysis requires the availability of polymorphisms in or near the rhodopsin gene. By using the DGGE method we have detected DNA polymorphisms in the 3' untranslated region of the rhodopsin gene as well as other gene sequences (32) that can be used for such experiments.

In summary, the assay described in this chapter provides a useful adjunct to the clinical diagnosis of retinitis pigmentosa (RP). It is especially useful for sporadic cases of RP. In addition, we are hopeful that correlations between genotype and phenotype will emerge that will allow patients to be given better prognostic information than is currently possible using clinical and electrophysiological methods alone.

Acknowledgments

We thank Drs. Alan Kimura and Gerald Fishman for sharing patients and expertise with us during the development of the assays described in this chapter. We also gratefully acknowledge three other colleagues for providing samples from affected patients for use in our comparative gels. Dr. S. Bhattacharya contributed samples from patients affected with mutations in codons 211 and 296; Dr. T. Dryja contributed samples from patients affected with mutations in codons 23, 125, 167, 181, 186, 188, 345, and 347; Dr. J. Nathans contributed samples from patients affected with mutations in codons 45, 87, 89, 106, 135, 178, 190, and 344. This work was supported in part by the Knight's Templar of Iowa, the National Retinitis Pigmentosa Foundation Fighting Blindness, and George Gund Foundation, the C. S. O'Brien Center for Macular Diseases, the Roy Carver Charitable Trust, U.S. Public Health Service Research Grants EY08426 (E.M.S.), P30HD27748 (V.C.S.), and HG00457 (V.C.S.), and an unrestricted grant from Research to Prevent Blindness, New York, New York.

References

1. P. McWilliam, G. J. Farrar, P. Kenna, D. G. Bradley, M. M. Humphries, E. M. Sharp, and D. J. Sharp, *Genomics* **5,** 619 (1989).
2. T. P. Dryja, T. L. McGee, and E. Reichel, *Nature (London)* **343,** 364 (1990).
3. T. P. Dryja, T. L. McGee, L. B. Hahn, G. S. Cowley, J. E. Olsson, E. Reichel, M. A. Sandberg, and E. L. Berson, *N. Engl. J. Med.* **323,** 1302 (1990).
4. C. F. Inglehearn, R. Bashir, D. H. Lester, M. Jay, A. C. Bird, and S. S. Bhattacharya, *Am. J. Hum. Genet.* **48,** 26 (1991).
5. V. C. Sheffield, G. A. Fishman, J. S. Beck, A. E. Kimura, and E. M. Stone, *Am. J. Hum. Genet.* **49,** 699 (1991).
6. T. P. Dryja, L. B. Hahn, G. S. Cowley, T. L. McGee, and E. L. Berson, *Proc. Natl. Acad. Sci. U.S.A.* **88,** 9370 (1991).
7. C. H. Sung, C. M. Davenport, J. C. Hennessey, I. H. Maumenee, S. G. Jacobson, J. C. Heckenlively, R. Nowakowski, G. Fishman, P. Gouras, and J. Nathans, *Proc. Natl. Acad. Sci. U.S.A.* **88,** 6481 (1991).
8. T. J. Keen, C. F. Inglehearn, D. H. Lester, M. Jay, A. C. Bird, B. Jay, and S. S. Bhattacharya, *Genomics* **11,** 199 (1991).

9. G. A. Fishman, E. M. Stone, L. D. Gilbert, and V. C. Sheffield, *Arch. Ophthalmol.* **110,** 54–62 (1992).

10. G. J. Farrar, P. Kenna, R. Redmond, D. Shiels, P. McWilliam, M. M. Humphries, E. M. Sharp, S. Jordan, R. Kumar-Singh, and P. Humphries, *Genomics* **11,** 1170 (1991).

11. K. Vandenburgh, G. A. Fishman, V. C. Sheffield, A. E. Kimura, and E. M. Stone, unpublished data (1992).

12. R. B. Wallace, M. J. Johnson, and T. Hirose, *Nucleic Acids Res.* **9,** 879 (1981).

13. R. M. Meyers, Z. Larin, and T. Maniatis, *Science* **230,** 1242 (1985).

14. R. M. Myers, V. C. Sheffield, and D. R. Cox, *in* "Genome Analysis: A Practical Approach" (K. E. Davies, ed.), p. 95. IRL Press, Oxford, 1988.

15. R. G. H. Cotton, N. R. Rodriquez, and R. D. Campbell, *Proc. Natl. Acad. Sci. U.S.A.* **85,** 4397 (1989).

16. R. G. H. Cotton, *Biochem. J.* **263,** 1 (1989).

17. M. Orita, H. Iwahara, and H. Kanazawa, *Proc. Natl. Acad. Sci. U.S.A.* **86,** 2766 (1989).

18. M. Y. Orita, Y. Suzuki, and T. Sekiya, *Genomics* **5,** 874 (1989).

19. M. Orita, T. Sekiya, and K. Hayashi, *Genomics* **8,** 271 (1990).

20. M. B. White, M. Carvalho, D. Derse, and S. J. O'Brien, *Genomics* **12,** 301 (1991).

21. J. Keen, D. Lester, C. Inglehearn, A. Curtis, and S. Bhattacharya, *Trends Genet.* **7,** 5 (1991).

22. S. G. Fischer and L. S. Lerman, *Proc. Natl. Acad. Sci. U.S.A.* **77,** 4420 (1980).

23. R. M. Myers, N. Lumelsky, L. S. Lerman, and T. Maniatis, *Nature (London)* **313,** 495 (1985).

24. R. M. Myers, T. Maniatis, and L. S. Lerman, *in* "Methods in Enzymology" (R. Wu, ed.), Vol. 155, p. 501. Academic Press, New York, 1987.

25. R. M. Myers and T. Maniatis, *Cold Spring Harbor Symp. Quant. Biol.* **51,** 275 (1986).

26. R. M. Myers, S. G. Fischer, and L. S. Lerman, *Nucleic Acids Res.* **13,** 3131 (1985).

27. R. M. Myers, S. G. Fischer, and T. Maniatis, *Nucleic Acids Res.* **13,** 3111 (1985).

28. V. C. Sheffield, D. R. Cox, and R. M. Myers, *Proc. Natl. Acad. Sci. U.S.A.* **86,** 232 (1989).

29. R. M. Myers, V. C. Sheffield, and D. R. Cox, *in* "PCR Technology" (H. A. Erlich, ed.), p. 71. Stockton, New York, 1989.

30. R. K. Saiki, S. Scharf, and F. Faloona, *Science* **230,** 1350 (1985).

31. V. C. Sheffield, unpublished data (1992).

32. V. C. Sheffield, J. S. Beck, B. E. Nichols, A. Cousineau, A. C. Lidral, and E. M. Stone, *Am. J. Hum. Genet.* **50,** 567–575 (1992).

33. J. Grimberg, S. Nawoschik, L. Belluscio, R. McKee, A. Turck, and A. A. Eisenberg, *Nucleic Acids Res.* **17,** 390 (1989).

34. R. F. Dubose and D. L. Hartl, *BioTechniques* **8,** 274 (1990).

Index